TOTAL HEALTH AND SAFETY FOR HEALTH CARE FACILITIES

Catalyzing Improvements in
Employee Safety, Patient Care,
and the Bottom Line

LINDA F. CHAFF

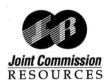

Joint Commission
RESOURCES

Health Forum, Inc.
An American Hospital Association Company
CHICAGO press

Discounts on bulk quantities of books published by Health Forum, Inc., are available to professional associations, special marketers, educators, trainers, and others. For details and discount information, contact Health Forum, Inc., One North Franklin, 28th Floor, Chicago, IL 60606-3421 (Phone: 1-800-242-2626).

Library of Congress Cataloging-in-Publication Data

Chaff, Linda F.
  Total health and safety for health care facilities : catalyzing improvements in employee safety, patient care and the bottom line / Linda F. Chaff.
     p. cm.
  Includes bibliographical references (p.).
  ISBN 1-55648-331-7
  1. Health facilities—Administration. 2. Medical care—Quality control. 3. Quality assurance.
4. Medical care—Evaluation. I. Title.
  RA971.C4553 2006
  362.1068—dc22
                    2006043660

Dedication

This book is dedicated to the author of *Guidelines for Protecting the Safety and Health of Health Care Workers*, published by the National Institute for Occupational Safety and Health in 1988.

A book so popular in the 1990s that health care safety professionals playfully dubbed it "The Blue Book," it was a regular in my courses and coaching sessions, its methodologies often quietly speaking for me.

That scientific work embodied leadership, technical knowledge, compassion, curiosity, and emotion—skills embraced among discerning health and safety professionals around the world and essential to keeping workers safe and healthy every single day of their lives.

Of course, my book is also for those discerning health and safety professionals who are the cornerstone of this vocation.

To the men and women of OSHA: Each day this agency makes me proud that we continue the journey begun by Bernardino Ramazzini 300 years ago to ease the suffering of workers in the health care industry—for without them this book would not exist.

Finally, to all the up-and-coming, discerning health and safety professionals—may this book help you as you set out to make your passion for the arena reality.

Contents

List of Figures

List of Tables

About the Author

Linda F. Chaff is president of Chaff & Co. Her understanding of organizational development and workplace safety and health derives from childhood and her experience in a wide range of organizations. Linda grew up on a farm in Washington State. Before there was an Occupational Safety and Health Administration (OSHA), her father experienced a debilitating injury, losing two fingers on his left hand while operating an unguarded saw to cut heavy logs. This experience, and the stories about her grandparents who suffered disabling workplace injuries, set her on a journey similar to those of Bernardino Ramazzini, MD, and Alice Hamilton, to try to ensure that everybody's husband, father, grandfather, wife, mother, and child can be in a workplace that is healthy and safe.

Following five years in the FBI's LA Field Office Laboratory, Linda served as the director of protection services for a medical facility. After she relocated to Louisville, Kentucky, Chaff & Co was born. One of Linda's first successes was the publication of *Progressive Waste Management: A Policy Guide for Healthcare* in 1988. Since then, Linda has written more than a dozen books that address various aspects of health and safety in the health care industry. These books have been published by the National Safety Council, the American Medical Association, and the American Hospital Association (AHA).

She has served as the Disaster Action Team Director for the American Red Cross in Monongalia County, West Virginia, where she developed a comprehensive disaster action team training program and trained volunteers to work at disaster sites. She also served on the Federal Emergency Management Agency's (FEMA) national committee for health care emergency preparedness. She also participated in the AHA video conference *Confronting the Risk: Hazardous Materials and Hospital Liability*.

Linda's credits include the Russell L. Colling Literary Award and appointments on committee and board positions with safety and civic councils, including the executive committee of the National Safety Council's Health Care Section. Linda has worked with the AHA, as well as with two of its personal membership groups—the American Society for Healthcare Engineering and the American Society for Healthcare Risk Management—on a number of successful projects.

With her experience in health care, passion for worker health and safety, and understanding of human values and how they affect our working lives,

Linda now presents *Total Health and Safety for Health Facilities: Catalyzing Improvements in Employee Safety, Patient Care, and the Bottom Line.*

Chaff & Co. is a corporate communications firm in Chattanooga, Tennessee, that develops ideas, training concepts, promotional campaigns, and programs to improve individuals' skills in ways that make an exciting difference in the profits and conduct of businesses. Chaff & Co.'s signature product line, *Valuing You*™, celebrates through dynamic and understandable messages that *people matter*.

Chaff & Co. operates on the principle that traditional workplace safety and health management is only a part of the solution for ensuring worker protection. Experience has demonstrated that working safely on the job is vastly improved by the catalyst of personal health and well-being. This idea of total health and safety is the core of Chaff & Co.'s business philosophy.

This new, broad-based approach was the cornerstone of the Tennessee Valley Authority's *MegaSafe*, a promotional and motivational workers' compensation reduction program that Chaff & Co. produced for over 18,000 employees. The program resulted in a 94 percent reduction in lost-time accidents, a 52 percent reduction in recordable accidents, and more than $3.5 million in annual savings. In this book, Chaff & Co. applies the lessons learned from that experience, along with the precepts of *Valuing You*, to the health care industry.

About the CD-ROM

The CD-ROM on the inside back cover contains the full text of standards, recommendations, guidelines, and other information described in this book. The documents identified in brackets in the book are on the CD-ROM (e.g., "[CD-ROM 1.1]") and are organized according to their corresponding book chapters.

In addition to the information from U.S. agencies and organizations such as the Centers for Disease Control and Prevention (CDC), the National Institute for Occupational Safety and Health (NIOSH), the Occupational Safety and Health Administration (OSHA), a number of OSHA state plan states, the Environmental Protection Agency, and several academic institutions, there are documents from a number of other countries and organizations, including Canada, Mexico, New Zealand, Puerto Rico, Switzerland, the United Kingdom, and the World Health Organization.

The CD-ROM contains additional resources for establishing and managing a cohesive program to reduce employee injuries and illnesses. Although most of the information is presented in English, there are a number of documents in Spanish, including selected OSHA standards from Puerto Rico and selected documents from other OSHA state plan states.

Three tables are provided in the appendix to serve as an index to the additional resources on the CD-ROM.

- ☐ Table A-1 lists additional resources organized by book chapter, although many of them can be helpful for understanding material in other chapters as well.
- ☐ Table A-2 provides text of selected portions of federal OSHA standards from Parts 1904, 1910, 1913, 1926, and 1960.
- ☐ Table A-3 provides selected NIOSH, federal OSHA, and state OSHA documents in Spanish. This table also includes selected OSHA Puerto Rico state plan regulations.

Foreword

Health care organizations are dedicated to curing and healing the ill and wounded. Simple consistency demands that they include in their mission the prevention of job-related illness and injury to their own workers. Health care workers are health care's single most important asset. Without the health care worker, patient care cannot occur. Yet according to the Bureau of Labor Statistics, more than 500,000 health care workers suffer work-related injuries annually, including back injuries and injuries associated with fire, hazardous chemicals, electrical shocks, and other risks. This does not even include the accidental needlestick injuries that occur in hospitals (estimated at 800,000 in a recent year), putting health care workers at risk for exposure to various bloodborne pathogens.

Through the publication of this book, Joint Commission Resources, the educational and publishing not-for-profit affiliate of the Joint Commission, is pleased to partner with Health Forum and the American Hospital Association to promote and ensure employee health and safety in health care facilities. We applaud the efforts of this book to champion total health and safety in health care facilities—not just for patients, but also for the employees who work tirelessly and devotedly to provide safe, quality care for patients.

Total Health and Safety for Health Care Facilities highlights the many challenges health care facilities face regarding employee health and safety. The book also provides practical solutions that show how to create, implement, and maintain comprehensive environmental health and safety programs that work in concert with and complement patient safety and risk management programs.

In the last 5 to 10 years or so, much attention has been given to patient safety. While patient safety has always been a goal and concern for health care facilities, the groundbreaking Institute of Medicine report of 1999 garnered much industry and media attention for patient safety. Consider the Joint Commission's own efforts in the patient safety arena over the last decade alone—the creation of the Joint Commission's Sentinel Event Database, the issuance of Sentinel Event Alerts, the inauguration of National Patient Safety Goals, and the creation of the Joint Commission International Center for Patient Safety, just to name a few. The Joint Commission recently even collaborated on a book to help patients engage as part of the health care team by becoming "Smart Patients."

The quality and safety initiatives of the American Hospital Association over its long history have recently evolved into the creation of the AHA Quality Center™. The Quality Center helps hospitals accelerate their quality improvement processes to achieve better outcomes and improve organizational performance. In collaboration with leading quality improvement stakeholders, the center brings together knowledge, expertise, and demonstrated methods in quality and patient safety from across the hospital field.

However, all of these efforts—by the Joint Commission, the American Hospital Association, and the myriad other health care associations and federal, state, and private agencies dedicated to patient safety—in no way diminish a very real and sincere concern for the safety and well-being of the health care employees.

This book explains how health care facilities can use a strong working knowledge of OSHA, Joint Commission, and other federal, state, and local requirements to improve health care employee health and safety. It also shows how the Joint Commission standards work in concert with OSHA standards and these other requirements. Both Joint Commission standards and OSHA requirements focus on ergonomics, bloodborne pathogen control, workplace violence prevention, emergency management, fire safety, hazardous materials management, and life safety. The Joint Commission and OSHA have long recognized their complementary goals regarding safety and have teamed up in an educational alliance centered on disseminating tools to improve and advance workplace safety and health. The overlap between the "environment of care" and the "environment of work" is very clear and real. It is hoped that this book will help health care facilities to manage and improve the safety of both environments for their patients and employees.

Karen H. Timmons, CEO
Joint Commission Resources

Preface

In 1970 the United States Congress passed the Occupational Safety and Health Act (Public Law 91-596). In the foreword to the legislative history of that act, the Chairman of the Committee on Labor and Public Welfare, Harrison A. Williams, wrote:

> To the tragedy of industrial accidents must be added the grim history of our failure to heed the occupational health needs of our workers. Not only are occupational diseases which first came to light at the beginning of the Industrial Revolution still undermining the health of workers, but new substances, new processes, and new sources of energy are presenting health problems of ever-increasing complexity.

This sentiment is reflected in the opening words of the Occupational Safety and Health Act:

> Sec. (2) The Congress finds that personal injuries and illnesses arising out of work situations impose a substantial burden upon, and are a hindrance to, interstate commerce in terms of lost production, wage loss, medical expenses, and disability compensation payments.
>
> (b) The Congress declares it to be its purpose and policy . . . to provide for the general welfare, to assure so far as possible every working man and woman in the Nation safe and healthful working conditions and to preserve our human resources. (Occupational Safety and Health Act of 1970 [CD-ROM P.1])

The Occupational Safety and Health Act created two separate agencies: the Occupational Safety and Health Administration (OSHA), which promulgates and enforces regulations, and the National Institute for Occupational Safety and Health (NIOSH), which conducts research and makes recommendations to OSHA for new and improved safety and health standards.

In 1988, following its congressional mandate, NIOSH published *Guidelines for Protecting the Health and Safety of Health Care Workers.*[1] In the introduction, NIOSH wrote:

> Health care facilities present workers with a myriad of potential health and safety hazards. Compared with the total civilian workforce, hospital workers have a greater percentage of workers' compensation claims for sprains and strains, infectious and parasitic

diseases, dermatitis, hepatitis, mental disorders, eye diseases, influenza, and toxic hepatitis.

As the twentieth anniversary of the publication of that seminal work approaches, it is reasonable to examine the progress that has been made in protecting this nation's health care workers. Unfortunately, that examination has proved disappointing. Despite the efforts of OSHA, NIOSH, health care organizations, accreditation organizations, safety councils and associations, insurance companies, consultants, and others, the picture painted in that introductory paragraph has not changed much. It can, in fact, be said with a high degree of certainty that we have failed to significantly reduce the number of work-related injuries and illnesses among America's health care workers. Much of what was written in 1988 remains true in 2006.

The current rate of injuries and illnesses among health care workers is one of the worst in all of private industry, according to the Bureau of Labor Statistics. Clearly, the prevailing system of safeguarding health care worker safety and health is not working. Health care workers remain at greater risk of incurring a work-related injury or illness than workers in other industries, including fabricated metal product manufacturing.

The majority of health care facilities operate under the notion that by complying with worker health and safety standards from accreditation organizations, primarily the Joint Commission on Accreditation of Healthcare Organizations, they are also complying with OSHA safety and health standards, but that is not the case. Certainly, there is some overlap between OSHA and Joint Commission requirements, but, as the Joint Commission points out, health care facilities are also responsible for complying with all applicable federal, state, and local regulations in addition to its accreditation standards. Unlike general industry, in which worker health and safety occupies a primary position in the corporate structure and business plan, in health care facilities the principal emphasis is on patient care and safety, accreditation requirements, and compliance with a host of federal regulations other than those governing employee health and safety. The employee health and safety functions are often scattered among several different departments. This approach may act as an impediment to improvements in employee well-being, patient care, and the corporate bottom line. This widely decentralized approach significantly reduces the likelihood that there will be a systematic collection and exchange of information needed to conduct epidemiological analysis or injury surveillance to identify and correct problems related to employee health and safety.

How has this happened? At whom do we point the finger? The comic strip hero Pogo gave us the answer: "We have met the enemy and he is us." Each person who works for a company bears a responsibility for the company's success or its failure. Ineffectual management, rotten customer service, poor product design, marketing failures, a lack of incentive to do quality work, injuries and illnesses, and finger pointing are all keys to failure. Put your finger in your pocket. We must start with a clean slate.

If you will allow the poets and philosophers to intervene, there is another way to approach this problem. Carl Sagan once said, "We are, all of us, made of star-stuff."[2] And John Donne wrote, "No man is an island, entire of itself; every man is a piece of the continent, a part of the main."[3] What were these two men, so separated in time and space, trying to tell us? We believe that their message is clear.

> *All* things are connected.
> Quality patient care requires quality employee care, and the emphasis on each should be equal. This philosophy forms the core of this book.

The intent of this book is to effect a culture change in the health care industry by demonstrating how health care workers' health and safety, the environment they work in, patient care, the well-being of health care workers' families, and the corporate bottom line are all connected.

This book presents a comprehensive program that creates a new dimension in health and safety for employees and their families and patients, and brings together three core elements for success: human values, regulatory and accreditation agencies, and business objectives.

The program is based on physical, emotional, and spiritual perspectives and incorporates two easily applied theories. One is a global, high-level communications concept while the other is specifically designed to improve the health and safety of patients, employees and their families, and all others who enter the facility. The first concept emphasizes human values; the second relies on data collection and problem solving. Taken together, these two concepts form a powerful tool to improve the health and safety experience of employees and patients in health care facilities and to have a positive effect on the bottom line. This holistic approach demonstrates how physical patterns and a healthy self-image are essential to reducing injuries and illnesses no matter where they occur.

The two concepts are *Valuing You*™ and *Total Health and Safety*™:

☐ *Valuing You* is a corporate communications program that instills confidence in people to help them handle the variety of activities, situations, and questions that arise at work, at home, and in everyday life. The program is based on the caring values that employees, their families, and patients deserve. This program also demonstrates how stress management, nutrition, basic hygiene, and physical fitness are essential to reducing injuries and illnesses in and outside the workplace.

☐ *Total Health and Safety* incorporates the concepts of *Valuing You* that affect safety and health with the concepts of occupational and environmental health and safety that have proven to reduce employee injuries and illnesses, enhance patient care, and increase the bottom line.

Total Health and Safety uses the very best elements of functional and motivational programs from around the world to bridge the gap between quality patient care and the safety and health of employees as well as their families.

No event is isolated. A work-related injury affects co-workers and families, and an accident or illness at home negatively affects that person's co-workers. With an understanding of the relationship between family safety and health and workplace safety and health, significant improvements in a person's work and personal life can be achieved.

This is not a "how-to" book, nor is it a checklist. The book provides guidance for establishing and managing a cohesive program to reduce employee injuries and illnesses. It presents core program components and resources needed to develop and advance an employee health and safety program. Therefore, the book serves as both a source of initial information for the beginner and a handy reference for the experienced health and safety professional. Each chapter provides a discussion of who should be involved, approaches for solving problems, solutions, and some examples of things facilities have tried that have been successful.

Used in conjunction with OSHA and other regulations, as well as Joint Commission worker health and safety accreditation standards, this book serves as an effective guide to implementing employee safety and health requirements in the facility. Therefore, a central theme is the necessity to become familiar with the requirements of those regulations and to show their connection to Joint Commission standards where applicable.

Another common thread that runs throughout the book is that information must be presented in a style that fits the communication expectations of the audience. Neither the housekeeping staff nor the COO wants to hear a science lecture. When such communications are presented, the goal must be to show how the health and safety concerns that have been raised relate to patient care and safety, and how corrective action will enhance the facility's ability to provide quality patient care and care for its employees, as well as contribute to the facility's economic well-being. The book shows how to convey this information in understandable, positive, and successful ways.

Key features of the book include:

- A model Environmental Health and Safety (EH&S) program
- Guidance for staffing the Environmental Health and Safety Department
- The relationship between employee health and safety and patient safety and health
- Information on how the Joint Commission is a significant partner in ensuring employee health and safety in health care facilities
- The significance of personal health and fitness and its relationship to workplace safety and health
- Guidance on marketing and positioning the department within the facility and community

- ☐ The role of the department in establishing a culture and climate of employee health and safety
- ☐ The importance of accurate data collection and surveillance
- ☐ Tools for hazard analysis, data analysis, and recordkeeping that reduce injuries and illnesses
- ☐ A CD-ROM with guidelines, regulations, tips, and other resources
- ☐ A process for ensuring that the facility is in continuous compliance with both OSHA (and other federal, state, and local) regulations and Joint Commission worker health and safety accreditation requirements

Simply complying with either regulatory agencies or accreditation standards or both does not mean that the facility has a strong, dynamic health and safety program. Both regulatory agencies and accreditation organizations are convinced that there is a direct relationship between strong leadership, effective management, and a reduction in the number and severity of injuries and illnesses in health care facilities.

But compliance with regulations and accreditation standards is not the sole burden of employers. Exceptional outcomes require a solid partnership between employers and employees, with each having equal responsibility for the program's performance. Employees must be active, informed participants in worksite health and safety. By encouraging employee involvement in the program's design and development, facilities will reap the benefits of employees' valuable ideas and their all-important support. This book describes how this culture can become a part of the daily routine of the health care facility.

By correcting the problems identified in this book, the health care industry can save tens of billions of dollars annually in direct and indirect costs. There will be better communications throughout facilities and enhanced relationships with local communities. Employee health and safety and patient care and safety will improve. There will be enhanced employee morale. This transformation positions and markets the health care industry's twenty-first–century Environmental Health and Safety program in ways that will lead to exceptional outcomes and notable recognition.

I hope you enjoy and benefit from reading *Total Health and Safety for Health Care Facilities*. If you have any thoughts or experiences you would like to share, please contact me. I would be delighted to hear from you.

Linda Chaff
Chaff & Co.
600 Republic Centre
Chattanooga, TN 37450
423-266-5541
linda@chaffco.com
www.chaffco.com

References

1. U.S. Department of Health and Human Services. *Guidelines for Protecting the Health and Safety of Health Care Workers*. DHHS (NIOSH) Publication No. 88-119. Washington, DC: U.S. GPO, September 1988.
2. Sagan, Carl. *Cosmos*. Novel and film series.
3. Donne, John. *The Complete Poetry and Selected Prose of John Donne* (Modern Library Series). New York: Random House, 1994.

Acknowledgments

I'd like to thank the many people without whose help you wouldn't be reading this book. As I began to think of all the people to whom I would like to express my appreciation for their support, suggestions, and hard work in making this book possible, the list continued to grow.

This book is truly a global effort, and therefore I want to acknowledge the contributions of the world's environmental health and safety community who made contributions from numerous countries, including Australia, Canada, Mexico, New Zealand, Puerto Rico, Switzerland, and the United Kingdom. I'm listing their websites because they have asked me to invite you to visit, and they encourage you to become familiar with and use their helpful documents, guidelines, and standards.

- Accident Compensation Corporation of New Zealand, www.acc.co.nz
- Alberta Human Resources and Employment, Workplace Health and Safety, www.whs.gov.ab.ca
- Canadian Centre for Occupational Health and Safety, www.ccohs.ca, especially Roger Cockerline
- European Agency for Safety and Health at Work, http://osha.eu.int, and Monica Azaola, for providing several documents, including *New Trends in Accident Prevention Due to the Changing World of Work*
- Health and Safety Executive, United Kingdom, www.hse.gsi.gov.uk
- Health Care Health & Safety Association of Ontario, www.hchsa.on.ca, especially Wendy Currie Mills
- International Labour Organization, www.ilo.org
- National Occupational Health and Safety Commission (NOHSC), www.nohsc.gov.au
- New Brunswick Family Violence and the Workplace Committee, www.toolkitnb.ca
- New Zealand Department of Labour, www.dol.govt.nz, especially Ben McFadgen
- Occupational Health and Safety Agency for Healthcare, www.ohsah.bc.ca, especially Tina Hancock
- Office of the Australian Safety Compensation Council, www.nohsc.gov.au

- Puerto Rico Department of Labor, Occupational Safety and Health Administration (PR OSHA), Puerto Rico state plan website: http://www.dtrh.gobierno.pr/osho.asp, especially Nilda Gonzalez
- World Health Organization, Switzerland, www.who.int, especially Dolores Campanario

Additional significant contributions were made by individuals and a number of agencies, organizations, associations, corporations, and academic institutions. I'm also listing their websites, and I feel certain you will find their information, membership opportunities, and guidance of value.

- American Medical Association, www.ama-assn.org, which provided *Report 12 of the Council on Scientific Affairs (A-97) Full Text* on the CD-ROM.
- American Nurses Association, www.ana.org, which participated in discussions regarding a survey.
- American Osteopathic Association, HFAP Program Education Specialist, www.hfap.org, in particular, Karen Y. Beem, MS, RN.
- American Society for Healthcare Engineering (ASHE), www.ashe.org, in particular Kate Wickham. Members reviewed the outline and participated in market research involved in planning the concept and direction of the book.
- American Society for Healthcare Risk Management (ASHRM), www.ashrm.org, especially Elizabeth Summy, executive director, and Pamela J. Para, RN, MPH, CPHRM, FASHRM. director of professional & technical services. The organization participated in market research involved in planning the concept and direction of the book, and members participated in surveys that assisted with the development of chapters.
- American Society for Safety Engineers, www.asse.org, and Tim Fisher, who provided *White Paper Addressing The Return on Investment for Safety, Health, and Environmental (SH&E) Management Programs.*
- American Society for Training and Development, www.astd.org, which provided *2005 State of the Industry: ASTD's Annual Review of Trends in Workplace Learning and* Performance.
- Association of periOperative Registered Nurses (AORN), www.aorn.org, and Annie Lenth, for two documents: *Advanced Practice Nurse Entrepreneurs in a Multidisciplinary Surgical-Assisting Partnership* and *Incident Reports: Correcting Processes and Reducing Errors.*
- Bureau of Labor Statistics (BLS), www.bls.gov, including numerous men and women who assisted with research and provided documents, studies, and data on injury and illness statistics.
- *Campus Safety* Magazine, campussafetymagazine@bobit.com, and Robin Hattersley Gray, for *How to Develop Your Own Hospital Fire Safety Plan,* written by Steve Ennis.

- Charlotte A. Smith, R.Ph., M.S., HEM, president of PharmEcology Associates, LLC, who updated the article *Managing Drug Waste Liabilities*, www.pharmacology.com.
- Compressed Gas Association, www.cganet.com, especially Mike Tiller, for providing safety alerts, M-x publications, and posters.
- Erlanger Health System, www.erlanger.org, and in particular Louise Bennett-Hall, BSN, MS, CPHQ, who furnished considerable assistance with Joint Commission standards.
- Health Facilities Management, www.hfmmagazine.com, for document approval.
- Healthcare Without Harm, www.noharm.org, for publications.
- Hospitals for a Healthy Environment (H2E), www.h2e-online.org, in particular, Laura Brannen, for discussion and document approval.
- International Association for Healthcare Security and Safety (IAHSS), www.iahss.org, whose members participated in market research involved with planning the concept and direction of the book, reviewed the outline and made suggestions, and participated in surveys that assisted with development of chapters.
- Joint Commission Resources, www.jcrinc.com, for document approval.
- Kentucky Pollution Prevention Center, www.kppc.org, and Donald P. Douglass, P.G., for numerous documents on the website.
- Montana Department of Labor & Industry, www.mt.gov, and Michelle Robinson, for providing *Compressed Gas Safety General Safety Guidelines*.
- Minnesota Department of Health, www.health.state.mn.us, for *Incidents of Jeopardy/Harm to Patient/Resident Health and Safety*.
- National Association of Psychiatric Health Systems (NAPHS), www.naphs.org, and Carole Szpak, for *Guidelines for the Built Environment of Behavioral Health Facilities*, by David M. Sine, CSP, OHST, and James M. Hunt, AIA.
- National Fire Protection Association, www.nfpa.org, for discussions involving health care facility fires, research, and guidance regarding publications.
- National Institutes of Health, Warren Grant Magnuson Clinical Center, for *Handling Chemotherapy Drugs Safely at Home*.
- National Safety Council, www.nsc.org, for articles from the library and the current *Injury Facts* CD. Also for research and statistics. Also, my thanks to Suzanne Powills, executive director of publications, for her assistance and support.
- Occupational Health and Safety Agency for Healthcare, www.ohsah.bc.ca.
- Occupational Safety and Health Administration (OSHA), www.osha.gov, and the numerous men and women who provided interpretations, expertise, and answered questions. Also, several OSHA state plan agencies provided consultation and publications.

- Scott Specialty Gases, Inc., www.scottgas.com, especially Jim Kraus, for *Design+Safety Handbook*.
- Smith Seckman Reid, Inc., www.ssr-inc.com, which provided *Is Your Fire Brigade Up to Snuff?*, written by Leo Old, P.E.
- Sustainable Hospitals, www.sustainablehospitals.org., and Catherine Galligan, for document approval.
- United States Fire Administration, www.usfa.fema.gov.
- Volunteers in Health Care at Memorial Hospital of Rhode Island, www.mhri.org and www.volunteersinhealthcare.org, in particular, Janet Walton, for providing *Overcoming Language Barriers, Part II: For Administrators*.
- Princeton University, www.princeton.edu; Virginia Tech, www.vt.edu; and West Virginia University, www.wvu.edu.

I am grateful to many other people for help with this book.

The following individuals assisted me in my scientific work and in the creation of this book. Many helped through reviewing, listening, and talking; some had suggestions and ideas for direction and information sources; many participated in developing surveys or agreed to answer surveys; many provided their expertise in specific areas, while others granted me interviews. Some provided data input.

Tim Buckley; Ray Cate; Connee J. Cantrill; Mark Chapman; Sherry T. Collura, RN, BSN, CHCM, CHSP; Frank Denny; Scott Dieter, Certified Fraud Examiner; Helen Gillespie, RN, MA, COHN-S; Jason Gunter; Jim Kendig; Wayne King; Eric Kirkland; several members of the executive committee of National Safety Council's Health Care Section; Marvin Lewiton, MS, CIH; Barbara McCarthy; Evelyn F. Meserve, CHPA; Ray Mulry, Ph.D., CSP; Jim Nash; Pamela Para, RN, MPH, CPHRM, FASHRM; Roger L. Pugh; Gerald M. Rakes; Robert Rettig; Don Robida; Joseph Saarinen; Thomas A. Smith, BS, HEM; Herman C. Statum, MS, CPP, CFE, CHS-V, PI; Karen Struck, RN, MS, CPHQ, CPHRM; Elizabeth Summy; Jerry Tatum; several individuals at the American Nurses Association; Jeffrey L. Weaver, OD; Donald White, CHSP, CHCM; Tom Zahorsky, CHSP

To all the people who have nurtured this project, "Thanks" isn't enough. This book was further made possible by a great team:

Health Forum, Inc. My editor, Richard Hill, for getting it all started. Many thanks for the enthusiasm and interest he has shown for this project. I have really enjoyed working with Rick and greatly appreciate his expertise. I also wish to thank Mary Grayson, publisher; Pat Foy, director of sales; and Peggy DuMais, production editor.

I am very grateful to Noemi Escutia with American Hospital Association, who assisted with title translations involving the Spanish documents for the CD-ROM. Thank you so much, Noemi, for all of your assistance with the Spanish documents and regulations.

Catherine C. Hinckley, Ph.D., executive director, publications, Joint Commission Resources. Cathy's vision and faith helped make this partnership possible.

David L. Woodrum, FAAHC, FACHE, my mentor and confidant, laid the groundwork many years ago.

My incredible staff at Chaff & Co., who worked hard under deadline pressures and made significant contributions. Denise Reed and Allison Todd suffered through reviews, research, editing, re-editing, and proofreading. They took on the Herculean task of developing the English and Spanish CD-ROM of resources. At the end of the project, Denise was certain she knew Spanish, without ever having uttered a word of it in her life.

I want especially to thank Steve Ennis, CHSP, CFPS; Linda Glasson, CHPA; Joseph S. McFadden, CHSP, MT; Evelyn F. Meserve, CHPA; Ray Mulry, Ph.D., CSP; and Peter Troy, CHPA, CIPS. They all listened patiently and contributed generously.

Charles Sexton, for his uplifting poems, words of wisdom, and his never-ending wellspring of creative ideas. You can find some of his poems on the CD-ROM that accompanies this book.

To those who helped keep me healthy and somewhat stress free during what seemed like a never-ending period of research and writing: Dr. Nancy Reinhardt and her office manager, Nancy Fletcher, at North River Chiropractic. Dr. Reinhardt also provided guidance in nutritional aspects of the *Total Health and Safety*™ concept. Priscilla Caine and Jenny Richards at Curves.

In memory of Al Kuntz, who worked tirelessly with me for several years and always willingly provided excellent data on medical equipment management systems. Randy Bullard of Modern Biomedical & Imaging, Inc. graciously stepped in and worked with me during this difficult time. Al was a good friend to both of us.

And finally, my husband, son, mom, and sister always. I owe a deep sense of gratitude to my family, who gave me my history and patiently endured the creation of this book.

TOTAL HEALTH AND SAFETY FOR HEALTH CARE FACILITIES

CHAPTER 1

THE CURRENT STATE OF HEALTH CARE EMPLOYEE SAFETY PROGRAMS AND A MODEL FOR THE FUTURE

Occupational injuries and illnesses have existed since Adam and Eve. Consider Noah—a lumberman, carpenter, painter, herdsman, and veterinarian. The men who built the pyramids were common laborers, stonemasons, engineers, and architects. Spend a few moments thinking about printers, painters, butchers, bakers, and candlestick makers, as well as the men who dug the Suez and Panama canals. Reflect on the lives of the men and women who built the subway system in Washington, DC, and the builders of the Golden Gate Bridge. Consider the experience of nuclear weapons workers, steel mill workers, miners, automakers, pipe fitters, electricians, plumbers, the rescuers of the injured and ill, and health care workers.

Among all those occupations, the health care worker is unique. When the steel worker is burned, the automaker cut, the painter dizzied, or the laborer crushed, it is the health care worker who soothes the burn, stitches the cut, provides respiratory therapy, and tries to save a finger, an arm, a life.

But there is a growing cost to those who would cure and heal. This chapter analyzes the numbers of health care workers who become sick or hurt while they are curing, healing, and saving, and it shows the cost of their sacrifice to the industry.

Hidden amidst all the high-tech medicine, equipment, and techniques are tens of billions of dollars in employee medical care, lost time, workers' compensation, and indirect costs incurred by the health care industry *every year*.

Although occupations assumed to be dangerous, such as metal fabrication and construction, have substantially improved their records over the last 20 years, the record of the health care industry in making health and safety improvements is a distant second. The kinds of injuries expected only in manufacturing and construction are also occurring regularly and at significant rates in health care facilities.

Furthermore, the scope and severity of risks have increased dramatically with the advent of HIV/AIDS and SARS and the threat of mass casualties from biological, chemical, radiological, and explosive weapons.

This book presents a philosophy of change. It is time to stop thinking of employee safety as separate and distinct from employee health, from the environment of health care workers, from its impact on patient care, and from the corporate bottom line. For that reason, what has been and may currently be referred to in health care facilities as a safety program needs a broader definition. This book uses the term *Environmental Health and Safety* (EH&S) to convey the idea that improving and maintaining a healthy and safe workforce requires more than simply having a safety program. (The term *occupational safety and health* is synonymous with Environmental Health and Safety.) This book describes the health and safety program in terms of the relationship between employees and their environment, families, patients, and visitors. Unless health care facilities adapt to the continuing and growing risk facing their employees, the cost of quality health care will increase and the number of qualified health care personnel will decrease through self-removal from the profession. The economic cost will continue to burden quality health care delivery.

If you will allow the poets and philosophers to intervene, you will discover another way to approach this problem. Carl Sagan once said, "We are, all of us, made of star-stuff,"[1] and John Donne wrote, "No man is an island, entire of itself; every man is a piece of the continent, a part of the main."[2] What were these two men, so separated in time and space, trying to tell us? Their message is clear:

> *All* things are connected.
> Quality patient care requires quality employee care, and the emphasis on each should be equal.

This book presents many regulations, standards, and guidelines. But beyond the "shalls" and "shoulds," it also presents a core philosophy that *all* workers have the right to return from their jobs as healthy as when they arrived at them. But those workers share the responsibility for doing their jobs safely with their employers. Employee health and safety is interactive. It is cooperative. It is a joint effort. It is the manifestation of the notion that "no man is an island."

EXTENT OF INJURIES AND ILLNESSES

Title 29 USC, Chapter 15, Article 651, Congressional statement of findings and declaration of purpose and policy:

> (a) The Congress finds that personal injuries and illnesses arising out of work situations impose a substantial burden upon, and are a hindrance to, interstate commerce in terms of lost production, wage loss, medical expenses, and disability compensation payments.[3]
> [CD-ROM 1.1]

According to the Bureau of Labor Statistics (BLS), the health care industry is the second-fastest-growing sector of the U.S. economy, with more than 13.7 million workers. Hospitals employ more than 4.2 million of those workers. Approximately 80 percent of all health care workers are women.[4]

The U.S. Standard Industrial Classification (SIC) defines industries in accordance with the composition and structure of the economy and covers the entire field of economic activities.[5] In 2003, the North American Industry Classification System (NAICS) replaced the U.S. Standard Industrial Classification system. Wherever possible, both the NAICS and the SIC codes are provided in this book.

Health care facilities have a single mission—the delivery of quality patient care. But hidden by the success of quality patient care is the toll paid by the caregivers. Hospital employee injuries and illnesses reported to the BLS in 2003 highlight that toll:[6,7]

- In 2003, there were 292,700 recordable injuries (219,000) and illnesses (73,400) among the 4,201,300 hospital workers (NAICS 622/SIC 806).
  - Of the 219,000 recordable injuries in 2003, 67,290 resulted in days away from work; 27,820 of those were due to overexertion, principally from lifting (12,130). An additional 10,670 were caused by falls on the same level.
  - The largest component of the 73,400 hospital illnesses was skin conditions (13,800), followed by respiratory illnesses (9,800).
  - Of the 292,700 recordable injuries and illnesses, 121,800 resulted in days away from work, job transfer, or restriction.
- Among all industries with at least 100,000 nonfatal injuries or illnesses reported in 2003, hospitals had the greatest number (292,700), followed by nursing and residential care facilities (221,500). (See figure 1-1.)
- In 2003, the rate of recordable injuries and illnesses in all of private industry fell from the 1994 rate by about 40 percent, to 5.0 per 100 full-time workers, while the rate in hospitals fell only about 24 percent, to 8.7 per 100 full-time workers.

The BLS has reported that in 2003, nonfatal injuries and illnesses in the health care industry contributed 15.0 percent of all nonfatal occupational injuries and 17.9 percent of all nonfatal occupational illnesses recorded among all workers in private industry in the United States.[8]

COST OF INJURIES AND ILLNESSES

As previously noted, hospitals recorded 121,800 injuries and illnesses in 2003 that resulted in days away from work, a job transfer, or restricted duties. For those injuries or illnesses that resulted in days away from work only (67,300), the median duration was six days, resulting in a total of about 403,800 days

Figure 1–1. Industries with at Least 100,000 Nonfatal Workplace Injuries and Illnesses (2003)

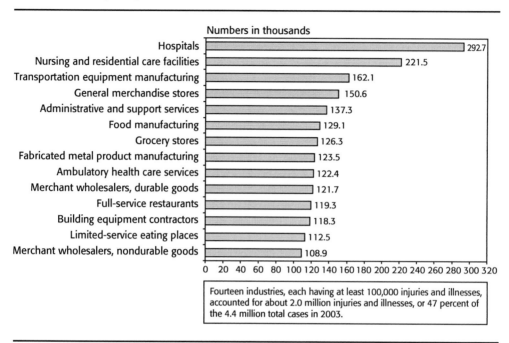

Numbers in thousands

Hospitals	292.7
Nursing and residential care facilities	221.5
Transportation equipment manufacturing	162.1
General merchandise stores	150.6
Administrative and support services	137.3
Food manufacturing	129.1
Grocery stores	126.3
Fabricated metal product manufacturing	123.5
Ambulatory health care services	122.4
Merchant wholesalers, durable goods	121.7
Full-service restaurants	119.3
Building equipment contractors	118.3
Limited-service eating places	112.5
Merchant wholesalers, nondurable goods	108.9

Fourteen industries, each having at least 100,000 injuries and illnesses, accounted for about 2.0 million injuries and illnesses, or 47 percent of the 4.4 million total cases in 2003.

Source: Bureau of Labor Statistics, U.S. Department of Labor (December 2004)

away from work. As a result of those days away from work, and assuming a 50-week work year and a 5-day workweek, the American hospital industry lost more than 1,600 full-time–equivalent employees in 2003, which is equivalent to one 1,600-employee hospital being closed for one year.

In 2003, the National Safety Council (NSC) reported that direct and indirect costs associated with the nation's 4,365,200 recordable workplace injuries and illnesses totaled $156.2 billion, or about $35,500 per case.[9] Thus, the recordable 292,700 injuries and illnesses among hospital employees cost the industry about $10.39 billion. Distributing that cost over the estimated 5,000 hospitals in the United States results in a cost of about $2.1 million per hospital.

Unfortunately, those numbers represent only the tip of the iceberg. Many public health professionals have expressed concern that the BLS estimates under-report the true number of workplace injuries and illnesses by perhaps 53 percent or more.[10] If this is correct, then the true number of injured and ill hospital workers in 2003 exceeded 448,000, and the associated industry cost was $15.9 billion, or about $3.2 million per hospital. It can also be assumed that the number of lost workdays would be similarly greater than reported and may have approached 600,000 days away from work, which is equivalent to a 2,400-employee hospital being closed for one year.

As this book was going to press, the BLS published the recordable injury and illness data for 2004. That data show that while full-time employment in hospitals increased about 1 percent (approximately 45,000 workers), the number of recordable injuries and illnesses increased about 20 percent from 292,700 in 2003 to 352,476 in 2004. Furthermore, hospitals remained first among those industry sectors having experienced 100,000 or more recordable injuries and illnesses in 2004. If that trend continues through 2005 and 2006, the cost per facility will exceed $3 million per year and cost to the industry will approach $15 billion.

TYPES OF INJURIES AND ILLNESSES HEALTH CARE FACILITIES REPORT TO THE BLS

The injury and illness data summarized above is available because the Occupational Safety and Health Administration (OSHA) requires health care facilities to prepare and maintain records of work-related injuries and illnesses using OSHA's Form 300, Log of Work-Related Injuries and Illnesses. [CD-ROM 1.2] These injuries and illnesses are called "recordable" and help OSHA and facilities keep track of the kinds of work-related injuries and illnesses in order to help prevent them in the future.

An injury or illness is recordable if it results in death, days away from work, restricted work or transfer to another job, medical treatment beyond first aid, or loss of consciousness. An injury or illness must also be recorded if it is diagnosed by a physician or other licensed health care professional, even if it does not result in death, days away from work, restricted work or job transfer, medical treatment beyond first aid, or loss of consciousness. All work-related needlestick injuries and cuts from sharp objects that are contaminated with another person's blood or other potentially infectious material must be recorded.[11]

HEALTH CARE HAZARDS THAT LEAD TO RECORDABLE INJURIES AND ILLNESSES

Health care facilities harbor an exhaustive list of hazards. Employees at risk range from caregivers to housekeeping staff. Categories of hazards that contribute to the high rate of injuries and illnesses are listed in figure 1-2.[12]

THE MOST FREQUENT OSHA NONCOMPLIANCE CITATIONS

OSHA inspects worksites for various reasons. Figure 1-3 lists the most common grounds for inspections in health care facilities.

For the period September 2003 through October 2004, there were 116 OSHA inspections in hospitals that resulted in 534 citations at a cost of more than $287,000. The most frequently cited standard was the Bloodborne pathogens (BBP) standard (29 CFR 1910.1030). In addition to those citations, the Centers for Disease Control and Prevention (CDC) estimates that each year there are 385,000 needlestick and other sharps-related injuries in hospitals, but because of under-reporting, the actual number may be 500,000 or more.[13]

Figure 1–2. Categories of Hazards That Contribute to the High Rate of Injuries and Illnesses

☐ Infectious hazards—Bloodborne pathogens (BBP) and tuberculosis (TB).

☐ Chemical hazards—Anesthetic agents, antineoplastic agents, cleaning and sterilizing agents, insecticides, solvents, and tissue fixatives.

☐ Physical hazards—Simply walking down a hospital corridor may be a challenge: housekeeping carts, wheelchairs, extra stretchers, and broken beds frequently clutter corridors. Sharps injuries, including needles, disposable syringes, and scalpel blades. Sprains and strains. Back injuries related to the lifting of patients and equipment. Electrical hazards related to the abundance of equipment with strong electrical charges. Patient assaults.

☐ Psychosocial/psychological health hazards—Emotional stress from constant demands from co-workers, physicians, and patients. Work patterns that do not allow for restful breaks. Substance abuse. Rotating shifts. Threats of terrorism.

☐ Environmental hazards—Radiation, noise pollution, and indoor air quality problems.

Following citations for violations of the Bloodborne pathogens standard were citations for violations of standards normally thought to be associated only with industrial environments[14] (table 1-1).

THE CURRENT ORGANIZATION OF HEALTH CARE EMPLOYEE HEALTH AND SAFETY

In an industrial environment, worker safety and health occupies a significant position within the corporate management structure and business plan. The relationship between productivity, product quality, and employee safety and health is well understood. A person in a senior position who is a direct report of senior leadership typically manages and has overall responsibility for all aspects of the workplace health and safety program. Further, industry often

Figure 1–3. The Most Common Bases for OSHA Inspections in Health Care Facilities

☐ Employee complaints

☐ Randomly planned inspections

☐ Anonymous reports from the public about an unsafe condition

☐ Historically higher injury or illness rates, as shown in the annual OSHA Form 300 logs and workers' compensation records

Table 1–1. The Most Frequently Cited OSHA Citations in Health Care Facilities Other than the Bloodborne Pathogens Standard

OSHA Standard	OSHA Standard Number	OSHA Requirement
The control of hazardous energy, lockout/tagout	29 CFR 1910.147	The source of energy must be turned "off," locked/tagged out, and verified to be in the "off" position prior to conducting assigned work. Lockout/tagout must be used whenever an employee performs service or maintenance around any machine where someone could be injured by unexpected start-up or release of stored energy.
Electrical systems design, general requirements	29 CFR 1910.303	The ability to work safely and reliably on electrical equipment systems.
Maintenance, safeguards, and operational features for exit routes	29 CFR 1910.37	When people need a safe and efficient means of leaving a building or facility under emergency circumstances, the means will be there and people will have minimal problems finding and using it.
Respiratory protection	29 CFR 1910.134	Employers must develop and implement a written respiratory protection program with required worksite-specific procedures and training.
Hazard communication	29 CFR 1910.1200	To help reduce the incidence of chemical-source illness and injuries, employers and employees must know about work hazards and how to protect themselves.
Abrasive wheel machinery	29 CFR 1910.215	Development of a written machine guarding program that includes training. The potential hazard is that an improperly mounted and used wheel can literally explode, causing serious or fatal injury to the operator.
Guarding floor and wall openings and holes	29 CFR 1910.23	Floor openings and holes, wall openings and holes, and the open sides of platforms must be protected using railings and guards that prevent people and equipment from falling through the openings.

works in labor-management partnership environments to solve health and safety problems.

However, in many health care facilities, the principal emphasis is on patient care and safety, accreditation requirements, and compliance with a host of federal regulations other than employee health and safety. This emphasis does not mean that health care facilities ignore employee safety and health. In fact, most health care facilities assign an individual to safety responsibilities. However, several factors contribute to the higher incidence of work-related injuries and illnesses in health care facilities when compared to the average of all other industries:

☐ The individual responsible for employee safety often has other areas of responsibility and is not able to devote the necessary time to employee health and safety.

☐ The safety professional may not have a leadership role and may report to any of several indirectly related departments, such as Human Resources or Engineering.

☐ The sphere of influence of the individual is often limited.

☐ The success of employee health and safety programs is judged almost entirely on the success of accreditation surveys.

☐ Health care facilities often overlook OSHA safety and health program guidelines that were developed to reduce accidents and illnesses.

In addition, health care facilities often maintain independent workers' compensation, public safety and security, and employee health programs. Further, OSHA Form 300 logs are often maintained in a department unrelated to health and safety. This functional separation of health and safety throughout health care facilities may at first seem rational based on the unique nature of those different areas. However, this approach may act as an impediment to improvements in employee well-being, patient care, and the corporate bottom line.

With this widely decentralized approach, what is the likelihood that there will be the systematic collection and exchange of information necessary to conduct epidemiological analysis or injury surveillance to identify and correct problems related to employee health and safety?

THE JOINT COMMISSION'S REQUIREMENTS FOR A HEALTHY AND SAFE WORK ENVIRONMENT

The Joint Commission on Accreditation of Healthcare Organizations is a significant advocate for the proposition that "health care organizations can and should minimize avoidable risks and injuries" not only to patients, but also to staff and others in the facility. In the "Management of the Environment of Care" chapter in its accreditation manuals, the Joint Commission articulates its expectations that health care organizations satisfactorily manage their safety risks for patients, staff, and visitors; maintain a safe and secure work environment and environment of care; and measure, monitor, and improve conditions in the health care environment for patients, staff, and visitors. The concept that patient safety and worker safety are inextricably bound and depend on strong leadership pervades Joint Commission standards, particularly in the "Management of the Environment of Care" and "Leadership" chapters.

There are many Joint Commission Leadership standards that are vital to the successful establishment and operation of the Environmental Health and Safety Department. For example, Leadership standard LD.1.30 requires that the health care facility comply with applicable laws and regulations; and LD.3.70 places the burden for adequate and competent staffing squarely on the health care facility's leadership, as it does for measuring and assessing safety improvement activities in LD.4.70.

Although the Joint Commission and OSHA share common goals and, in many cases, approaches to reducing work-related injuries and illness, they are not identical. Achieving Joint Commission accreditation is not equivalent to OSHA compliance. By the same token, compliance with OSHA regulations alone does not ensure that the requirements of the Joint Commission have been met.

ENVIRONMENTAL HEALTH AND SAFETY: THE CORNERSTONE OF THE ENVIRONMENT OF CARE

As described earlier in this chapter, one of the costs of providing patient care is an above-average rate of recordable injuries and illnesses compared with all private industry sectors. The critical role that employee health and safety plays in patient health and safety may be overlooked, not out of a callous disregard for employees but because of an assumption that the guidelines and standards established by accreditation organizations to improve patient health and safety satisfy federal regulations for protecting employee health and safety as well.

Recordable injuries and illnesses in the health care industry exceed the average for all of private industry. Although these rates have declined over the last decade in the health care industry, they have done so at a slower rate than in other industry sectors. These data demonstrate that a sole emphasis on compliance with accreditation guidelines and standards does not adequately protect employees even though there are many accreditation standards that address employee health and safety. This pattern can be changed if health care facilities elevate the status of their employee safety program within the corporate structure. The first step in the process is to understand the nature of the problem and to adopt a functional concept of employee health and safety that encompasses all aspects of the facility's operations.

Until health care facilities begin to understand that a safe and healthy workforce is essential to quality patient care, the present pattern of injuries, illnesses, and accidents will continue. To improve their workers' compensation record and reach the next level of performance in patient care, health care facilities need to recognize that employee safety and health has a significant impact on each department's overall performance as well as on the cost of providing patient care.

CHANGING THE CULTURE

It is not enough that management commits itself; they must know what it is that they are committed to.

J. Edward Deming

The complaint is often voiced that management is not committed to the facility's safety and health program. However, what is perceived as a lack of commitment may actually be a lack of understanding of the details of an effective employee health and safety program and the role it plays in quality patient care.

In most cases, senior leadership does not understand the process of industrial hygiene monitoring or the details and basis of the standards and regulations that apply to employee health and safety. That does not mean they are not committed to the health and safety of their employees, but "they must know what they are committed to." For administrators to have an active commitment to employee health and safety, they need to understand the extent and nature of that commitment.

Environmental Health and Safety should be a driver of patient safety as well as employee safety and health, and should operate as a profit center rather than a cost center. The truly visionary Environmental Health and Safety program will also recognize the relationship between personal well-being and workplace health and safety. The Environmental Health and Safety professional must find ways to convey this vision to the facility's administration.

The *Total Health and Safety*™ Program

The *Total Health and Safety*™ program presented throughout this book is one way to convey this vision to administrators. It provides the facility with an understanding of the reason for federal regulations and guides the development of plans and procedures to build a comprehensive health and safety management program. While each element of the total program is a distinct unit (e.g., hazardous chemicals, fire safety, medical surveillance, and data collection), together the components form a continuous system that has a positive influence on the operation of the facility and on the health and well-being of employees and patients alike. *Total Health and Safety* adds a new dimension to a facility's safety and health effort by serving as the cornerstone of the facility's employee and patient safety and health programs. [CD-ROM 1.3]

The *Total Health and Safety* program is a broad-based initiative that uses the very best elements of functional and motivational programs from around the world to bridge the gap between the safety and health program for employees and that for patients, as well as for their families (see figure 1-4).

The program is based on the concept that exceptional workplace health and safety programs and outcomes rely on the partnership of management and employees, who share equal responsibility for the program's success. The program integrates traditional workplace safety and health principles with those of stress management, proper body mechanics, and standard concepts of basic hygiene and nutrition.

Quality-of-life issues, such as respect, courteous treatment, and attitude, also affect safety and health and patient care. A positive atmosphere results

Figure 1–4. The *Total Health and Safety*™ Program

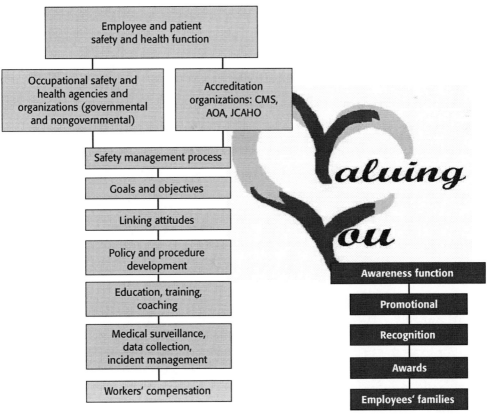

in employees who take greater pride in their work, and that pride is reflected in their patient care. *Total Health and Safety* helps to instill this positive attitude through hands-on activities that teach the skills needed to ensure that patients receive safe, compassionate, and quality care. Patients and employees will communicate their positive experiences to their friends and families when they return home.

Conveying the Vision of Health and Safety

It is the Environmental Health and Safety director's responsibility to understand the impact of occupational illnesses and injuries and to be positioned to explain that impact to administrators in terms they are familiar with, specifying what it is they should be committed to and why. Unless the Environmental Health and Safety professional can clearly communicate the needs of the department in terms that the chief financial officer (CFO) or chief operating officer (COO) can understand, the chances of success are limited. The Environmental Health and Safety director must be able to reach out to senior leadership and impart a sense of what the department is doing that has a positive impact on the day-to-day operations of the facility.

The most effective communications are those that are supported by data. The administration must be presented with summary data that includes the following:

- ☐ Recent monitoring results for chemical substances and agents covered by standards and regulations
- ☐ Data from OSHA Form 300 logs
- ☐ The incidence of recordable injuries and illnesses
- ☐ The causes of injuries and illnesses
- ☐ The costs, both direct and indirect, of those injuries and illnesses
- ☐ Recent requests for health and safety assistance and the disposition of those requests
- ☐ Findings from in-house audits and inspections
- ☐ Current and planned training and why it is needed
- ☐ A plan for correcting any problems, including the anticipated expense and return on investment

When such presentations are made, the goal must be to show how the health and safety concerns that have been raised relate to patient care and how corrective action will enhance the facility's ability to provide quality care. For example, if it can be demonstrated that the training of department liaisons to recognize health and safety hazards they encounter in their departments leads to quicker, less costly corrective action and a safer environment for employees, patients, and the general public, it will become easier to show that the ultimate outcome is fewer accidents, lower risk exposure, fewer days away from work, and a decrease in workers' compensation costs. Presentations must be made in a style that fits the communication expectations of the audience. Neither the housekeeping staff nor the COO wants to hear a science lecture.

HIRING AND PLACEMENT CONSIDERATIONS

For the administration, the most important staffing considerations for the Environmental Health and Safety Department should be qualifications and location within the structure of the organization. Qualifications should be based on a combination of education, experience, and training and be appropriate to the complexity and size of the facility's operations. While it is true that the senior leader of the facility sets the tone for what is important, Environmental Safety and Health professionals also have a major responsibility to senior leadership, employees, and patients throughout the facility. The person in charge of Environmental Health and Safety is responsible for the well-being of each employee, contractor, volunteer, vendor, patient, and visitor.

Because of the complexity of a health care facility, the person in charge of Environmental Health and Safety should have the following qualifications, skills, and values:

- ☐ Strong technical knowledge of Environmental Health and Safety and a passion for the arena.
- ☐ A demonstrated knowledge of federal, state, and local regulations and accrediting organization standards.
- ☐ A balanced and thorough knowledge of the health and safety aspects of the profession.
- ☐ A commitment to safety and health that is based on caring.
- ☐ Flexibility and the ability to think quickly.
- ☐ A superior knowledge of the technical aspects of the job, as well as a solid understanding of business processes.
- ☐ The ability to professionally communicate verbally and in writing, including the ability to determine how to effectively communicate with staff having a wide range of education, training, and language backgrounds.
- ☐ A philosophy based on the principle that risk and safety can be managed.
- ☐ Excellent analytical and problem-solving skills.
- ☐ Effective project management skills and the ability to set effective goals.
- ☐ Negotiation skills and the ability to win the support of certain individuals for projects. Environmental Health and Safety professionals negotiate for many reasons. Style is critical.
- ☐ Facilitation skills and active listening skills.
- ☐ A willingness to take risks and try new methodologies.

To be valued by the administration, the Environmental Health and Safety professional must be positioned in the facility as an authority with adequate resources and direct access to senior leadership.

A MODEL ENVIRONMENTAL HEALTH AND SAFETY DEPARTMENT: ORGANIZATIONAL AND FUNCTIONAL DESCRIPTION

Employee health and safety is unlike any other activity in the health care facility. Although it deals with workers' compensation issues, it is not a Human Resources activity. And while it addresses issues of emergency management, it is not a Security activity. Similarly, employee health and safety is concerned with preventing diseases, but it is not a clinical activity.

Figure 1-5 presents the organizational chart of a model Environmental Health and Safety Department.

Even though it may be argued that many of the functions described in this model are already being performed within the facility and are fully staffed, they may be distant from senior management and have little interaction with each other. This model unifies the various activities that are vital to a cohesive, efficient employee health and safety program. In addition, the model relies on a strong relationship between the Environmental Health and Safety Department and the facility's infection control coordinator, patient safety officer, and risk manager.

This model is applicable to a facility of any size, although small facilities may need to arrange for external support for some of the environmental monitoring activities. The intent of this model is not to add staff where needed but to consolidate the various functions of a first-tier Environmental

Figure 1–5. Model for an Environmental Health and Safety Department

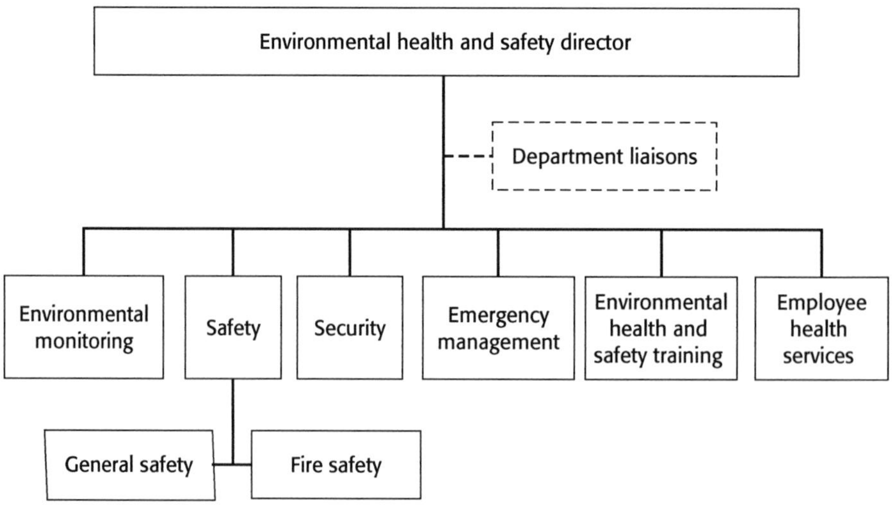

Health and Safety program. In this model, the Environmental Health and Safety director is positioned to fully manage the department, with direct access to senior leadership. The director is a senior-level position, with no responsibilities other than the leadership and direction of the department.

Teams derived from the appropriate functions within the department will conduct some activities. In some cases, it will be necessary to seek the expertise of staff from other departments. For example, team approaches are effective in conducting a job hazard analysis (JHA) to identify work-related hazards and take measures to eliminate or control them, because the team members will have different areas of expertise that are all essential to a thorough JHA. [CD-ROM 1.4] Additional team activities may include incident investigations, emergency management, policy development, ergonomics, hazard surveillance, and program evaluation.

Environmental Health and Safety intersects with every aspect of the facility's operations, from the administration to the kitchen, and includes the following major functions:

> Environmental Health and Safety Director
> Environmental Monitoring
> Safety (General Safety and Fire Safety)
> Security
> Emergency Management
> Environmental Health and Safety Training
> Employee Health Services
> Department Liaisons

Environmental Health and Safety Director

The model organization chart demonstrates the scope of responsibility of the Environmental Health and Safety director. This function requires a senior manager who has broad experience in occupational health and safety and a thorough knowledge of federal, state, and local regulations and worker health and safety accreditation standards governing the facility's operations. This individual must also have excellent communication and analytical skills. The Environmental Health and Safety director determines who will be the "competent person," as defined by OSHA.

The Environmental Health and Safety director has overall program responsibility, providing technical and policy direction. Among the responsibilities are:

> □ Leadership and direction
> □ Current knowledge and oversight of regulatory requirements, including the Occupational Safety and Health Act of 1970 (OSH Act) [CD-ROM 1.5]

☐ An understanding of how to implement OSHA's *Safety and Health Program Management Guidelines*[15] [CD-ROM 1.6]

☐ A current library of recognized health and safety reference texts, journals, standards, regulations, and guidelines

☐ Adherence to regulatory and accreditation guidelines and standards under the responsibilities of the department

☐ Chairing the Environmental Health and Safety Committee

☐ Serving as the facility's community liaison on Environmental Health and Safety issues

☐ Budget preparation, presentation, and management

☐ Communicating existing and emerging health and safety issues to senior leadership

☐ Marketing the department to employees and their families

☐ Measuring the program's success

☐ Producing annual reports and other department documentation

Environmental Monitoring

An individual knowledgeable in industrial hygiene should perform the Environmental Monitoring function, which includes the following responsibilities:

☐ Chemical, biological, radiological, and noise monitoring

☐ Periodic environmental audits and mandatory inspections to recognize, evaluate, and control chemical releases or exposures to hazardous substances

☐ Ensure compliance with OSHA health regulations and Joint Commission monitoring standards not required by OSHA or other federal, state, and local regulatory agencies

☐ Periodic JHAs for health-related issues

☐ Administering the respiratory protection program

☐ Protective clothing and equipment, including the OSHA-required hazard assessment

☐ Hazardous and medical waste management

☐ Hazard communication program

☐ Serves as a resource to other departments for occupational health-related issues

Safety

The Safety function is split into a General Safety function and a Fire Safety function.

The General Safety function is performed by an individual who is knowledgeable in worker safety standards and regulations and in the recognition of safety hazards. This function is responsible for the following:

□ Compliance with workplace safety standards and guidelines

□ Undertake periodic JHAs for safety-related issues

□ Confirm that identified safety-related maintenance and repair needs have been completed

□ Department activities involving incident investigations, root cause analyses, and corrective actions

□ Serve as a resource to other departments for safety-related information

□ Administer driver safety program for facility vehicles, use of personal cars on company business, and use of rented vehicles on company business

The Fire Safety function is performed by an individual who is knowledgeable in fire safety, hazards, and standards and regulations, and includes:

□ Maintaining compliance with fire codes and accreditation standards related to fire and life safety

□ Overseeing the fire prevention and control program

□ Liaison with the local fire department

Security

By virtue of their service, Security staff can serve as the first line of surveillance for emerging safety and health problems, if they have been trained to recognize them. Security also acts as liaison with the local Police Department and is an essential element of any emergency response. Security staff also address workplace violence issues.

Although the Security function is included in the model for those reasons, valid arguments exist for maintaining Security as a separate department. Regardless of where the Security function resides administratively, security officers should be trained in the recognition and evaluation of health and safety issues.

Emergency Management

An Emergency Management function is also included in the model. The Emergency Management function:

□ Ensures that the facility is prepared for either natural or man-made disasters by ensuring compliance with federal, state, and local regulations and accreditation standards related to emergency management

□ Provides liaison with state, county, and local emergency management activities

□ Directs hazardous materials (HAZMAT) teams and responses in coordination with other functions of the department, and decontamination teams in coordination with state and local emergency response organizations

Environmental Health and Safety Training

The Training function is responsible for planning and directing Environmental Health and Safety training for the facility. This function also:

□ Develops and trains the department liaisons and the Security staff to carry out their responsibilities for health and safety

□ Assists other departments with in-service training programs in all areas of health and safety

□ Provides support to other departments regarding personal protective equipment training

□ Encourages employee and family participation in health and safety activities

□ Participates in new-employee orientation specific to worker health and safety issues

□ Performs group training sessions relating to the prevention of specific injuries

□ Ensures that a competent person, as defined by OSHA, is available when required

This individual should have broad experience with and knowledge of Environmental Health and Safety and be a skilled trainer.

Employee Health Services

The Employee Health Services function has responsibility for:

□ Pre- and post-employment medical examinations required by regulatory agencies

□ Periodic medical examinations

□ Medical surveillance activities required by OSHA standards[16]

□ Recordkeeping, including maintenance of OSHA Form 300 logs

□ Epidemiological analysis of injury and illness data

□ Liaison with state and local health departments

□ Management of workers' compensation cases and return-to-work programs

□ Distribution of publications and pamphlets on workplace health and safety

□ Awareness programs involving personal and family safety and health

Department Liaisons

The Environmental Health and Safety department liaison is a new function for each department but does not require a new position. An essential condition for the success of this model is that each department liaison receive training in at least the following areas:

- ☐ The OSH Act
- ☐ Principles of Environmental Health and Safety
- ☐ Applicable worker health and safety accreditation standards from the Joint Commission
- ☐ How to recognize, evaluate, and control workplace health and safety hazards in their departments
- ☐ Risk communication

The department liaisons serve as the connection between the Environmental Health and Safety Department and the other departments in the facility. The principal activities of the liaison function are to:

- ☐ Routinely interact with department managers and staff to identify existing or emerging problems
- ☐ Work with department managers and staff to develop a plan to resolve problems
- ☐ Represent their respective departments on the Environmental Health and Safety Committee
- ☐ Identify the department's training needs and work with the Environmental Health and Safety Training function to implement the training

In this model, the department liaison function is not a direct report of the Environmental Health and Safety Department. The duties of the liaisons should be included in the job description along with the specific percentage of time allocated to Environmental Health and Safety. In addition to other positions, the facility's hazardous drug officer, chemical hygiene officer, biological safety officer, and radiation safety officer are ideally suited to serve as department liaisons to the Environmental Health and Safety Department.

BENEFITS OF THE MODEL DEPARTMENT

Earlier in this chapter, data from the BLS and the NSC was presented that documented the human and capital costs of recordable injuries and illnesses. The safety and health function is centralized in most businesses other than health care facilities, and the health care industry is urged to follow suit in order to reduce work-related injuries and illnesses. This centralized approach has met with great success in many different industries, and the same success can be realized in health care facilities.

In 2002, the American Society of Safety Engineers (ASSE) published a white paper addressing the return on investment for effective Environmental Health and Safety management programs.[17] [CD-ROM 1.7] ASSE documented the success stories of businesses that made a commitment to investing in Environmental Health and Safety management programs:

☐ In 1994, 178 companies that participated in an OSHA program designed to reduce injuries and illnesses reported that overall they experienced only 45 percent of the injuries expected based on data from prior years.

☐ Implementation of an improved safety and health program reduced one company's workers' compensation costs by $2.4 million over a two-year period.

☐ A coal mining company reported a workers' compensation rate of $1.28 per $100 in payroll, compared with its competitor's rate of $13.78.

☐ A manufacturer saved $61,000 on its workers' compensation insurance premiums and saved $130 million in direct and indirect injury and illness costs in 1999.

The ASSE also cited *Forbes* magazine's 1999 financial rankings, which concluded that 10 of the most successful U.S. businesses were participants in an OSHA program designed to reduce worker injuries and illnesses. Finally, the ASSE cited a report by the OSHA Office of Regulatory Analysis: "Our evidence suggests that companies that implement effective safety and health (programs) can expect reductions of 20% or greater in their injury and illness rates and a return of $4 to $6 for every $1 invested."

If health care facilities achieve the same 45 percent reduction in injuries and illnesses, the industry-wide savings could amount to between roughly $5 billion and $10 billion in the first year.

There are a host of intangible benefits as well. By centralizing the facility's Environmental Health and Safety activities, there will be:

☐ Better communications
☐ Improved data collection and recordkeeping
☐ More comprehensive medical and safety surveillance
☐ A more precise understanding of the direct and indirect costs of injuries and illnesses
☐ An enhanced relationship with the local community
☐ Improved employee morale
☐ Enhanced patient care and safety

In addition, if each of the functions in the model performs properly, the information and data needed from the Environmental Health and Safety Department to support an accreditation survey will be readily available to the facility's accreditation coordinator. By understanding the interrelationship between worker safety and health and patient safety and health, and by giving them equal emphasis, the health care facility can ensure that it is in continuous compliance with all federal, state, and local regulations as well as accreditation standards for worker health and safety.

References

1. Sagan, Carl. *Cosmos*. Novel and film series.
2. Donne, John. *The Complete Poetry and Selected Prose of John Donne* (Modern Library Series). New York: Random House, 1994.
3. Occupational Safety and Health Act of 1970 (OSH Act), Title 29, Chapter 15, Article 651. Available at http://www.osha.gov/pls/oshaweb/owadisp.show_document?p_table=OSHACT&p_id=2743 (accessed 3/28/2006).
4. NIOSH, www.cdc.gov/niosh.
5. *Standard Industrial Classification Manual 1972*. Washington, DC: U.S. Government Printing Office.
6. Table SNR08, "Incidence Rates of Nonfatal Occupational Illness, by Industry and Category of Illness, 2003." Available at http://www.bls.gov/iif/oshwc/osh/os/ostb1350.pdf (accessed 3/28/2006).
7. Table R4, "Number of Nonfatal Occupational Injuries and Illnesses Involving Days Away from Work by Industry and Selected Events or Exposures Leading to Injury or Illness, 2003." Available at www.bls.gov/iif/oshwc/osh/case/ostb1159.txt (accessed 3/28/2006).
8. *Percent of Nonfatal Workplace Injuries and Illnesses by Industry, 2003*. Available at http://www.bls.gov/iif/oshwc/osh/os/ossm0014.pdf (accessed 3/28/2006).
9. National Safety Council. *Injury Facts*. Itasca, IL: National Safety Council, 2004.
10. Leigh, J.P., et al. *Costs of Occupational Injuries and Illnesses*. Ann Arbor: University of Michigan Press, 2000. Available at http://www.pbs.org/wgbh/pages/frontline/shows/workplace/etc/cost.html (accessed 3/28/2006).
11. OSHA. *Recordkeeping Policies and Procedures Manual*. Directive CPL 02-00-135. December 30, 2004. Available at http://www.osha.gov/pls/oshaweb/owadisp.show_document?p_table=DIRECTIVES&p_id=3205 (accessed 3/28/ 2006).
12. Behling, D., and J. Guy. Adapted from: "Industry Profile: Healthcare Hazards of the Healthcare Profession," *Occupational Health & Safety*, February 1993.
13. CDC. *Workbook for Designing, Implementing, and Evaluating a Sharps Injury Prevention Program*. Available at http://www.cdc.gov/sharpssafety/workbook.html (accessed 3/28/2006).
14. Bureau of Labor Statistics, www.bls.gov.
15. OSHA. *Safety and Health Program Management Guidelines; Issuance of Voluntary Guidelines* (54 FR 3904–3916). Available at http://www.osha.gov/pls/oshaweb/owadisp.show_document?p_table=FEDERAL_REGISTER&p_id=12909 (accessed 3/28/2006).

16. OSHA. *Access to Medical and Exposure Records*. Publication 3110 (revised). Washington, DC: U.S. Department of Labor, Occupational Safety and Health Administration, 2001. Available at http://www.osha.gov/Publications/osha3110. pdf#search='Access%20to%20Medical%20and%20Exposure%20Records% 20 OSHA%203110.2001' (accessed 3/28/2006).

17. American Society of Safety Engineers. *White Paper Addressing the Return on Investment for Safety, Health, and Environmental (SH&E) Management Programs.* 2002. Available at http://www.asse.org/prac_spec_cops_issues10.htm (accessed 3/28/2006).

CHAPTER 2

GETTING THE ENVIRONMENTAL HEALTH AND SAFETY PROGRAM STARTED

The rabbit-hole went straight on like a tunnel for some way, and then dipped suddenly down, so suddenly that Alice had not a moment to think about stopping herself before she found herself falling down what seemed to be a very deep well.

Lewis Carroll, *Alice's Adventures in Wonderland*[1]

The first step in getting started on an Environmental Health and Safety program is to find out where you are and decide where you want to go before you fall into what may seem to be "a very deep well." How do you find out where you are? If you were driving across the country, you might stop every now and then to ask a gas station attendant or even a friendly-looking stranger, "Where am I? Where am I going? How do I get there?" However, once you got tired of other people giving you the information that they thought you needed, you'd probably find your own road map. The situation is not much different in the world of health and safety. You can ask around, but until you examine the historic performance of the existing program, you will have no idea where you are, where you have been, or what your goal is.

To get started, find out where you are by asking:

- ☐ What is the facility's record of work-related injuries and illnesses?
- ☐ Do any trends in the types of injuries or illnesses emerge when the data is examined?
- ☐ Has there been a sudden increase in a certain type of injury or illness over the past few weeks, months, or years?
- ☐ Is there one department, one task, or one process in which the injury rates seem to be unusually high?

- What is the facility's lost-time record?
- How much has been spent on workers' compensation during the last three years?
- Is there an existing Environmental Health and Safety program that includes major functions such as environmental monitoring, safety, emergency management, training, and employee health?
- How often are employees being trained, what is the level of training, and in what are they being trained?

RECORDKEEPING: THE ROAD MAP TO DEVELOPING AN ENVIRONMENTAL HEALTH AND SAFETY PROGRAM

The development of a successful Environmental Health and Safety program, requires that both a needs assessment and a worksite analysis be conducted. Reviewing prior records and building a foundation for future recordkeeping are essential to conducting the needs assessment and worksite analysis [CD-ROM 2.1] for several reasons:[2]

- Tracking work-related injuries and illnesses allows them to be prevented in the future.
- The use of injury and illness data helps identify problem areas and trends. The more that is known, the more effectively hazardous workplace conditions can be identified and corrected.
- With accurate records, health and safety programs can be administered more effectively.
- As employee awareness about injuries, illnesses, and hazards in the workplace improves, employees are more likely to follow safe work practices and report workplace hazards.

The Bureau of Labor Statistics (BLS) uses injury and illness records as the source of data for the *Annual Survey of Occupational Injuries and Illnesses*,[3] a report that summarizes safety and health trends nationwide and industry-wide. [CD-ROM 2.2]

THE NEEDS ASSESSMENT

An essential component of the needs assessment is an on-site evaluation of the current health and safety program. Needs assessments are generally carried out in three phases:

Preliminary data gathering
Facility tour and meetings with key people
Written report

Preliminary Data Gathering

Prior to the facility tour, the following information needs to be collected and reviewed:

☐ The status of the health and safety training program
☐ The written health and safety program
☐ Health and safety goals of the facility
☐ Minutes of the Health and Safety Committee meetings for the last two years
☐ Appropriate regulatory reports for the last three years, including loss control inspections from the insurance company
☐ Copies of Occupational Safety and Health Administration (OSHA) inspections and citations
☐ OSHA Form 300 injury and illness logs for the last three years
☐ Workers' compensation loss summaries for the last three years
☐ The workers' compensation return-to-work program
☐ Safety budget requests and approvals for the last two years
☐ Safety management reports for the last two years
☐ A copy of the new-employee orientation program
☐ The facility's mission statement, vision statement, and current business objectives

Facility Tour and Meetings with Key People

After a review of the preliminary data, meetings should be scheduled with senior leadership and key people to gain a more in-depth understanding of the facility's health and safety program. During this review:

☐ Talk with senior leadership and employees to obtain their perspective on the program and to evaluate attitudes, roles, and obstacles.
☐ Analyze the health and safety program organization and implementation.
☐ Evaluate health and safety procedures, employee training, and the application of regulatory requirements that relate to the safety program.
☐ Review the injury and illness incident reporting program.
☐ Evaluate the process for collecting data and taking actions to solve problems.
☐ Conduct a walk-through of selected departments to identify visible areas of risk.
☐ Review how the current program relates to employees and patients.

Written Report

Using the data and information that have been collected, a written report should be prepared that presents the findings, along with recommendations for program improvement. The report should include the following:

- ☐ Identification of the problems associated with the program as well as the aspects of the program that are successful
- ☐ Recommendations for remediation of identified problems
- ☐ Order-of-magnitude estimate of the cost to implement the recommendations
- ☐ Estimate of the time required to implement the recommendations
- ☐ Resources and skills necessary to implement the recommendations
- ☐ Expected outcomes based on the extent and nature of identified problems

A prioritized list of recommendations and suggestions for implementation should be developed. Once an element has been chosen for implementation, the facility's leadership should decide on the actions to be implemented and the resources to be allocated.

THE WORKSITE ANALYSIS

Once the needs assessment is complete, the worksite analysis can be started. The worksite analysis is essential to helping the administration focus on existing and emerging hazards or any changes in conditions or operations that may result in an increased hazard. The disciplines of industrial hygiene and epidemiology serve as powerful tools in the worksite analysis for identifying the causes and the extent of workplace injuries and illnesses.

> **Industrial hygiene.** Industrial hygiene is the science of recognizing, evaluating, and controlling workplace conditions that may cause employee injuries or illnesses. Industrial hygienists use environmental monitoring and analytical methods to determine the extent of worker exposure and to apply engineering solutions, work practices, and other methods to control potential health hazards. [CD-ROM 2.3]
>
> Hazards in health care facilities that require industrial hygiene expertise include air contaminants such as construction dust, airborne biological hazards, and potentially hazardous chemicals such as waste anesthetic gases, ethylene oxide, solvents, and aerosols generated during respiratory therapy.
>
> **Epidemiology.** Epidemiology is the study of epidemics, and it has been one of the most important and successful tools in the identifica-

tion of occupational injuries and illnesses and their causes. The methods of epidemiology can be applied to the injury and illness data collected by the health care facility to identify trends and excesses in the rates of specific injuries and illnesses—for example, an outbreak of respiratory illnesses among employees, an increase in the number of skin diseases and disorders in a particular department, and, in some cases, an analysis of workplace injuries.

Conducting the Worksite Analysis

A team consisting of individuals knowledgeable in industrial hygiene, epidemiology, and safety and that is educated and trained to identify, analyze, and measure workplace hazards should conduct the worksite analysis. The team can identify hazards and propose solutions for their remediation. The most effective worksite analyses examine processes, operations, jobs, and tasks.

The following steps form the basis of a good worksite analysis:[4]

□ Conduct a comprehensive baseline health and safety survey. For the industrial hygiene survey, at a minimum, all chemicals and hazardous materials in the facility should be inventoried, the hazard communication program should be reviewed, and air samples should be analyzed. The respirator program should also be examined, and a review of the ergonomic risk factors is needed. For some health care facilities, the noise levels in certain areas should be surveyed.

□ Analyze the potential health and safety hazards of planned additions and new processes, materials, and equipment (e.g., new patient care equipment, new cleaning solutions, scheduling changes in the nursing staff).

□ Identify hazards associated with job tasks. One of the most commonly used techniques is a job hazard analysis (JHA).[5] [CD-ROM 2.4] Jobs that were initially designed with safety in mind may now pose hazards. The most effective job hazard analysis will include information from employees performing the jobs.

□ Conduct periodic safety and health inspections of the workplace. Routine site safety and health inspections are sometimes known as "hazard surveillance" and are designed to identify new hazards or hazards that were missed at earlier stages. In addition, procedures should be established for conducting a daily inspection of work areas.

Although there are pre-designed checklists for worksite analyses, Environmental Health and Safety professionals should develop checklists specific to their own facilities.

In a health care facility, the worksite analysis may focus on some of the areas listed in figure 2-1.

Figure 2–1. Potential Health and Safety Hazards Confronting Health Care Workers

---

- ☐ Needlestick incidents
- ☐ Back injuries
- ☐ Work-related stress
- ☐ Lockout/tagout (LOTO)–related accidents
- ☐ Slips, trips, and falls
- ☐ Ergonomics
- ☐ Respiratory illnesses
- ☐ Skin diseases and disorders
- ☐ Introduction of new chemicals
- ☐ Chemical exposures
- ☐ Modifications to heating or ventilation systems

HOW THE JOINT COMMISSION SUPPORTS ENVIRONMENTAL HEALTH AND SAFETY PROGRAM DEVELOPMENT

Both OSHA and the Joint Commission require that health care facilities have written programs for protecting the health and safety of health care workers. The Joint Commission has made this a requirement of the accreditation process and fully supports the concept that a written program is essential to reducing work-related injuries and illnesses:

> In order to reduce employee injuries, health care organizations need to define, initiate, and maintain programs and procedures designed to prevent these injuries from occurring.[6]

Like OSHA, the Joint Commission understands that the effectiveness of any health and safety program relies fully on the commitment and leadership of the organization's management. That understanding is reflected in its Environment of Care standard, safety management (EC.1.10).

DESIGNING AND WRITING THE ENVIRONMENTAL HEALTH AND SAFETY PROGRAM

The most effective programs are designed based on the information gathered during the needs assessment and worksite analysis. Furthermore, for the program to continue to operate effectively, its performance must be routinely analyzed for successes and failures. No matter how sophisticated the health and safety efforts are, they can always be improved. Regardless of the facility's size, a systematic approach to developing an Environmental Health and Safety program will work.

Written health and safety programs can document good practices in such tasks as inspecting equipment, conducting training, evaluating contractors, and performing job observations. Establishing and implementing written health and safety procedures and guidelines should be viewed as an enhancement to health care facilities, not a hindrance, and are important in preventing incidents that cause personal injury, loss of assets, or business interruption. Procedures and guidelines are a moral obligation and a sound business practice. There is no conflict between operating safely and operating efficiently: injuries cause both human suffering and financial loss, neither of which is acceptable to a well-managed facility.

An assessment or analysis can be used to determine when written procedures and guidelines are necessary. Information is gathered by asking questions: Which employees work on electrical equipment that requires a lockout/tagout program? Which employees are required to wear personal protective equipment (PPE)? Which chemicals require industrial hygiene monitoring? Which employees need to enroll in a safe-driving program? Which employees require medical surveillance? Figure 2-2 lists some of the critical elements of a written Environmental Health and Safety program.

In order for written health and safety procedures to be successful, health and safety responsibilities should be included in each job description. The administration, department heads, and supervisors must also be assigned specific responsibilities to ensure a safe and healthful workplace. Individual performance and participation in the overall health and safety process should be considered an essential part of every employee's total job performance and be included in the performance evaluation program. The ultimate responsibility for injury and illness prevention rests with each employee.

As is the case with the worksite analysis, there are pre-designed safety and health programs available, but Environmental Health and Safety professionals should design one specific to their facility.

ESTABLISHING AND LEADING A PRODUCTIVE HEALTH AND SAFETY COMMITTEE

The Health and Safety Committee is essential to the success of the Environmental Health and Safety program. There are many different types of Health and Safety Committees. Some facilities base the committee primarily on the Joint Commission Environment of Care (EC) standards and thus call it the Environment of Care (EC) Committee. Other facilities design the committee to be a management Health and Safety Committee. Some facilities with unions have joint labor/management Health and Safety Committees. Some facilities that are not unionized have joint employee/management Health and Safety Committees.

Figure 2–2. Critical Elements of a Written Environmental Health and Safety Program

---

☐ Introduction to the program

☐ Goals of the program

☐ Structure and function of the Environmental Health and Safety Department

☐ Contact information for the Environmental Health and Safety Department

☐ Types of records to keep, the importance of keeping them, and the system used for recordkeeping

☐ Procedure for reporting an injury or illness

☐ Function of the department liaisons

☐ Standards and regulations that apply to the entire health care facility

☐ Standards and regulations that apply to specific departments

☐ Requirements for training

☐ Requirements for personal protective equipment (PPE)

☐ Organization and function of the Environmental Health and Safety Committee

☐ Awards and incentives programs

☐ Copy of written health and safety procedures and plans as required by regulatory agencies and/or accreditation organizations, including waste management, hazard communication, respiratory protection, emergency management, fire prevention, hazardous waste operations and emergency response (HAZWOPER), personal protective equipment (PPE) hazard assessment, chemical hygiene, bloodborne pathogen (BBP) exposure control, construction, and violence

☐ Copy of the safety and health program required for federal health care facilities (Section 19 of the Occupational Safety and Health Act of 1970 and 29 CFR 1960), if appropriate

---

Regardless of the type of committee that is established, the most effective one will have management and employees working together toward the goal of a workplace free from hazards. It is the administration's overall responsibility to provide resources and implement policies and procedures. It is the department's responsibility to promote health and safety policies and procedures to its employees. Employees and management must demonstrate their commitment in many ways to achieve success. Required resources may vary from money to personnel to time.

Other elements that are necessary for establishing and leading an effective Health and Safety Committee include the following:

☐ Technical knowledge

☐ Program management skills

☐ Knowledge of organizational behavior
☐ Understanding that health and safety is another tool for business decision making
☐ Understanding that health and safety is not simply an add-on program or a requirement for regulatory compliance or accreditation

A successful Health and Safety Committee also considers:

Organizational structure
Communications
Training
Meeting conduct

Organizational Structure

The organizational structure of a Health and Safety Committee is essential to its operation. The committee should be comprised of representatives from each department, including clinical and nonclinical staff, union members (if applicable), the administration, and the department liaisons. The Environmental Health and Safety director should chair the committee. The committee should have a recording secretary, and it should be a mix of managerial and non-managerial staff.

Communications

Effective communication is key to a successful Environmental Health and Safety Committee and program. Committee minutes should be posted and made available for employee review, and they should be used to track action items and their closure dates.

Training

Training for Environmental Health and Safety Committee members should be designed to assist both management and employee representatives. Members should learn their roles and responsibilities as health and safety representatives in the health care facility. Training topics should include the following:

☐ The principles of health and safety
☐ A basic understanding of the Occupational Safety and Health Act of 1970 (OSH Act) and the responsibilities assigned to all employees
☐ Accreditation organization standards that relate to the Environmental Health and Safety program

☐ A guide to safety committee meetings, describing how a Health and Safety Committee should operate, responsibilities of all committee members, and the process of making and following up on recommendations

☐ How to recognize, evaluate, and control workplace hazards

☐ Accident investigation techniques

Meeting Conduct

The most effective committees encourage a free flow of ideas and make decisions based on data and objective information. In addition, they observe the following operating principles:

☐ Meetings are held at regularly scheduled times and places.

☐ Ground rules are established for how the meetings will proceed.

☐ An agenda is prepared and distributed prior to the meeting.

☐ The agenda is followed.

☐ Official notes are taken.

☐ Members agree on a decision-making process.

☐ Timelines are established for implementing decisions.

☐ Individuals are assigned action items and are held accountable for completion of those items.

DEPARTMENT HAZARD SURVEILLANCE

The successful Environmental Health and Safety program is led from the top but built from the bottom up. To keep from falling down the same "deep well" as Alice, the Environmental Health and Safety Department must have the active participation of each department of the health care facility. Each department must, at a minimum, know:

☐ Which OSHA and other federal, state, local, and Joint Commission standards apply to the activities within the department

☐ Whether the department is currently in compliance with the applicable standards

☐ The department's injury and illness experience

☐ The status of the department's medical surveillance activities

Every six months, each department head and department liaison should conduct an audit to determine the compliance status of the department and its injury and illness experience. The results of these audits should be presented at the Health and Safety Committee meetings.

When department audits are conducted, appropriate staff from the Environmental Health and Safety Department should be involved. The audit should address not only the appropriate OSHA, Environmental Protection Agency (EPA), National Fire Protection Association (NFPA), and other regulatory standards, guidelines, and recommendations, but the standards and survey recommendations of accreditation organizations as well. The concept of the biannual department-level audit is consistent with OSHA standards requiring biannual air monitoring for chemicals that are regulated under the OSH Act. [CD-ROM 2.5–2.8]

Such proactive surveillance will, in conjunction with the concepts presented in this chapter, prevent injuries, illnesses, and deaths from work-related causes; minimize losses of material resources; and prevent service interruptions in both work-related and other activities.

Each department faces unique employee health and safety challenges, including ever-increasing compliance requirements from OSHA, EPA, NFPA, other agencies, and accreditation organizations. By understanding the potential hazards in their departments, the department heads and department liaisons are well positioned to identify potential hazards and to correct them before an injury or illness occurs.

There are many types of hazards, including environmental (unlabeled containers that may contain hazardous chemicals), physical (damaged sidewalks), and unsafe practices (using ladders with broken rungs). Alternative work arrangements, such as job sharing, assigning part-time employees, scheduling longer shifts, and employing temporary workers, are common responses to rapid technological and economic changes. The unintended consequences of these alternative work arrangements can include fatigue and hectic work environments that can lead to injuries and illnesses and may compromise patient safety. In addition, cultural differences and language barriers presented by non–English-speaking workers can create stressful situations among employees and patients.[7]

Additional observations should be noted during departmental audits, such as the attitudes of employees, the condition of the physical facility, compliance with the elements of the existing health and safety program, and, in some cases, the condition of the equipment.

Hazard surveillance is the first step in the ongoing three-step process of recognition, evaluation, and control. Whether the hazard surveillance inspections are conducted by the Environmental Health and Safety Department, by the Health and Safety Committee, or by department liaisons, department heads, and employees, data must be collected that can be measured and tied in with the facility's health and safety program goals. The successful hazard surveillance program is dynamic and changes with the work environment. Furthermore, the list of items to be considered may change with each inspection because the problems that had been identified and corrected will have been removed and new areas of interest identified.

It is pointless to send teams to conduct surveillance activities if the list of items to be examined is not customized to the department or doesn't address the concerns of the employees or the facility. Typically, such completed forms are simply turned in to the Health and Safety Committee with few or no results.

Figure 2–3. Hazard Surveillance Planning

1. What is the primary job function of each department, and what are the potential hazards for each department?
2. What injuries or illnesses occur most frequently (e.g., strains, sprains, abrasions)?
3. What department(s) had the most injuries or illnesses?
4. What job(s) resulted in the most injuries or illnesses (e.g., nurse, maintenance worker, housekeeper, cook)?
5. What caused the most injuries or illnesses (e.g., being struck by an object, slipping on wet floors, lifting objects)?
6. What injuries or illnesses cost the most in workers' compensation claims?
7. What "recommendations to prevent future accidents" appear most frequently on the accident investigation form (e.g., training, wearing proper PPE, addressing worker fatigue, correcting unsafe methods)?
8. What safety and health suggestions have employees submitted?
9. What do the safety and health committee minutes identify as prominent issues?
10. Review the specialized programs required for compliance with OSHA regulations, such as lockout/tagout, PPE hazard assessment and training, the BBP exposure control plan, the chemical hygiene plan, the respiratory protection program, and ergonomics.
11. Review training records against the OSHA Form 300 logs and workers' compensation reports.
12. Submit baseline surveys for safety and health hazards, including industrial hygiene sampling records and material safety data sheets.
13. Complete OSHA-required monitoring and medical surveillance records. What hazardous chemicals are employees exposed to in each department and at what concentrations? This portion of the inspection/surveillance focuses on air quality, noise level, exposure to toxic and hazardous substances, and ergonomics.
14. Consider breaking the inspections down through the use of teams or scheduling several mini-inspections throughout the year instead of performing two full-scale inspections each year.

Figure 2-3 provides examples of situations to consider in the design of the surveillance or inspection form.

Table 2-1 is an example of the data to include on a checklist to document problems and record actions taken as well as observations and action taken after follow-up visits.

Table 2–1. Examples of Data Types to Include on a Hazard Surveillance Checklist

Location	Topic, Item, or Subject	Date Observed	Comments	Immediate Action Taken	Follow-up Action Taken

Table 2-2 provides a partial list of items and standards that will govern the majority of health care facilities and that should be considered in hazard surveillance planning. Each facility must carefully review its operations to determine which items and standards apply. Training must be provided to the appropriate staff before any hazard surveillance inspections so that employees understand the requirements of the standards that apply to their jobs. Some items and standards on the list apply to more than one department. For example, "Hand and portable power tools and other handheld equipment" applies to the Engineering, Dietary, and other departments. "Fire prevention plans" applies to every department in the facility. Many of the government standards are provided on the CD-ROM accompanying this book.

Table 2-2 lists specific state and federal laws, standards, recommendations, and guidelines that apply to health care facilities. The Joint Commission also has a series of standards that apply to health care worker health and safety. However, the Joint Commission standards are performance oriented and thus have wider applicability than the specific federal laws and standards listed here. For example, EC.1.10, "The hospital manages safety risks," and EC.1.20, "The hospital maintains a safe environment," apply to each of the specific standards in table 2-2. Furthermore, the Joint Commission has parallel Leadership, Human Resources, and Management of Information standards that apply to specific elements of the individual federal standards. Compliance with the Joint Commission standards does not ensure compliance with any state or federal standard or regulation, which is required by law. For the sake of clarity, table 2-2 lists only state and federal laws, standards, recommendations, and guidelines.

OSHA Hazard Awareness Advisor, Version 1.0[8]

The Occupational Safety and Health Administration's Hazard Awareness Advisor is a powerful, interactive software program. It can help facilities identify and understand common occupational safety and health hazards in the workplace. It will query the user about activities, practices, materials, equipment, and policies at the workplace. Most questions have follow-up questions (depending upon the previous answers). The Hazard Awareness Advisor uses the answers to these questions to determine the hazards that are likely to be present. Then it prepares a customized report briefly describing

Table 2–2. Items and Standards to Consider in Hazard Surveillance Planning

Topic, Item, or Subject	Standard
Abrasive wheel machinery (see also Machinery and machine guarding)	29 CFR 1910.215
Access to employee exposure and medical records	29 CFR 1910.1020
Accident reporting and investigation	29 CFR 1904
Air contaminants (toxic and hazardous substances)	29 CFR 1910.1000 29 CFR 1910.1200
Asbestos (older facilities)	29 CFR 1910.1001
Bloodborne pathogens	29 CFR 1910.1030
Chemicals, hazardous (also known as Hazard communication)	29 CFR 1910 Subpart I 29 CFR 1910.132–.138 29 CFR 1910 Subpart I Appendix A 29 CFR 1910 Subpart I Appendix B 29 CFR 1910.1200
Color code for marking physical hazards	29 CFR 1910.144
Competent person (for construction)	29 CFR 1926.700–.706
Compressed gases	29 CFR 1910.101 Compressed Gas Association
Confined spaces	29 CFR 1910.146
Construction	29 CFR 1910.26
Contractor safety	Occupational Safety and Health Act, Sec. 4., Applicability of This Act
Corrosives	29 CFR 1910.1200
Disaster recovery plans	Several federal and state laws and regulations
Distances for access and clearance (i.e., storage, fire extinguishers, eye washes, exits)	Several OSHA standards
Electrical safety and protective devices (includes dangers such as electric shock, electrocution, fires, and explosions)	29 CFR 1910.137 29 CFR 1910 Subpart S NFPA 70 NFPA 70E
Emergency response plan	EPA 29 CFR 1910.120
Emergency action plans	29 CFR 1910.38 NFPA 1600
Ergonomics	No specific standard Occupational Safety and Health Act, Sec. 5(a), Duties (known as the OSHA general duty clause)
Ethylene oxide	29 CFR 1910.1047
Exits	29 CFR 1910.34–.37
Eye and face protection	29 CFR 1910.133
Fire brigades	29 CFR 1910.156

(Continued on next page)

Table 2–2. *(Continued)*

Topic, Item, or Subject	Standard
Fire extinguishers	29 CFR 1910.157
Fire prevention plans	29 CFR 1910.39
Fire and life safety	NFPA 99 NFPA 101 Over 60 other NFPA standards
Flammable and combustible liquids	29 CFR 1910.106–.108
Floor and wall openings and holes	29 CFR 1910.23
Foot protection	29 CFR 1910.136
Formaldehyde	29 CFR 1910.1048
Gases, vapors, fumes, dusts, and mists (for construction)	29 CFR 1926.55 Appendix A 29 CFR 1910.103 29 CFR 1926.1101 (if appropriate) 29 CFR 1910.1048 (if appropriate)
HACCP (Hazard Analysis and Critical Control Point; a Total Quality Management program)	FDA
Hand and portable power tools and other hand-held equipment	29 CFR 1910 Subpart P 29 CFR 1910.242–.244
Hand and portable power tools (for construction)	29 CFR 1926.300
Hand protection	29 CFR 1910.138
Hazard assessment	Several OSHA standards
Hazardous waste	40 CFR 261
Hazardous waste operations and emergency response (HAZWOPER) (applies to hospital patient decontamination and some chemical spills)	29 CFR 1910.120
Head protection	29 CFR 1910.135
Helicopters (includes equipment hazards, noise levels, debris on helipads, ergonomics, and fueling hazards)	29 CFR 1910.183 29 CFR 1910.95
Housekeeping	No specific OSHA standard OSHA general duty clause Several OSHA standards
Indoor air quality	No general OSHA standards OSHA general duty clause Specific issues addressed in various standards 29 CFR 1910.1000 (Air contaminants) 29 CFR 1910.94 (Ventilation)
Infection control	29 CFR 1910.1020 29 CFR 1910.1030 29 CFR 1910.1904 CDC
Ionizing radiation	29 CFR 1910.1096

(Continued on next page)

Table 2–2. *(Continued)*

Topic, Item, or Subject	Standard
Job hazard analysis (also known as Job safety analysis or Hazard assessment)	No specific standards OSHA general duty clause Several OSHA standards
Laboratory standard (hazardous chemicals in laboratories)	29 CFR 1910.1450
Ladders	29 CFR 1910.25–.27
Lasers	No specific OSHA standard OSHA general duty clause 29 CFR 1910.132 (Face and eye protection) FDA Standard Number 21 21 CFR 1040.10–.11 ANSI Z136 (series of laser safety standards) NFPA 99 Product performance regulated by the Center for Devices and Radiological Health (CDRH) and the FDA
Laundry machinery and operations	29 CFR 1910.264
Lifting patients	No specific standard OSHA general duty clause Ergonomics guidelines
Control of hazardous energy (lockout/tagout)	29 CFR 1910.147
Machinery and machine guarding (general requirements for all machines)	29 CFR 1910.211 29 CFR 1910.212 29 CFR 1910.213 29 CFR 1910.215 29 CFR 1910.217
Materials handling and storage	29 CFR 1910.176 NIOSH lifting equation
Medical surveillance	29 CFR 1910.120 (HAZWOPER) Several OSHA standards relating to chemical and physical stressors listed in 29 CFR 1910 Subpart Z and 29 CFR 1926.55
Medical equipment management	FDA Safe Medical Device Act (SMDA) of 1990 No specific OSHA standard OSHA general duty clause 29 CFR 1910.301–.399
Medical waste	29 CFR 1910.1030 State regulations
Nitrous oxide	29 CFR 1910.105
Noise exposure	29 CFR 1910.95

(Continued on next page)

Table 2–2. *(Continued)*

Topic, Item, or Subject	Standard
Oxygen	29 CFR 1910.104
Personal protective equipment	29 CFR 1910 Subpart I 29 CFR 1910.132–.138 NIOSH respirator requirements ANSI requirements
Pharmaceutical waste	40 CFR 261 State regulations
Powered industrial trucks (also known as forklifts)	29 CFR 1910.178
Radioactive waste	Nuclear Regulatory Commission (NRC) Environmental Protection Agency (EPA) Department of Energy (DOE) Department of Transportation (DOT) State regulations
Recordkeeping	29 CFR 1904
Respiratory protection	29 CFR 1910.134 NIOSH respirator requirements required by OSHA
Risk management program	No federal requirements for health care facilities
Safety and health programs	Several OSHA standards, including 29 CFR 1960 (OSHA requirements for federal employees)
Sanitation	29 CFR 1910.141
Scaffolding (for construction)	29 CFR 1926.450–.454
Signs and tags	29 CFR 1910.144–.145 Several OSHA standards
Site safety plan (for construction)	29 CFR 1926.20
Slips, trips, and falls (e.g., housekeeping, aisles and passageways, covers and guardrails, floor loading protection, ladders, scaffolding)	OSHA general duty clause 29 CFR 1910.21–.30
Substance abuse program	No standard
Temperature extremes	No specific standard OSHA general duty clause
Universal waste	40 CFR Part 273 State regulations
Ventilation	29 CFR 1910.94 American Society of Heating, Refrigerating and Air-Conditioning Engineers (ASHRAE)

(Continued on next page)

Table 2–2. *(Continued)*

Topic, Item, or Subject	Standard
Walking-working surfaces (see also Slips, trips, and falls)	29 CFR 1910.21–.22
Welding, cutting, and brazing	29 CFR 1910.251–.255
Workplace violence	No specific OSHA standard OSHA general duty clause OSHA 3148-01R 2004
Waste management (see also Hazardous waste, Medical waste, Pharmaceutical waste, Radioactive waste, and Universal waste)	40 CFR 261 40 CFR 273 29 CFR 1910.1030 DOE DOT NRC State regulations

the likely hazards and indicating the OSHA standards that address those hazards. The Hazard Awareness Advisor can be used online or downloaded and run in a Windows environment.

The Hazard Awareness Advisor is a useful introduction to hazard recognition, but it is not able to identify all hazards. It is not a substitute for safety and health professionals. It will not determine whether the facility is in compliance with OSHA standards. It is designed for beginners, not experts, although experts can also use it. Figure 2-4 lists the Hazard Awareness Advisor's capabilities.

MANAGING THE ENVIRONMENTAL HEALTH AND SAFETY PROGRAM

The information in this chapter is based on and consistent with OSHA's *Safety and Health Program Management Guidelines.*[9] [CD-ROM 2.9] This chapter is also consistent with EPA, NFPA, other regulatory standards, and with accreditation

Figure 2–4. Features of OSHA's Hazard Awareness Advisor

- □ Asks the user questions about workplace situations, including activities, equipment, and materials
- □ Analyzes the user's answers with expert decision logic
- □ Alerts people in general industry to common occupational hazards
- □ Explains briefly the nature of common occupational hazards
- □ Points out applicable OSHA standards
- □ Identifies consultation offices for the user's state
- □ Provides definitions of keywords and phrases via a "keyword" button

standards that are designed to protect employees, as well as patients. However, simply complying with regulatory standards, accreditation standards, or both does not mean that the facility has a strong, dynamic health and safety program.

Both regulatory agencies and accreditation organizations are guided by the conviction that effective management is essential to reducing the number and severity of injuries and illnesses in health care facilities. That conviction is based on their separate experiences in evaluating worksites during compliance inspections, state-run consultation service site visits, Voluntary Protection Program (VPP) visits, and accreditation surveys.

In general industry, there is a direct relationship between effective management and a reduction in the number and severity of injuries and illnesses. But compliance with OSHA regulations or accreditation standards is not the sole burden of employers. Employees must also be active, informed participants in worksite health and safety. By encouraging employee involvement in the program's design and development, a facility will reap the benefits of the employees' valuable ideas and their all-important support.

The most successful programs recognize that to achieve the next level of performance, worker health and safety must be integrated with personal wellness, family safety and well-being, a commitment to human values, and sound business practices. Health care facilities that can successfully integrate these components into their health and safety programs will experience a reduction in the number of recordable injuries and illnesses, improved employee and patient relations, heightened morale, enhanced patient care and safety, and reduced costs.

References

1. Carroll, Lewis. *Alice's Adventures in Wonderland*. New York, 1941, p. 3.

2. U.S. Department of Labor. *Recording and Reporting Occupational Injuries and Illnesses* (29 CFR 1904). Available at http://www.osha.gov/pls/oshaweb/owadisp.show_document?p_table=STANDARDS&p_id=9631 (accessed 2/16/2006).

3. U.S. Department of Labor. *Recordkeeping Policies and Procedures Manual* (CPL 02-00-135). Available at http://www.osha.gov/pls/oshaweb/owadisp.show_document?p_table=DIRECTIVES&p_id=3205 (accessed 2/16/2006).

4. U.S. Department of Labor. *Industrial Hygiene* (OSHA 3143). Available at http://www.osha.gov/Publications/OSHA3143/OSHA3143.htm (accessed 2/16/2006).

5. U.S. Department of Labor. *Job Hazard Analysis* (OSHA 3071). Available at http://www.osha.gov/Publications/osha3071.pdf (accessed 2/16/2006).

6. *Protecting Those Who Serve: Health Care Worker Safety*. Oakbrook Terrace, IL: Joint Commission on Accreditation of Healthcare Organizations, 2005, p. 8.

7. New York City Office of the Comptroller. *Getting in the Door: Language Barriers to Health Services at New York City's Hospitals* (January 2005). Available at http://www.comptroller.nyc.gov/bureaus/opm/reports/jan10-05_geting-in-the-door.pdf (accessed 2/16/2006).

8. U.S. Department of Labor. *OSHA Hazard Awareness Advisor, Version 1.0* (September 1999). Available at http://www.osha.gov/dts/osta/oshasoft/hazexp.html (accessed 2/16/2006).

9. U.S. Department of Labor. *Safety and Health Program Management Guidelines; Issuance of Voluntary Guidelines* (54 FR 3904-3916). Available at http://www.osha.gov/pls/oshaweb/owadisp.show_document?p_id=12909&p_table=FEDERAL_REGISTER (accessed 2/16/2006).

CHAPTER 3

POSITIONING AND MARKETING THE ENVIRONMENTAL HEALTH AND SAFETY PROGRAM AND ACHIEVING NATIONAL RECOGNITION

Thus I discovered the basic truth on which The Fuller Brush Company was to be founded. . . . Whenever a housewife saw that I had a superior brush or mop that she needed, at a price she could pay, she bought it. The trick was not to make her buy, but to show her what the brush could do. This required actions rather than words. I washed babies with a back brush, swept stairs, cleaned radiators and milk bottles, dusted floors—anything that could prove the worth of what I had to sell.

Alfred C. Fuller[1]

In 1906, 21-year-old Alfred Fuller began manufacturing brushes in his house and selling them door to door. Today the Fuller Brush Company manufactures more than 2,000 separate items in a 12-acre manufacturing facility in Kansas.

In the retail industry, a manufacturer who wants to consistently increase sales and profits must make sure that two conditions are satisfied: the consumer must preferentially identify the product, and the consumer must purchase the product because it is superior to competing products. True success is attained when the consumer allocates a progressively greater percentage of the budget to purchase more of the product.

This same strategy can be applied to elevate the status of the health and safety program within a health care facility. First, departments and employees must know who the individuals are on the Environmental Health and Safety staff, what their functions are, and how to contact them. Second, departments and employees must be able to trust that the "product" of the Environmental Health and Safety Department is a superior one, and that supporting it will enhance their work experience.

Visibility can be achieved only if the Environmental Health and Safety staff routinely visit different departments of the facility and solicit input from the departments' staff about their health and safety concerns. By acting on those concerns promptly and effectively, the Environmental Health and Safety Department will earn the employees' confidence that its product is worth supporting.

This approach is precisely what made the Fuller Brush Company so successful, and it is embodied in the corporate motto:

> To provide a combination of excellent products and excellent service to distributors and customers through education and information on ways in which our products can enhance their quality of life.

POSITIONING AND LEADING THE ENVIRONMENTAL HEALTH AND SAFETY PROGRAM

Effective protection from workplace hazards takes commitment from top management. That commitment is essential, and it must be visible. The administration must provide support and leadership so that all employees know of its commitment to a safe and healthful workplace.

If employees can see the emphasis that the administration puts on health and safety, they are more likely to emphasize it in their own activities. The leaders must demonstrate to everyone in the facility that they are vitally interested in employee health and safety. This can be accomplished in several ways, including the following:

- Encouraging employees to speak up about safety and health problems in their units or departments
- Providing adequate budgets and resources
- Listening carefully to employee concerns and then taking appropriate action to resolve them
- Promoting a dynamic Environmental Health and Safety Department and culture within the facility

Regardless of the facility's formal system of accountability, hourly employees and managers will watch the administration for clues as to what is important. If the subject of health and safety is never raised, they will assume that it does not matter. The administration should require department heads and supervisors to implement and monitor the facility's Environmental Health and Safety program as it applies to them.

Achieving Success and Maintaining the Program

A successful health and safety program is one that is marked by achievement and strives to maintain a safe and healthful workplace. Administration commitment as well as employee training, involvement, and accountability, plus routine program evaluation, characterize the successful health and safety program.[2]

Commitment from the Administration

Simply stating one's commitment is not enough. The successful program will demonstrate that words of commitment are linked to actions. The administration can demonstrate its proactive commitment:

- □ By developing and making available to all employees a written mission statement and policy that emphasizes the importance the facility places on employee health and safety
- □ By actively working to understand the nature and causes of accidents, and to see that action is taken to prevent them in the future
- □ By participating in Environmental Health and Safety Committee meetings and responding appropriately to the committee's recommendations
- □ By encouraging their staff to follow safe and healthful work practices and leading by example

Employee Accountability

Just as the administration's commitment is essential to achieving and maintaining a safe and healthful workplace, employees must also be committed and understand that they will be accountable for functioning in a safe manner. Employee accountability is an essential element of the Occupational Safety and Health Act (OSH Act) [CD-ROM 3.1] and of any employee health and safety program.

Employee accountability can be reinforced by:

- □ Having written job descriptions that clearly state employees' health and safety responsibilities
- □ Having the training and authority to recognize and report hazards
- □ Ensuring that the employees they supervise perform their jobs in a safe manner
- □ Understanding that failing to work safely can cause harm to themselves or others and may lead to disciplinary action

Employee Involvement

Effective Environmental Health and Safety programs involve employees who have a stake in the program's success. Employees may feel more vested in a program that they are responsible for. That responsibility should include participation in program evaluation, health and safety training classes, and the Environmental Health and Safety Committee.

Education and Training

Employees need to know about the workplace hazards to which they may be exposed—how to recognize them, how to evaluate the extent or nature of the hazard, and the controls needed to reduce or eliminate their potential exposure. The best way to gain this knowledge is through education and training. At a minimum, education and training should cover the following topics:

- □ Intentions and principles of the OSH Act
- □ Recognizing, evaluating, and controlling physical, chemical, biological, and radiological hazards
- □ Safety and health issues specific to their duties
- □ Occupational Safety and Health Administration (OSHA) and other federal, state, and local regulations as well as Joint Commission standards they are expected to comply with while performing their duties
- □ Proper use of personal protective equipment (PPE) specific to their duties
- □ Routes of exposure to chemicals, and the signs and symptoms of chemical exposure
- □ Hazards specific to their environment

Recognizing and Reporting Hazards

Before hazards can be controlled, they must be recognized. Once they are recognized, they must be reported as quickly as possible. Successful programs train employees to recognize and report workplace hazards in the following ways:

- □ Knowing how to operate and maintain equipment properly, and when it should be taken out of service for repair
- □ Knowing when help is needed to perform a task and then obtaining that help
- □ Ensuring that any PPE required for their job is in good working order and is used appropriately
- □ Refraining from performance of a task until the hazard has been eliminated
- □ Ensuring that equipment safeguards are not overridden
- □ Encouraging employees to report hazards or problems with equipment

Reviewing and Modifying the Program

At least once a year, the program should be reviewed for strengths and weaknesses. However, if it becomes apparent that program modification is needed based on surveillance data or reports of other health and safety problems in the facility, a review should occur immediately and appropriate modifications made.

Building Relationships with Other Departments

There are many challenges to the future of health and safety. It is crucial to break down the barriers that separate individual professional efforts. The Environmental Health and Safety Department should join other departments in a partnership to achieve a safer, healthier health care industry. Partnership efforts should be aimed at information dissemination among departments, mutual participation at Environmental Health and Safety Committee meetings, and promotion of the mutual goal of employee and patient quality care.

The Environmental Health and Safety Department must assist other departments in taking steps to impart a strong health and safety attitude among employees and managers. Activities that the Environmental Health and Safety director can help departments implement to educate their employees include:

- Talking about the human and economic consequences of not working safely
- Including employees in incident investigations
- Having regular meetings with employees to drive home the point that health and safety is a personal matter
- Insisting on proper reporting of all incidents, no matter how minor they may seem, to assist in the identification of problems
- Making health and safety an important factor in employee performance appraisals
- Maintaining strict safety discipline, being consistent in enforcing the rules, and applying the facility's disciplinary procedures fairly
- Talking with employees when unsafe actions have been identified

While the backbone of the health and safety program is a detailed manual with a regulatory focus, the more practical, day-to-day emphasis should be on values that reflect the facility's philosophy. Sometimes a slogan can be used to achieve this goal:[3]

- "Our commitment to health and safety is based on caring."
- "Nothing we do is worth getting hurt for."
- "Every job can be done safely."
- "Risk and safety can be managed."
- "Safety is everyone's responsibility."

Departments can incorporate these values into health and safety communications. They can be included in new-employee orientation, posted in offices and break rooms, discussed when an incident occurs, and mixed into everyday conversation.

Environmental Health and Safety staff should be responsive to those who need the resources of the department, even on short notice. The ability to be flexible and to respond to various requests and concerns is a key element in affecting the lives of others. Flexibility is a business skill and a basic factor in management, training, and strategic thinking.

Employee Involvement

The best protection occurs when everyone at the worksite shares responsibility for health and safety. For that to occur, employees must know that they are instrumental in shaping the program. Employees at all levels should be actively involved in identifying and correcting health and safety problems. However, this does not mean that senior leadership gives up responsibility and authority. The Occupational Safety and Health Administration places the responsibility for employee protection from workplace hazards squarely on the employer and the employee. The wise employer, however, uses employees' unique knowledge and experience to help identify and resolve problems. Wise employees will understand that regulations, Joint Commission standards, and the employer's health and safety policies are intended to protect them from potential hazards.

Employer Involvement

Employers should provide for and encourage employee involvement in the structure and operation of the program, and in decisions that affect employees' health and safety. Employees will then be more likely to commit their insight and energy to achieving the Environmental Health and Safety program's goals and objectives and understand that their participation and suggestions will be welcomed and not discouraged.

Responsibilities for every aspect of the Environmental Health and Safety program should be assigned and communicated to all department heads, supervisors, and employees so they will know what is expected of them. Performance objectives should be action oriented and measurable.

MARKETING THE PROGRAM

Successful Environmental Health and Safety programs are based on the concept that exceptional outcomes require strong leadership, superior technical knowledge and skill, and a solid partnership between department managers and employees. Enhancements in patient care and safety and in the business aspects of the health care facility also require effective communication among the administration, department managers, employees, physicians, and patients and their families. But before this culture can become a part of the daily routine, the administration, department managers, and employees must understand its value. There are a number of national awareness and recognition programs available to health care facilities. Following is an example of an awareness program that recognizes health care facilities that operate an exemplary health and safety management system.

An Awareness Program

Once the organizational backbone of the Environmental Health and Safety program is in place and is functional, an awareness program can serve as a public relations tool to build broad participation. (See figure 1-4.)

The Environmental Health and Safety staff should be recognizable and visible throughout the facility. Color-specific clothing, in-house newsletters, and creative, fun health and safety educational activities can promote program recognition. The contribution of an awareness program to the facility's vision of improved health and safety encompasses more than a reduction in liability exposure or workers' compensation costs. The program will encourage and catalyze broad-based team efforts; boost morale; and increase cooperation among employees and their families, patients, and the general public. This enhanced awareness will carry over to and have a positive influence on other health care facility programs.

An awareness program should be built on caring attitudes and values that have a positive effect on safety and health, and that embrace and encourage the respect and courtesy that employees, patients, and the general public deserve. [CD-ROM 3.2] Such values affect patient care and also enhance relationships among employees and their families. Additionally, employees will understand that they are:

□ Valued
□ Treated fairly and equitably
□ Treated as individuals
□ Entitled to courteous treatment
□ Well informed about issues of concern to them
□ Given prompt explanations of issues in an understandable manner
□ Recognized, acknowledged, and thanked for good performance
□ Entitled to raise issues of concern and have those concerns addressed

A successful awareness program will lead to an increased understanding of the value of a successful Environmental Health and Safety program and its relationship to quality care. Improved health and safety performance will lead to enhanced relationships among employees, patients, and the general public as well as increased patient satisfaction. The awareness program will also demonstrate to employees how the principles and practices of workplace Environmental Health and Safety apply to their home life and will have the added benefit of reducing the number and severity of workplace injuries and illnesses.

A hospital in Ohio has incorporated an awareness program into its Environmental Health and Safety activities by extending the program to include patients and families of employees. Although this is only one element of the Environmental Health and Safety program, the Environmental Health and Safety staff believe that it is a significant contributing factor to the facility's record of no lost-time injuries in more than five years.[4]

A successful awareness program consists of the following activities and extends to the employees' families, patients, and the general public:

Promotional activities
Recognition activities
Reward programs
Involving employees' families
Involving patients

Promotional Activities

Promotional activities can expand employees' awareness and increase their interest and involvement. These programs are commercials for safety and health and are intended to:

□ Educate employees about Environmental Health and Safety
□ Advance understanding of the need for a strong commitment to health and safety
□ Establish a culture in which all jobs are expected to be performed in a safe and healthful manner

Elements of successful promotional activities may include the following:

□ A symbol that anchors the program and that is distinctive and clearly represents the program and its goals
□ Promotional products such as shirts and caps
□ Annual safety planning meetings with kickoff celebrations
□ Safety suggestion programs
□ Memberships in national and international organizations that promote safety and health
□ Community-wide programs to generate publicity and good public relations
□ Poster campaigns
□ Awareness agenda items for Environmental Health and Safety Committee meetings
□ Programs to promote health and fitness
□ New-employee orientation presentations that reflect the facility's safety commitment to employees, patients, and their families

Recognition Activities

Recognition activities are designed to recognize employees for specific behaviors. Elements of recognition activities may include:

- ☐ Safety recognition pins
- ☐ On-the-spot awards
- ☐ Certificates of achievement
- ☐ Team trophies
- ☐ Department-specific recognition
- ☐ Newsletter publicity
- ☐ Safety messages and interviews with employees on in-house communication networks

Reward Programs

Another way of promoting the program and increasing participation is through reward programs that recognize the efforts of individual employees or groups of employees who have met or exceeded the health and safety goals of the facility. Examples of targeted activities for reward programs are:

- ☐ Environmental Health and Safety Committee members competing toward the achievement of a facility goal
- ☐ Vice presidents challenging their departments to compete against other vice presidents' departments
- ☐ Winners from individual departments competing for an annual award

Involving Employees' Families

Family involvement in safety and health is key to reducing employee injuries and illnesses both on the job and off the job. As employers and employees begin to experience the benefits of safe and healthful work practices, they will extend those practices into their personal lives to the benefit of themselves and their families. Family safety and health activities include the following:

- ☐ Learning about vacation safety
- ☐ Home fire safety lessons
- ☐ Educating children who stay home alone
- ☐ Electrical safety instruction
- ☐ Including stories and pictures of family health and safety experiences in newsletters
- ☐ Utilizing local recreation programs to promote swimming classes or courses in boating safety

- ☐ Distributing magazines devoted to family safety and health
- ☐ Increasing ergonomic awareness (e.g., eye rest breaks from computer monitors)
- ☐ Nutrition, exercise, and fitness programs
- ☐ Awareness of chemical hazards
- ☐ Promoting caring values among family members (e.g., handling difficult situations, increasing communication, enhancing awareness of how our own behavior affects the way others see us, and practicing respect for others)
- ☐ Integrating traditional workplace health and safety principles with those of home safety, health, and personal care

Involving Patients

Once Environmental Health and Safety becomes an integral part of the facility's vision, patient incidents and illnesses decrease. Quality-of-life issues and caring values, such as respect, courtesy, and compassion have a positive effect on patient care. When patients see or understand that the facility's employees are truly concerned about their well-being, and then discover that they are being encouraged to participate in the facility's Environmental Health and Safety program, it will create a partnership consisting of patients, staff, and family all working toward the goal of a favorable patient experience with the added benefit of increased awareness for Environmental Health and Safety from each partner. One way patients can become involved in a facility's Environmental Health and Safety program is by being encouraged to report obvious hazards, such as broken equipment, spills on floors, or power cords that pose a tripping hazard.

PROMOTING PROGRESS

Commitment to the Environmental Health and Safety program can also be demonstrated by advertising its successes in the health care facility's annual report and on its website. These and other types of public presentations clearly demonstrate that the facility is being proactive, and that it is concerned about the health and well-being of its patients, employees, and visitors. How the department's annual report is read depends on the reader's purpose. The chief executive officer's purpose may be to assess performance and to learn of problems, risks, and other factors that may affect the facility's management systems. An annual report is not read like a normal book. There is no single author, no plot, no requirement that the text be read cover to cover, no beginning, and no end. Putting annual reports together year after year creates a kind of "never-ending story" as the department progresses.

The challenge in designing annual reports is to turn summaries of health and safety performance into a visually appealing package. The report should be well written, interesting, and graphically appealing to the senior administration and board members. The report should discuss the goals of the Environmental Health and Safety program and the progress that has been made toward meeting those goals. It may also be useful to describe how the facility's program compares with other successful programs in the health care industry.

The facility's annual report should present an overview of its health and safety policy and those areas in which it has made improvements over the prior year. Do not focus too much on the consequences of failures; rather, report on developments toward the achievement of improved health and safety performance. The executive summary should cover changing conditions, goals, and actions taken or not taken. Is the document written in clear language? Read between the lines—what is being apologized for? The report should include the following information, or give an indication of the steps that the facility is taking to gather the information for publication in later reports:

- ☐ The broad context of the facility's policy on health and safety, and its relationship to patient safety
- ☐ The significant risks faced by employees and others, and the strategies and systems in place to control them
- ☐ The facility's health and safety goals as they relate to the facility's health and safety policy, with specific and measurable targets for the future
- ☐ OSHA (and other federal, state, and local regulations) and accreditation standards for worker health and safety (e.g., EC, HR, LD) and how outcomes contribute to employee injury and illness reduction
- ☐ Any benchmarking initiatives the department has undertaken, and any performance improvements resulting from the initiatives

The report should provide summaries of data that is already available from the facility. New procedures or information gathering systems should not need to be set up. The following data should be included:

- ☐ Summaries of the effectiveness of the department's core functions (Environmental Monitoring, Safety, Emergency Management, Security, Training, Employee Health Services, and department liaisons) as they relate to worker health and safety federal, state, and local regulations and accreditation standards
- ☐ A summary of the department's strengths, weaknesses, opportunities, and threats (SWOT) analysis, if one has been undertaken
- ☐ The number of injuries and illnesses reported on the OSHA Form 300 logs
- ☐ Brief details of the circumstances of any fatalities and of the actions taken to prevent a recurrence
- ☐ Milestones that have been reached in the past year or over any other appropriate period of time
- ☐ The total number of employee-days that were lost and the total number of employee-days that were restricted due to all causes of injuries and illnesses

☐ The number of health and safety enforcement notices sent to the facility and information on what actions the notices required the facility to take

☐ The number and nature of the citations and penalties for health and safety offenses that were sustained by the facility, their outcome in terms of penalties and costs, and steps taken to prevent recurrences

☐ The total cost to the facility of the occupational injuries and illnesses suffered by employees during the reporting period

☐ Summaries of active and reactive monitoring activities

☐ Information on the outcomes of hazard surveillance inspections and health and safety audits

☐ A comparison of the present year's data with data obtained from the prior five years

ACHIEVING NATIONAL ENVIRONMENTAL HEALTH AND SAFETY PROGRAM RECOGNITION

An effective Environmental Health and Safety program is an investment in employees and in the future of quality patient care. Investment in health and safety is a sound business strategy for any health care organization, regardless of size, and will have a positive impact on the facility's bottom line. In the past, most improvements in health and safety were driven by regulations, but in today's highly competitive market, and with all of the pressures on the health care industry, the relationship between a strong Environmental Health and Safety program and the financial well-being of the industry must be understood. National recognition for a facility's Environmental Health and Safety program can be acquired by successful participation in one of the following OSHA programs.[5]

The Safety and Health Achievement Recognition Program (SHARP)

The SHARP program recognizes small employers (250 employees or fewer) who operate an exemplary safety and health management system. [CD-ROM 3.3] Acceptance into SHARP by OSHA is an achievement of status that will single out a small health care facility as a model for worksite safety and health relative to its peers. Upon receiving SHARP recognition, the health care facility is exempted from programmed inspections during the period over which the SHARP certification is valid. SHARP success stories include:

☐ One company reduced its lost-workday incidence rate from 28.5 to 8.3 and reduced its insurance claims from $50,000 to $4,000 through decreases in direct and indirect losses as a result of reducing the number of employee back and shoulder injuries.

□ A custom woodworking company saved as much as $60,000 a year in workers' compensation premiums and now often goes 90 consecutive days without a workplace injury.

Voluntary Protection Program (VPP)

The Voluntary Protection Program (VPP) is OSHA's premier recognition program for worksites that do an excellent job of protecting their employees. [CD-ROM 3.4] Sites are approved based on their written safety and health program and their overall performance in meeting the standards set by the program.

OSHA keeps VPP application information confidential. Sites participating in VPP have become safer and more healthful places to work. Injury and illness rates have dropped among participating companies, and employees and managers are working together more than ever before to promote workplace safety and health.

□ Participation in OSHA's VPP has allowed one company to save $930,000 per year and to experience 450 fewer lost-time injuries than its industry average.

□ A manufacturing company increased production by 97 percent in five years, and its injury rate fell from 3.8 to a low of 0.9 during this same time period.

□ A national park's lost-time rate dropped 10 percent, to its lowest level in five years, and its incident rate declined 40 percent. No workers died on the job during the term of the partnership—compared with five deaths within a period of three and a half years immediately before the partnership.

□ A health care facility has not had a lost-time incident in five years, and its incidence rate is 0.2 percent.

USING JOINT COMMISSION RESOURCES TO HELP POSITION AND MARKET THE ENVIRONMENTAL HEALTH AND SAFETY PROGRAM

Joint Commission Resources (JCR) is an affiliate of the Joint Commission on Accreditation of Healthcare Organizations, which disseminates information regarding accreditation, standards development and compliance, good practices, and health care quality improvement. Joint Commission Resources is a client-focused, expert resource for health care organizations that provides consulting services, educational services, and publications to assist in improving the quality, safety, and efficiency of health care services. Joint Commission Resources also assists health care facilities as they work toward meeting the accreditation standards of the Joint Commission. Because of their relationship to the Joint Commission and its expertise, JCR is uniquely qualified to assist in the positioning and internal marketing of a facility's Environmental

Health and Safety program. Therefore, it can be a valuable asset in establishing a new program or redefining an existing one.

References

1. *The History of Fuller Brush.* Available at http://home.att.net/~homebusiness/fullerbrush/history.htm (accessed 3/6/06).
2. Oregon Occupational Safety & Health Division (OR-OSHA). *Developing Your Safety and Health Program: Suggestions for Business Owners and Managers.* Available at www.cbs.state.or.us/external/osha/pdf/pubs/expired%20pubs/2293.pdf (accessed 3/6/06).
3. "Safety is the Flavor Every Day at Edy's," *Compliance Magazine* (July 2004).
4. Samaritan Regional Health System, Ashland, OH.
5. U.S. Department of Labor. *OSHA Cooperative Programs* (SHARP and VPP). Available at http://www.osha.gov/dcsp/compliance_assistance/index_programs.html (accessed 2/21/2006).

CHAPTER 4

OCCUPATIONAL SAFETY AND HEALTH AGENCIES AND ORGANIZATIONS

Every night we go to sleep with the expectation that we will wake up in the morning in the same condition as when we went to bed. We flip a switch on a light that has been wired by a qualified electrician whose work has been verified by a building inspector. We eat a breakfast that has been inspected according to the regulations and standards of the U.S. Department of Agriculture (USDA). We use personal care products, and perhaps medication, that has been approved by the Food and Drug Administration (FDA). We drive to work in an automobile that has been built to increase our safety, through the efforts of automobile manufacturers, the National Highway Traffic Safety Administration (NHTSA), and a number of insurance companies. We may stop to buy gasoline for the car from a pump that is designed to reduce the risk of fire and the release of fumes that adversely impact our air. All of these efforts, however, rely on us to do our part—by not overloading the electrical system, by storing and preparing our food properly, by using our personal care products and medications as directed and prescribed, by driving according to the rules, and by dispensing gasoline as instructed. In most cases, we don't think about the electricians, the USDA inspectors, the traffic engineers, or the Environmental Protection Agency (EPA) scientists who developed and enforce those regulations. We simply go about our daily routine, expecting to be protected.

The workplace is no different. It is governed by a myriad of rules and regulations designed to protect us and others from harm. However, it is not enough to trust that others will ensure our health and safety. Just as we are responsible for knowing how to store and prepare our food and drive safely, we are also responsible for knowing something about the rules and regulations that govern our work experience.

To effectively administer compliance activities in a health care facility, the Environmental Health and Safety director must have a solid knowledge of at least the following information:

☐ The Occupational Safety and Health Act of 1970 (OSH Act)[1] [CD-ROM 4.1] and other appropriate federal and state regulations that govern workplaces and the equipment therein.

☐ Why regulations are written in certain ways. For example, the OSHA standard 29 CFR 1910.147[2] is designed to control the short-term high exposures to ethylene oxide that have been associated with adverse health effects among health care facility employees. [CD-ROM 4.2]

☐ The OSH Act general duty clause,[3] which applies to hazards not addressed by any specific OSHA standard. For example, there is no federal standard specifically covering glutaraldehyde. However, both employers and employees must be aware that glutaraldehyde has very serious adverse health effects. In fact, other countries have recommended banning it from health care facilities.

☐ The potential hazards of chemicals in the workplace. Having a material safety data sheet (MSDS) on file is not sufficient to acquire a thorough understanding of the potential health and safety hazards posed by a chemical. When a new chemical is introduced into the facility, it is the Environmental Health and Safety professional's responsibility to determine if there is a standard that covers it, acquire detailed knowledge of the hazards posed by the substance, and effectively communicate the resulting information.

☐ The necessity for rigorous medical surveillance. Medical surveillance is necessary to ensure that the Environmental Health and Safety program is functioning as designed. Certain OSHA and Nuclear Regulatory Commission (NRC) standards contain specific requirements for medical surveillance. In order to conduct adequate surveillance activities, there must be a thorough understanding of the potential adverse health effects posed by the substances used in the facility. The Occupational Safety and Health Administration requires careful recordkeeping and periodic review of medical surveillance records. Properly conducted surveillance activities can identify existing or emerging problems that can be corrected to prevent further harm.

☐ The basis for health care facility fire and life safety policies. In general, these policies are based on nationally recognized codes and standards promulgated by OSHA and issued by the National Fire Protection Association (NFPA). Components of fire protection include construction, protection, and occupancy features that are necessary to minimize life-threatening dangers arising from fire, smoke, fumes, or panic.

☐ The requirements for personal protective equipment (PPE), which is regulated by OSHA, the American National Standards Institute

(ANSI), and the National Institute for Occupational Safety and Health (NIOSH). PPE is an essential part of many jobs and may be required in order to reduce an employee's risk of exposure to—by contact with, or inhalation or ingestion of—an infectious agent, toxic substance, or radioactive material. Health care facilities must document in writing that a PPE workplace hazard assessment has been performed.

☐ The OSHA regulations that are most commonly violated in the health care industry, and the facility's record of compliance. The four most commonly violated regulations in health care facilities include OSHA Standard CFR 1910.1030, Bloodborne pathogens [CD-ROM 4.3], OSHA Standard CFR 1910.303, Electrical—general requirements [CD-ROM 4.4], OSHA Standard CFR 1910.147, The control of hazardous energy (lockout/tagout) [CD-ROM 4.5], and OSHA Standard CFR 1910.134, Respiratory protection[4] [CD-ROM 4.6].

☐ Understand the requirements for environmental protection training and worker safety and health training, how they overlap, how they relate to Joint Commission standards, and which regulations include specific requirements for trainers. The Occupational Safety and Health Administration, the EPA, and the NFPA are the primary sources for health and safety training requirements. Knowledge of these requirements includes understanding how to properly use packaged programs, self-paced training programs, and employee group/marathon-type training programs. Effective safety and health training includes a combination of activities that involve instructor participation, the opportunity for questions, and learning by doing.

☐ Effective communication and risk communication techniques. Though it is not required by statute or regulation, the Environmental Health and Safety director must be able to communicate effectively with all levels of personnel within an organization. Such communication skills are essential when one is discussing risk and risk management concepts.

This chapter lists government agencies, legislation, as well as non-governmental organizations and agencies that have a role in health care facilities. Table 4-1 lists the agencies and organizations discussed in this chapter along with a brief description of the scope of their services. The guidelines, standards, and regulations described in this chapter are easy to obtain from the agencies that developed them. These agencies should be checked periodically for new information. To operate effectively, the Environmental Health and Safety director must have a copy of the complete standards and guidelines that apply to the facility, understand how to read them and apply them to the workplace, and know when to cross-reference information with that obtained from another agency.

Table 4–1. Summary of Agencies, Legislation, and Organizations and Their Scope of Services

Agency/Organization	Abbreviation	Scope
Federal Compliance Agencies Americans with Disabilities Act	ADA	Helps protect the civil rights of disabled Americans (divided into five federal categories)
Centers for Medicare & Medicaid Services	CMS	Develops standards of quality and safety for health care facilities that must be met for participation in the Medicare and Medicaid programs
Department of Transportation	DOT	Develops and coordinates policies that support public transportation safety and reduce environmental impact
Drug Enforcement Administration	DEA	Enforces controlled-substances laws and regulations
Environmental Protection Agency	EPA	Regulates of the release of harmful materials into the environment
Food and Drug Administration	FDA	Supervises the development, testing, and monitoring of food, drugs, and medical devices
Nuclear Regulatory Commission	NRC	Oversees the handling, use, and disposal of radiological materials
Occupational Safety and Health Administration	OSHA	Regulates workplace safety and health by setting and enforcing standards
Office of Justice Programs	OJP	Provides federal leadership in developing the nation's capacity to prevent and control crime
Other Federal Agencies Bureau of Labor Statistics	BLS	Serves OHSA as an independent national statistical resource
Centers for Disease Control and Prevention	CDC	Provides for disease research, prevention, and control
Department of Homeland Security	DHS	Works to secure the nation from terrorist attacks
Federal Emergency Management Agency	FEMA	Protects the nation's infrastructure from all types of hazards through a risk-based emergency management program

(Continued on next page)

Table 4–1. *(Continued)*

Agency/Organization	Abbreviation	Scope
National Institute for Occupational Safety and Health	NIOSH	Evaluates scientific data, conducts direct studies, and provides valid scientific recommendations to prevent worker exposure to hazards
State and Local Agencies State OSHA offices, other regulatory bodies, such as state and local hazardous and medical waste management and workers' compensation agencies, and fire and health codes		
Nongovernmental Organizations and Agencies American Conference of Governmental Industrial Hygienists	ACGIH	Collects, investigates, and reviews information on air contaminants; develops Threshold Limit Values (TLVs) for chemical exposures
American Institute of Architects	AIA	Represents the professional interests of American architects
American National Standards Institute	ANSI	Works to provide continuity and conformity standards according to specific requirements
American Society for Testing and Materials International	ASTM	Sets voluntary standards
American Society of Heating, Refrigerating and Air-Conditioning Engineers	ASHRAE	Advances the arts and sciences of heating, ventilation, air conditioning, and refrigeration internationally via research, standards writing, continuing education, and publications
Compressed Gas Association	CGA	Develops and promotes safety standards wherever compressed gases are used; advises the NFPA in developing standards
National Fire Protection Association	NFPA	Reduces worldwide burden of fire and other hazards, develops scientifically based codes, standards, research, training, and education
Accreditation Organizations American Osteopathic Association's Healthcare Facilities Accreditation Program	HFAP	Accredits qualified health care facilities through safety and quality standards

(Continued on next page)

Table 4–1. *(Continued)*

Agency/Organization	Abbreviation	Scope
Commission on Accreditation of Rehabilitation Facilities	CARF	Accredits qualified facilities that provide adult day services, assisted living, behavioral health, medical services, and employment and community services through service and quality standards
Joint Commission on Accreditation of Healthcare Organizations	JCAHO	Accredits qualified health care facilities through safety and quality standards; also provides certification to disease management companies and health care staffing agencies

FEDERAL COMPLIANCE AGENCIES AND LEGISLATION

The following federal compliance agencies and legislation address the issue of health and safety in the workplace:

> Americans with Disabilities Act (ADA)
> Centers for Medicare & Medicaid Services (CMS)
> Department of Transportation (DOT)
> Drug Enforcement Administration (DEA)
> Environmental Protection Agency (EPA)
> Food and Drug Administration (FDA)
> Nuclear Regulatory Commission (NRC)
> Occupational Safety and Health Administration (OSHA)
> Office of Justice Programs (OJP)

Americans with Disabilities Act (ADA)

To help the disabled live independently and become economically self-sufficient, Congress passed the Americans with Disabilities Act (ADA) in July 1990. [CD-ROM 4.7, 4.8] The ADA prohibits prospective employers from discriminating against the disabled. According to the ADA, a qualified individual with a disability is one who satisfies the requisite skill, experience, education, and other job requirements and can perform the essential functions of the position, with or without reasonable accommodation.

The ADA also states that any business or industry hiring the disabled must make reasonable structural or other process changes (such as ramps and wider doorways that enable wheelchair accessibility) to allow a disabled person to perform the essential job functions. The ADA further provides that those alterations should not cause undue hardship or expense to the employer.

Under the ADA, job descriptions must clearly define the actual physical and mental requirements needed to perform the job. For instance, a written job description that states, "lifting required" does not provide sufficient information. The maximum amount of weight that may need to be lifted must be provided with the description.

If an applicant is denied employment because the prospective employer or designated hiring authority has decided that the applicant cannot perform the necessary task or tasks, the job description can become a critical document in case of legal action against the employer. Job descriptions require analysis of the minimum physical capabilities and mental acumen required to perform the task successfully and safely. A job description must clearly explain the steps necessary to perform the job's function (e.g., physical positioning, repetitions, and torso movements). Trained professionals should perform the job function analysis, which may require the services of a consultant.

It is essential that health care facilities have written policies and procedures that comply with the ADA guidelines, which protect not only the rights of the disabled but also their health and safety while helping to prevent legal action.

U.S. Department of Justice
950 Pennsylvania Avenue NW
Washington, DC 20530-0001
Telephone: (202) 514-2000
Website: www.usdoj.gov

Centers for Medicare & Medicaid Services (CMS)

Centers for Medicare & Medicaid Services (CMS) develops Conditions of Participation (CoPs) and Conditions for Coverage (CfCs) that health care organizations must meet to participate in the Medicare and Medicaid programs. These standards are used to improve quality and protect the health and safety of beneficiaries. Centers for Medicare & Medicaid Services also ensures that the standards of accrediting organizations recognized by CMS (through a process called *deeming*) meet or exceed Medicare standards. Centers for Medicare & Medicaid Services also enforces fire safety requirements for patients and staff in health care facilities through the National Fire Protection Association's *Life Safety Code*.

Centers for Medicare & Medicaid Services is responsible for implementing the provisions of the Health Insurance Portability and Accountability Act of 1996 (HIPAA) [CD-ROM 4.9], including the HIPAA Administrative Simplification provisions. The Administrative Simplification provisions in Title II of the HIPAA address the security and privacy of health data.

Centers for Medicare & Medicaid Services
7500 Security Boulevard
Baltimore, MD 21244-1850
Telephone: (877) 267-2323
Website: www.cms.hhs.gov

Department of Transportation (DOT)

The Department of Transportation (DOT) was established by an act of Congress and signed into law in 1966. The DOT develops and coordinates policies that support public transportation safety and environmental protection. The Research and Special Programs Administration (RSPA) operates the Office of Hazardous Materials Safety and provides services pertaining to safety, compliance, training, and research, including protecting the public from the dangers inherent in the transportation of hazardous materials by air, rail, highway, and water. State hazardous-waste transportation guidelines fall under the rules and regulations of the DOT.

> U.S. Department of Transportation
> 400 7th Street SW
> Washington, DC 20590
> Telephone: (202) 366-4000
> Website: www.dot.gov

Drug Enforcement Administration (DEA)

The mission of the Drug Enforcement Administration (DEA) is to enforce the controlled-substances laws and regulations of the United States. The Controlled Substances Act (CSA), Title II of the Comprehensive Drug Abuse Prevention and Control Act of 1970, is the legal foundation of the government's fight against drug and substance abuse. This is a consolidation of numerous laws that regulate the manufacture and distribution of narcotics, stimulants, depressants, hallucinogens, anabolic steroids, and chemicals used in the illicit production of controlled substances. [CD-ROM 4.10]

> Drug Enforcement Administration
> U.S. Department of Justice
> 950 Pennsylvania Avenue NW
> Washington, DC 20530-0001
> Telephone: (202) 305-8500
> Website: www.dea.gov

Environmental Protection Agency (EPA)

The mission of the Environmental Protection Agency (EPA) is to protect human health and to safeguard the air, water, and land. Many of the EPA's activities impact health care facilities, including enforcement of air quality standards; controls on the disposal of toxic chemicals; strict regulation of pollutant emissions; banning the use of chemicals with the potential to cause cancer or harm the environment, such as pesticides; and controlling the quality of the public water supply.

While the OSHA Hazard communication standard addresses the use and handling of hazardous chemicals in the workplace, the EPA addresses how those chemicals should be handled and disposed of upon removal from the workplace.

U.S. Environmental Protection Agency
Ariel Rios Building
1200 Pennsylvania Avenue NW
Washington, DC 20460
Telephone: (202) 272-0167
Website: www.epa.gov

Food and Drug Administration (FDA)

Few government departments are more closely associated with a health care facility than the Food and Drug Administration (FDA). The FDA Modernization Act of 1977 affirmed the FDA's public health protection role and defined the agency's mission. Included in its mission is the responsibility to oversee the safety of food and drug products, medical devices, and electronic products that emit radiation. The FDA promotes the public health by promptly and efficiently reviewing clinical research and taking appropriate action on the marketing of regulated products in a timely manner. With respect to such products, the FDA protects the public health by ensuring that drugs are safe and effective, providing a reasonable assurance of the safety and effectiveness of devices intended for human use, and protecting the public health and safety from electronic product radiation.

Under the FDA's requirements, health care facilities must assume corrective action to ensure the safety and well-being of patients if a hazardous substance or product is brought to their attention. A health care facility must accept the responsibility to obtain, evaluate, and act on any information pertaining to hazards related to its equipment or the medications it dispenses.

Safe Medical Devices Act (SMDA)

In 1990 Congress passed the Safe Medical Devices Act (SMDA) [CD-ROM 4.17, 4.17a], which narrows the responsibilities of the FDA to certain fundamental activities, including:

☐ Reporting any incident of death, serious injury, or illness if it is suspected that a medical device was a contributing factor
☐ Conducting postmarket surveillance of permanent implants
☐ Instituting recalls or stop-use notices on medical devices

In order for the FDA to keep accurate records on the performance of drugs as well as biological and medical devices, reports from manufacturers and user facilities are mandatory. However, reporting by health care professionals is voluntary.

MedWatch, the Medical Products Reporting Program

The FDA is responsible for ensuring the safety and efficacy of all regulated marketed medical products.

MedWatch, the FDA's Safety Information and Adverse Event Reporting program, serves both health care professionals and the medical product–using public. MedWatch provides important and timely clinical information about safety issues involving medical products, including prescription and over-the-counter drugs, biologics, medical and radiation-emitting devices, and special nutritional products (i.e., medical foods, dietary supplements, and infant formulas).

Medical product safety alerts, recalls, withdrawals, and labeling changes that may affect the health of Americans are quickly disseminated to the medical community, thereby improving patient care.

MedWatch encourages health practitioners to promptly and voluntarily report any serious adverse health or product problems. Nurses, doctors, or other health care professionals are often the first to witness when a drug or device is not performing as anticipated. [CD-ROM 4.18]

Center for Devices and Radiological Health (CDRH)

Another program within the FDA's jurisdiction is the Center for Devices and Radiological Health (CDRH). This program protects the public's health by providing a reasonable assurance of the safety and effectiveness of medical devices and by eliminating unnecessary human exposure to radiation emitted from electronic products. The CDRH implements the SMDA and runs the MedWatch program. The CDRH provides workshops and develops documents such as information updates on breast implants.

> U.S. Food and Drug Administration
> 5600 Fishers Lane
> Rockville, MD 20857-0001
> Telephone: (888) 463-6332
> Telephone (Medical Device Office): (800) 332-1088
> Website: www.fda.gov

Nuclear Regulatory Commission (NRC)

The Nuclear Regulatory Commission (NRC) oversees the operation of nuclear power facilities and regulates the handling, use, and disposal of radioactive materials. The NRC is an independent agency that was established by the U.S.

Congress under the Energy Reorganization Act of 1974 to ensure adequate protection of public health and safety, the common defense and security, and the environment in connection with the use of nuclear materials in the United States.

The extent of radiological hazard varies according to the type of radionuclide, as do disposal techniques. In certain cases contaminated materials may be incinerated, but in other cases they may be left to decay in approved storage sites or disposed of through the sanitary (sewer) system. The NRC has published regulations governing these practices in 10 CFR Part 20, Standards for Protection against Radiation. [CD-ROM 4.19]

U.S. Nuclear Regulatory Commission
One White Flint North
11555 Rockville Pike
Rockville, MD 20852-2738
Telephone: (800) 368-5642
Website: www.nrc.gov

Occupational Safety and Health Administration (OSHA)

As the technology of the twentieth century progressed, so did the understanding that occupational injuries and illnesses could be prevented. While some worker protection laws were enacted at the state and local levels, they were often limited to specific industries or diseases. There was no single federal law directed toward improving the general health and welfare of all workers.

In response to a long history of serious workplace injuries, fatalities, and debilitating illnesses, and in recognition of the economic impact this set of conditions had on American commerce, the federal government moved to establish uniform rules and regulations to ensure worker health and safety in American workplaces. In 1970 the Occupational Safety and Health Act (OSH Act) created the Occupational Safety and Health Administration (OSHA) within the U.S. Department of Labor to help employers and employees reduce the number of work-related injuries, illnesses, and deaths in America. (See figure 4-1.) Since then, workplace fatalities have been cut by 62 percent, and occupational injury and illness rates have declined 40 percent. At the same time, U.S. employment has doubled and now includes nearly 115 million workers at 7 million worksites.[5] The Occupational Safety and Health Administration is now the centerpiece of an extensive array of public health agencies and organizations, all of which are dedicated to enhancing the safety and health of workers and the public at large.

The Occupational Safety and Health Administration provides national leadership in occupational safety and health. The agency seeks to find and share the most effective ways to get results to advance its mission to save lives and prevent injuries and illnesses. The message is simple: safety and health add value to your business, to your workplace, and to your life.

Figure 4–1. Workplace Safety Requirements

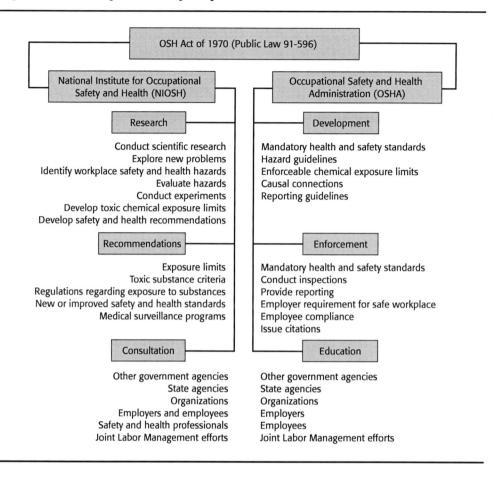

To achieve its objective of enabling all workers to return home safely every day, OSHA established performance goals to guide the development of programs and activities. These goals include improving workplace safety and health, changing workplace culture, and securing public confidence in OSHA's programs and services.

The Occupational Safety and Health Administration has long recognized that it cannot achieve its goals through enforcement alone. Thus, OSHA reaches out to partner with employers and employees to teach, train, and inspire people to work in safer ways.

Customer interactions and staff professionalism are also among OSHA's top priorities. Many customer outreach programs (presented in both English and Spanish) include:

☐ An extensive publications program. Many of these publications can be downloaded from OSHA's website.

☐ Electronic products for compliance assistance, including safety and health topics, slide presentations, targeted CD-ROMs, and eTools.

eTools are stand-alone, interactive, web-based training tools that cover occupational safety and health topics. They are heavily illustrated and utilize graphical menus.

☐ Enhanced training, education, and assistance outreach efforts, including technology-enabled training. These advances in communications technology promise to help OSHA enhance its education and compliance assistance activities.

☐ Web-based training and satellite teletraining initiatives. These allow OSHA to deliver more training to employers and workers at their job sites.

☐ Web-based expert advisors and technical advisors. These tools help users identify workplace hazards that are unique to their situations.

☐ Electronic complaint filing for workers.

☐ The Voluntary Protection Program (VPP), which is designed to recognize and promote effective worksite safety and health. In the VPP, members of management, labor, and OSHA work together to establish cooperative relationships in workplaces that have implemented a comprehensive safety and health management system. Acceptance into the VPP represents OSHA's official recognition of the outstanding efforts of employers and employees who have achieved exemplary occupational safety and health.

☐ The OSHA Strategic Partnership Program (OSPP), which departs from traditional enforcement methods and embraces collaborative agreements. Through OSPP, OSHA and its partners work cooperatively to address critical safety and health issues. This very different approach is proving to be an effective tool for reducing fatalities, injuries, and illnesses in the workplace. Participation in OSPP enables employers to view OSHA as a willing listener and a useful ally rather than an adversary.

☐ The Alliance Program, created in March 2002. This program enables organizations committed to safety and health to work with OSHA to prevent injuries, illnesses, and fatalities in the workplace. OSHA and its Alliance Program partners work together to advance workplace safety and health by reaching out to, educating, and leading the nation's employers and their employees.

☐ The Safety and Health Achievement Recognition Program (SHARP). This program recognizes employers who operate an exemplary safety and health management system. Acceptance into SHARP is an achievement of status singling out health care facilities among their business peers as models for worksite safety and health.

☐ Special liaisons. These individuals work to assist victims and families of workers who are hurt or killed on the job.

☐ Standards that are written in plain language to make them more understandable. Resources also include interpretations, enforcement guides, and other enforcement-related information that is cross-referenced with regulatory requirements using hypertext links.

☐ Public participation, submitted via the Internet. This participation is taken into consideration in the standards development process.

Each of the 115 million American workers and their families, and the more than 7 million businesses that employ them, is directly or indirectly affected by OSHA activity.

The OSH Act requires employers to comply with the safety and health standards issued by OSHA. In addition, the OSH Act includes the general duty clause, which applies to hazards not addressed by any specific OSHA standard. The general duty clause requires employers to provide their employees with a workplace free from recognized hazards that are causing or are likely to cause death or serious physical harm. For a more detailed summary of the OSH Act, see the U.S. Department of Labor's *Employment Law Guide: Occupational Safety and Health*.[6] [CD-ROM 4.11]

While some OSHA regulations specifically address health care facilities, others are general in their application. For example, OSHA enacted the Hazard communication standard in 1983 to help control exposure to hazardous chemicals and to ensure worker access to important information concerning the effects of exposure. Later dubbed *Right-to-Know*, it called for all employees to be informed about the hazards of the chemicals with which they work and how best to protect themselves.

Certain standards of organizations that are not agencies of the federal government are incorporated by reference into OSHA Standard 29 CFR 1910.6. They have the same force and effect as OSHA standards and are adopted as standards under the OSH Act. [CD-ROM 4.12]

To enforce its standards, OSHA is authorized under the OSH Act to conduct workplace inspections, write citations, issue penalties, or impose civil or criminal fines for noncompliance. Every establishment covered by the OSH Act is subject to inspection by OSHA compliance safety and health officers. Similarly, states with their own occupational safety and health programs conduct inspections using qualified compliance safety and health officers. OSHA has established the following system of inspection priorities:

Imminent Danger Situations—Imminent danger situations are given top priority because there is reasonable certainty that a danger exists that can be expected to cause death or serious physical harm. Compliance officers will ask employers to correct these hazards immediately or remove the endangered employees.

Fatalities and Catastrophes—Second priority is given to incidents that involve a death or catastrophes that result in hospitalization of three or more employees. Employers must report such catastrophes to OSHA within eight hours.

Employee Complaints—Third priority is given to employee complaints of alleged violations of standards or of unsafe or unhealthful working conditions. Employees may request anonymity when they file complaints.

Referrals—Hazard information received from individuals, organizations, the media, or other federal, state, or local agencies is also considered in determining whether an inspection is needed.

Unprogrammed Related—Inspections of employers at multi-employer worksites whose operations are not directly affected by the subject of the conditions identified in the complaint, accident, or referral are designated as unprogrammed related.

Follow-up Inspections—In certain circumstances, follow-up inspections are conducted to determine whether previously cited violations have been corrected.

Planned or Programmed Investigations—Specific high-hazard industries, and individual workplaces that have experienced high rates of injuries and illnesses, also receive priority.

There are special circumstances under which OSHA may give notice of an inspection to an employer, but even then such notice will be given less than 24 hours in advance of the inspection. Employers receiving advance notice of an inspection must inform their employees' representative or arrange for OSHA to do so. The OSH Act permits appropriate legal action if an employer refuses to admit an OSHA compliance officer or if an employer attempts to interfere with the inspection. Employers have the right to require compliance officers to obtain an inspection warrant before entering the worksite.

In some states, it is not the federal OSHA that regulates workplace safety and health; rather, a state-run occupational safety and health administration operates under the approval of the federal agency. Such states are referred to as State Plan states. [CD-ROM 4.13, 4.14, 4.15] Although these state agencies must meet federal OSHA standards, they may tailor their regulations to the most prevalent type of industry within their borders.

U.S. Department of Labor (OSHA)
200 Constitution Avenue
Room N3647
Washington, DC 20210
Telephone: (800) 321-6742
Website: www.osha.gov

Office of Justice Programs (OJP)

In 1994 Congress passed the Violence Against Women Act (VAWA), which has been administered by the Office on Violence Against Women (OVAW) since 1995. The purpose of this program is to prevent domestic violence, sexual assault, and the stalking of women. [CD-ROM 4.16]

The OVAW works closely with other Department of Justice programs, including the Office of Justice Programs, the Office of Legal Policy, the Office of Legislative Affairs, the Office of Intergovernmental Affairs, the Immigration and Naturalization Office, the Executive Office for United States Attorneys, U.S. Attorneys' Offices, and state, tribal, and local jurisdictions to implement the mandates of the Violence Against Women Act and subsequent legislation.

Community-based agencies and state, tribal, and local governments receive grants from OVAW that can be used to train personnel, establish specialized domestic violence and sexual assault units, assist victims of violence, and hold perpetrators accountable. More than 6,500 such grants have supported community partnerships among police, prosecutors, victim advocates, and others to address violence against women.

> Office of Justice Programs
> U.S. Department of Justice
> 810 Seventh Street NW
> Washington, DC 20001
> Telephone: (202) 307-5933
> National Domestic Violence Hotline: (800) 799-7233
> Website: www.ojp.usdoj.gov

Other Federal Agencies

Some federal agencies that lack the authority to promulgate or enforce laws may issue guidelines and recommendations in response to emerging health and safety problems. This section describes the federal agencies whose guidelines and recommendations can impact a health care facility:

> Bureau of Labor Statistics (BLS)
> Centers for Disease Control and Prevention (CDC)
> Department of Homeland Security
> Federal Emergency Management Agency (FEMA)
> National Institute for Occupational Safety and Health (NIOSH)

Bureau of Labor Statistics (BLS)

The Bureau of Labor Statistics (BLS) is the principal fact-finding agency of the federal government in the broad field of labor economics and statistics. The BLS is an independent national agency that collects, processes, analyzes, and disseminates essential statistical data to the American public, the U.S. Congress, other federal agencies, state and local governments, businesses, and labor organizations.

The BLS also serves as a statistical resource for OSHA and annually reports on the number of workplace injuries, illnesses, and fatalities in its section on safety and health. The BLS uses the information that health care facilities report on OSHA's Form 300, Log of Work-Related Injuries and Illnesses, to sample and report data.

Nonfatal Injuries and Illnesses

Summary data identifying the total number and rate of injuries and illnesses by industry are released first, usually in December. After more analysis has been completed, case and demographic data are released early in the following spring. For those cases that involve one or more days away from work, the data provide additional details on the workers injured, the nature of the disabling conditions, and the events and sources that produced those conditions.

Fatalities

Fatality data encompass 28 separate elements, including information on the workers, the fatal incidents, and the machinery or equipment involved.

> U.S. Department of Labor
> Bureau of Labor Statistics
> Postal Square Building
> 2 Massachusetts Avenue NE
> Washington, DC 20212-0001
> Telephone: (202) 691-5200
> Website: www.bls.gov

Centers for Disease Control and Prevention (CDC)

Agencies such as OSHA and the EPA as well as accreditation organizations routinely rely on research results and published recommendations and guidelines from the Centers for Disease Control and Prevention (CDC). The CDC is an agency of the Department of Health and Human Services and exists to promote human health and quality of life by preventing and controlling diseases, injuries, and disabilities.

Through the CDC's weekly scientific publication, *Morbidity and Mortality Weekly Report* (*MMWR*), health care facilities can stay informed about specific diseases and health and safety topics. The data provided include reports on infectious and chronic diseases, environmental hazards, natural or human-generated disasters, occupational diseases and injuries, and intentional or un-intentional injuries. Also included are reports on topics of international interest and notices of events of interest to the public health community.

Since communicable diseases have become more easily spread as a result of modern transportation and a far more mobile society, the research conducted by the CDC becomes increasingly valuable. In its attempt to battle disease, the CDC has established a number of mission-specific centers, including the National Institute for Occupational Safety and Health (NIOSH), the National Center for Infectious Diseases, and the National Center for Injury Prevention and Control.

> Centers for Disease Control and Prevention
> 1600 Clifton Road
> Atlanta, GA 30333
> Telephone: (404) 639-3311
> Website: www.cdc.gov

Department of Homeland Security (DHS)

The National Strategy for Homeland Security and the Homeland Security Act of 2002 are intended to mobilize and organize the United States to secure the nation from terrorist attacks. [CD-ROM 4.20] To accomplish this exceedingly complex mission, a focused effort from all of society is required. A primary reason for the establishment of the Department of Homeland Security (DHS) was to provide a single federal agency having overall responsibility for coordinating the activities of federal and nonfederal assets to provide for the security of the nation as well as to assist in any recovery efforts.

Vision statements, mission statements, and strategic goals and objectives provide the framework for the actions that make up the daily operations of the department.

U.S. Department of Homeland Security
Washington, DC 20528
Telephone: (202) 282-8000
Website: www.dhs.gov

Federal Emergency Management Agency (FEMA)

The Federal Emergency Management Agency (FEMA) is part of the Department of Homeland Security's Emergency Preparedness and Response Directorate. Since its founding in 1979, FEMA's mission has been to limit the loss of life and property and to protect our nation's critical infrastructure from all types of hazards through a comprehensive, risk-based emergency management program of mitigation, preparedness, response, and recovery. Often FEMA works in partnership with other organizations that are part of the national emergency management system. These partners include state and local emergency management agencies, 27 federal agencies, and the American Red Cross. The primary responsibilities of FEMA are:

□ *Response and recovery*—When it is clear that a hurricane or other potentially catastrophic disaster is about to occur, FEMA pre-positions equipment, supplies, and people in areas adjacent to those that are likely to be affected. Once it is safe to operate, FEMA moves its assets directly into the affected areas. FEMA is also responsible for providing this same service following an unforeseen catastrophe.

□ *Disaster aid programs*—The two types of aid that FEMA provides are government assistance and individual assistance.

□ *Mitigation*—FEMA implements measures to limit the effects of floods, earthquakes, hurricanes, and other hazards.

□ *Preparedness, training, and exercises*—Survival and quick recovery from a disaster depend on planning, such as designing and equipping emergency centers, training professionals, developing courses, sponsoring exercises, and coordinating emergency plans.

☐ *Federal Insurance Administration (FIA)*—This program administers the self-supporting National Flood Insurance Program.

☐ *U.S. Fire Administration (USFA)*—Through USFA's National Fire Academy, new fire management technologies are developed, firefighters and emergency medical professionals are trained, the public is educated on how to lower the risk of fire, and fire statistics are collected and analyzed.

☐ *Crisis and communication technologies*—When normal systems are crippled, emergency teams must quickly set up operations, gather information, and maintain or restore communications.

Federal Emergency Management Agency (FEMA)
500 C Street SW
Washington, DC 20472
Telephone: (202) 566-1600 or (800) 621-FEMA
Website: www.fema.gov

National Institute for Occupational Safety and Health (NIOSH)

The Occupational Safety and Health Act of 1970 also established the National Institute for Occupational Safety and Health (NIOSH). (See figure 4-1.) NIOSH is one of the centers within the CDC and is the only government agency established to conduct research and provide scientifically valid public health recommendations to OSHA and others to prevent worker exposure to hazards. NIOSH is responsible for conducting research on the full scope of occupational diseases and injuries, ranging from lung disease in miners to carpal tunnel syndrome in computer users. In addition to conducting research, NIOSH:

☐ Investigates potentially hazardous working conditions as requested by employers or employees

☐ Makes recommendations and disseminates information on preventing workplace diseases, injuries, and disabilities

☐ Provides training to occupational safety and health professionals

Although the OSH Act created both NIOSH and OSHA, they are two distinct agencies with separate responsibilities, and they operate out of separate cabinet-level departments. OSHA operates out of the Department of Labor, and NIOSH operates out of the Department of Health and Human Services. NIOSH conducts its mandated scientific research based on the overall health and safety of the American worker, without concern for the economic impact of their recommendations. While OSHA often incorporates NIOSH research and data into its regulations, this is done only after consideration of the economic impact and technological feasibility of its standards.

National Institute for Occupational Safety and Health
Hubert H. Humphrey Building
200 Independence Avenue SW
Room 715H
Washington, DC 20201
Telephone: (800) 356-4674
Website: www.cdc.gov/niosh

STATE AND LOCAL AGENCIES

Individual states have requirements for health care facilities on many of the same topics as federal agency regulations. However, state requirements may be more rigorous or extensive than federal standards. Complying with state and local regulations can provide a strong foundation for compliance with federal and voluntary standards.

The individual states may regulate practices, enforce regulations, and develop programs in many areas. Figure 4-2 lists examples of these practices, regulations, and programs.

Because state and local requirements on these and other subjects may differ from or expand on national standards, it is crucial that health care facilities know the regulations that affect them. As with federal mandates, facilities should be aware that regional or state requirements can change as new information becomes available.

NONGOVERNMENTAL ORGANIZATIONS AND AGENCIES

Standards and guidelines from nongovernmental organizations and agencies can become part of occupational safety and health regulations. Some standards can also be interpreted as implicit regulations through the legal system, which means that health care facilities that do not comply have a potential liability exposure. Available information may be used as the basis for a new regulation, or an existing standard may be incorporated by reference.[7] The following are the agencies and organizations most often used by health care facilities as sources for the guidelines and standards used as reference codes by authorities and federal agencies:

American Conference of Governmental Industrial Hygienists (ACGIH)
American Institute of Architects (AIA)
American National Standards Institute (ANSI)
American Society of Heating, Refrigerating and Air-Conditioning Engineers (ASHRAE)
American Society for Testing and Materials International (ASTM)
Compressed Gas Association (CGA)
National Fire Protection Association (NFPA)

Figure 4–2. Examples of Practices, Regulations, and Programs Often Administered by Individual States

---

□ *Occupational Safety and Health Administration*—This federal agency gives states the option of implementing their own workplace safety and health programs instead of adopting the federal program. State OSHA regulations must be at least as stringent as those of the federal program.

□ *Hazardous waste*—States may establish their own hazardous waste management agencies to assist in compliance with EPA and DOT rules. Requirements include proper storage, disposal, preparation for shipment, and transportation of hazardous materials, and training employers in the proper identification and control of hazardous substances.

□ *Medical waste*—Although this practice is beginning to change, state agencies usually create the rules concerning the handling of medical waste. Usually either the state board of health or the state equivalent of the EPA issues the regulations. In addition, local sanitation districts may have rules about the disposal of hazardous or infectious materials through the sewer.

□ *Workers' compensation*—A common denominator among most states is the existence of workers' compensation laws. These laws are generally enforced by the state attorney general or an agency that handles similar matters. The penalties for failure to comply with these laws, as well as the actual compensation amounts to injured employees, are cumulative and can cause financial hardship for a facility of any size. Effective accident prevention and comprehensive safety programs can minimize the cost of workers' compensation.

□ *Fire codes*—The state or local fire authority, usually the fire marshal's office, verifies that fire safety requirements are met according to state codes, OSHA regulations, and NFPA codes.

□ *Health codes*—The health department or other authority having jurisdiction verifies compliance with requirements governing infection control techniques and sanitation practices.

American Conference of Governmental Industrial Hygienists (ACGIH)

When writing the OSH Act, Congress recognized that it would take some time for the standards setting process to begin working, so it allowed OSHA to adopt guidelines for air contaminant concentrations from lists produced by nongovernmental consensus organizations. Therefore, the first OSHA standards governing chemical exposures were, in fact, the threshold limit values (TLVs) published by the American Conference of Governmental Industrial Hygienists (ACGIH) in 1960. The TLVs were renamed permissible exposure limits (PELs) and can be found in OSHA Standard 29 CFR 1910 Subpart Z, Toxic and Hazardous Substances, 1910.1000, table Z-1. There are about 400 chemicals listed in table Z-1.

For more than 60 years, ACGIH has been an organization with the purpose of encouraging the exchange of experience among industrial hygiene workers and of collecting and making information and data accessible to them. The Threshold Limit Values for Chemical Substances Committee was established in 1941 as a subcommittee of the Committee on Technical Standards. This group was charged to investigate, recommend, and annually review exposure limits for chemical substances. Today's list of TLVs includes more than 700 chemical substances and physical agents, as well as 50 biological exposure indices (BEI) for selected chemicals.

The American Conference of Governmental Industrial Hygienists also provides publications and professional reference texts. In addition to its publications, ACGIH supports educational activities that facilitate the exchange of ideas, information, and techniques.

For a variety of reasons, at the present time many of the ACGIH TLVs and their documentation are more current than either the PELs listed in 29 CFR 1910.1000 tables Z-1 through Z-3 [CD-ROM 4.21, 4.22, 4.23] or the recommended exposure limits (RELs) published by NIOSH.

American Conference of Governmental Industrial Hygienists
1330 Kemper Meadow Drive
Cincinnati, OH 45240
Telephone: (513) 742-6163
Website: www.acgih.org

American Institute of Architects (AIA)

Since 1857 the American Institute of Architects (AIA) has represented the professional interests of architects in the United States. Members adhere to a code of ethics and professional conduct that assures the client, the public, and colleagues of an AIA-member architect's dedication to the highest standards of professional practice.

In 2001 the AIA and the Facility Guidelines Institute (FGI) introduced *Guidelines for Design and Construction of Hospital and Health Care Facilities*. The AIA guidelines specify minimum program and equipment needs for clinical and support areas of health care facilities, and they expand on the planning process by establishing an infection control risk assessment (ICRA), which first appeared in the 1996–1997 AIA guidelines. As a consensus guideline, it relies heavily on input from groups including the American Society for Healthcare Engineering (ASHE) and the American Society of Heating, Refrigerating and Air-Conditioning Engineers (ASHRAE), and it maintains consistency with published guidelines from the CDC. Authorities, accreditation organizations, and federal agencies have adopted the AIA guidelines as a reference code or standard when reviewing construction designs and plans for health care facilities.

The American Institute of Architects
1735 New York Avenue NW
Washington, DC 20006-5292
Telephone: (800) AIA-3837
Website: www.aia.org

American National Standards Institute (ANSI)

The American National Standards Institute (ANSI) was founded more than 80 years ago by five engineering societies and three governmental agencies as a private, nonprofit, membership organization serving as an umbrella for the U.S. standardization community. At the time, agencies with similar responsibilities had overlapping and sometimes conflicting standards. The mission of ANSI is to enhance the global competitiveness of U.S. businesses and the American quality of life by promoting and facilitating voluntary consensus standards and conformity assessment systems and ensuring their integrity. Conformity assessment involves evaluating products, processes, or services to determine whether they adhere to a set of specific requirements.

The American National Standards Institute itself does not develop standards. Rather, technical societies, trade associations, and other groups are accredited by ANSI to coordinate and lead technical development efforts. Accredited developers voluntarily submit the results of their work as candidate standards to ANSI for approval as "American National Standards." The ANSI designation signifies that ANSI criteria for due process have been met and that a consensus for approval exists among those directly and materially affected who choose to participate in the approval process.

Just as Congress incorporated ACGIH TLVs into the Occupational Safety and Health Act, it also allowed the incorporation of certain ANSI standards because they were considered to represent the best practices at the time.[8,9]

The standards of the American National Standards Institute can also be interpreted as implicit regulations through the U.S. legal system. The American National Standards Institute and OSHA formalized their relationship in a memorandum of understanding. The American National Standards Institute furnishes assistance and support and continues to encourage the development of national consensus standards for occupational safety and health issues for use by OSHA and other groups.

The standards of the ANSI apply to all areas of industry, including health care; one example is the safe use of medical lasers and personal protective equipment (PPE).

American National Standards Institute
Washington, DC, Headquarters
1819 L Street NW
6th Floor
Washington, DC 20036
Telephone: (202) 293-8020
Website: www.ansi.org

American Society of Heating, Refrigerating and Air-Conditioning Engineers (ASHRAE)

The American Society of Heating, Refrigerating and Air-Conditioning Engineers (ASHRAE) is an international organization that consists of 50,000 members. The society's sole purpose is to advance the arts and sciences of heating, ventilation, air-conditioning, and refrigeration (HVAC&R) for the public's benefit through research, standards writing, continuing education, and publication.

Through its membership, ASHRAE writes standards that set uniform methods of testing and rating equipment, and it establishes accepted practices for the HVAC&R industry worldwide, including the design of energy-efficient buildings. Contractors use the established standards and accepted practices of this organization when building new facilities or remodeling health care facilities to ensure that ventilation systems are adequate and support the intended use of the facility.

> American Society of Heating, Refrigerating and Air-Conditioning
> Engineers (ASHRAE)
> 1791 Tullie Circle NE
> Atlanta, GA 30329
> Telephone: (800) 527-4723
> Website: www.ashrae.org

American Society for Testing and Materials International (ASTM)

The American Society for Testing and Materials International (ASTM) is one of the largest voluntary standards development organizations in the world. The society's standards have an important role in the information infrastructure that guides design, manufacturing, and trade in the global economy. The American Society for Testing and Materials International develops consensus standards that have made products and services safer, better, and more cost-effective.

> American Society for Testing and Materials International (ASTM)
> 100 Barr Harbor Drive
> West Conshohocken, PA 19428-2959
> Telephone: (610) 832-9585
> Website: www.astm.org

Compressed Gas Association (CGA)

Health care facilities routinely use a number of compressed gases, including carbon dioxide, anesthetic gases, and oxygen. Because these gases are stored under tremendous pressure, the slightest disturbance can cause this pressure to be released in a destructive or deadly manner. If not handled and stored with great caution, compressed gases pose a serious threat of explosion, fire, injury, and property damage.

Since 1913 the Compressed Gas Association (CGA) has been dedicated to the development and promotion of safety standards and safe practices in the industrial gas industry. It provides technical advice and safety coordination for businesses in these industries. However, the CGA is also concerned with the handling of compressed gases wherever they are used, including health care facilities that use them to treat patients.

Hospital personnel must be apprised of the potential dangers of mishandling compressed gases, and the CGA offers technical publications and audiovisual materials to safeguard the facility's staff, visitors, and premises. It also advises the NFPA in developing compressed gas standards.

Compressed Gas Association
4221 Walney Road
5th Floor
Chantilly, VA 20151-2923
Telephone: (703) 788-2700
Website: www.cganet.com

National Fire Protection Association (NFPA)

For more than a century, the National Fire Protection Association (NFPA) has been dedicated to protecting people and their property from the devastating effects of fire. In some way, virtually every building, process, service, design, and installation in today's society is affected by codes and standards developed through NFPA's true consensus system. Through its National Fire Codes, as well as its education and community outreach programs, NFPA is a membership organization that is recognized throughout the world as the leading authority for technical background, data, and consumer advice on fire problems, protection, and prevention. The federal government and many state and local governments accept NFPA codes and standards as the basis for fire prevention and construction. The association publishes 300 codes and standards, of which more than 60 directly affect health care facilities.

When tragedies do occur, investigations invariably reveal serious life safety code violations. An important fire safety resource for health care facilities is the *NFPA 101®: Life Safety Code®*. It is the cornerstone of life safety in new and existing structures and has protected countless lives during the past 80 years.

The *NFPA 101®: Life Safety Code®* also includes requirements for emergency preparedness plans and drills, exit arrangements, and portable fire extinguishers. The emergency preparedness section provides information necessary for the preparation and implementation of a hospital's individual plan. Another source of overall information on the latest developments in fire protection systems, equipment, and techniques is the latest edition of the *NFPA Life Safety Code Handbook.*

The NFPA also works to make health care facilities safer for patients and staff by providing the *NFPA 99: Standard for Health Care Facilities.* Continuing developments in medical equipment and processes create new opportunities for improved health care delivery, as well as new methods to mitigate fire, explosion, and electrical hazards. The *NFPA 99* presents rules for the safe application of electrical and gas vacuum systems, environment systems, and materials and emergency management practices.

The *NFPA 70: National Electrical Code* (NEC) provides practical rules to help safeguard persons and property from hazards arising from the use of electricity. Adoption and enforcement of the NEC protects public safety by establishing requirements for electrical wiring and equipment in virtually all buildings.

NFPA
1 Batterymarch Park
P.O. Box 9101
Quincy, MA 02169-7471
Telephone: (617) 770-3000
Website: www.nfpa.org

ACCREDITATION ORGANIZATIONS

Every hospital and health system is responsible for developing and implementing a comprehensive and systematic quality management system. Such a system is directed at continually improving care provided to patients and preventing harm or injury to patients and all who work in the hospital environment.

Many hospitals and health care systems utilize external standards, often developed by peers within the health care professions, to assess or enhance the comprehensiveness of the organization's quality management structure and its ability to ensure the safety and quality of care provided to patients.

One application of external standards is *accreditation.* Accreditation is a voluntary process by which a health care facility demonstrates that it meets the standards established by its professional peers. Accreditation has also been used by state and regulatory agencies to confer *deemed status.* Deemed status in the context of health care organizations originated with the creation of the Medicare program in 1965. Under the authority of Section 1865 of the Social Security Act, hospitals accredited by the American Osteopathic Association (AOA) or the Joint Commission on Accreditation of Healthcare Organizations (JCAHO) are automatically "deemed" to meet all health and safety requirements, except the utilization review requirement, the psychiatric hospital special conditions, and the special requirements for hospital providers of long-term care services.

The "deeming" concept is also utilized by a large number of states as the criterion for meeting state health and safety requirements. Organizations that have "deeming" status vary from state to state.

American Osteopathic Association Healthcare Facilities Accreditation Program (HFAP)

The Healthcare Facilities Accreditation Program (HFAP) of the American Osteopathic Association has been in existence since 1945. This program accredits acute care, critical access, physical rehabilitation, and psychiatric hospitals; clinical laboratories; ambulatory care, urgent care, and occupational health centers; single- and group-practice physician offices; ambulatory surgery, eye surgery, outpatient surgery, and plastic surgery centers; behavioral health residential and day centers; psychological counseling, substance abuse, mental health, and opioid treatment centers; and physical rehabilitation centers.

> Healthcare Facilities Accreditation Program (HFAP)
> 142 East Ontario Street
> Chicago, IL 60611-2864
> Telephone: (312) 202-8060
> Website: www.hfap.org

Commission on Accreditation of Rehabilitation Facilities (CARF)

The Commission on Accreditation of Rehabilitation Facilities (CARF) was founded in 1966. Since that time, it has developed accreditation programs for adult day care services, assisted-living services, behavioral health services, employment and community services, and medical rehabilitation services. More than 25,000 programs and services in more than 3,500 organizations in the United States, Canada, and Sweden have been accredited by CARF. The American Hospital Association (AHA) is a sponsor member of CARF.

> CARF International
> 4891 E. Grant Road
> Tucson, AZ 85712
> Telephone: (520) 325-1044 or (888) 281-6531
> Website: www.carf.org

Joint Commission on Accreditation of Healthcare Organizations (JCAHO)

The Joint Commission on Accreditation of Healthcare Organizations is focused on improving the safety and quality of the care provided to the public. It accomplishes this goal by accrediting health care organizations and offering health care performance improvement services.

Since 1951 the Joint Commission has maintained performance-based standards and evaluated the quality and the safety of care by assessing the compliance of health care organizations with these national standards. A not-for-profit organization, the Joint Commission is the oldest and largest health care accrediting body. The Joint Commission accredits and certifies more than 15,000 health care organizations and programs.

The Joint Commission accredits hospitals, critical access hospitals, ambulatory care organizations, office-based surgery practices, behavioral health care facilities, home care agencies, hospices, home medical equipment companies, long-term care facilities, and laboratories. It also certifies disease management companies and health care staffing agencies.

The Joint Commission's manuals of accreditation standards are designed to aid a facility's continuous operational improvement, as well as the self-assessment of its performance against Joint Commission standards. One key chapter of the standards manual, "Management of the Environment of Care (EC)," addresses employee safety and health.

Joint Commission on Accreditation of Healthcare Organizations
One Renaissance Boulevard
Oakbrook Terrace, IL 60181
Telephone: (630) 792-5000
Website: www.jcaho.org

GUIDELINES FOR REGULATORY INSPECTIONS

Inspections are an integral element of regulatory oversight. Regulatory agencies are committed to the strict, fair, and effective enforcement of safety and health requirements in the workplace. Inspectors are experienced, well-trained professionals whose goal is to ensure compliance with requirements and to help employers and workers reduce on-the-job hazards in order to prevent injuries, illnesses, and deaths in the workplace.

Most agencies conduct inspections without advance notice. Health care workers face a wide range of hazards on the job, and the facility should develop procedures for dealing with inspections. Management should develop a call list containing the names and telephone extensions of all individuals to be notified in the event of an inspection. Facilities can be perpetually prepared for inspections if the needs assessments and the worksite analyses are conducted on a regular basis and any problems that are identified are corrected as soon as possible.

A typical inspection involves the following four steps:

1. *Arrival*—A management representative should greet the inspectors as promptly as possible, make them comfortable, and confirm that the inspectors are at the correct location. If they are not, the representative should give the inspectors directions to the proper

site, if known. The representative should ask to see credentials, if they are not already visible, and, if the inspectors are responding to a specific complaint, copies of any warrants or other documents.

2. *Opening conference*—The opening conference is a meeting where the inspectors state the reason for the inspection and describe its scope, the walk-around procedures, and the handling of employee interviews. The representative should supply any information requested by the inspectors but volunteer nothing else.

3. *Inspection tour*—A staff member should accompany the inspectors. If the same person cannot serve as a guide throughout the inspection, then someone in each department should be asked to assist. Make certain that the inspectors are provided with any necessary equipment and that all safety procedures are adhered to during the inspection. Take notes detailing the exact areas inspected, which employees were interviewed, and any comments made by the inspectors with regard to the inspection itself.

4. *Closing conference*—After the walk-around, there is usually a closing conference with the employer and the employee representatives, during which the compliance officers discuss their findings. Compliance officers discuss possible courses of action that an employer may take following the inspection. The person or persons responsible for health and safety for the facility should be present. If there are unanswered questions, those best able to clarify the issues should attend as well. As the closing conference draws to an end, the inspectors should be asked for a copy of the report. Based on the information in that report, an in-house closing report is prepared detailing all items requiring improvement. This report should also include any notes taken, any relevant photographs, and the names of the employees who were interviewed. If the inspectors made any comments during the inspection that may prove useful in the improvement of the facility, these comments should be included as part of the in-house report. The administration should receive all of this information as promptly as possible.

It is reasonable to attempt to replicate any documentation by the inspectors. If photographs were taken, then the same subjects should be photographed. The time, location, and date should be noted for each photograph. If the inspector used a camcorder instead of a camera, it would probably be best to videotape the same areas.

If staff members are cooperative, friendly, and prepared to accompany an inspector through an inspection, the integrity of the facility can only be enhanced.

During the walk-around, compliance officers may point out some apparent violations that can be corrected immediately. Although the law requires that these hazards still be cited, prompt correction is a sign of good faith on the part of the employer. Compliance officers seek to minimize work interruptions during the inspection and will maintain the confidentiality of any trade secrets they observe.

Follow-up Inspections

Sometimes agencies conduct follow-up inspections to determine whether previously cited violations have been corrected. If an employer has failed to correct a violation, the agency informs the employer of the situation and the consequences of the failure, which could include the daily assessment of penalties while such failure or violations continue.

Citations and Penalties

Following an inspection, the agency will determine whether citations will be issued and, if so, what penalties will be assessed. The health care facility will be informed of any citations or violations within the time frames established by the agency.

Appeals Process

Appeals processes are established separately by the agencies and usually follow specific formats that may include informal conferences, written reviews, or notices of contest from the employer. Agencies have legally established time limits for appeals.

GUIDELINES OF THE JOINT COMMISSION

Outside of regulations and guidelines established by the federal government, the most significant contribution to ensuring quality health care delivery, patient care and safety, and employee health and safety are the standards inherent in the Joint Commission's accreditation process. In 1996 the Joint Commission and OSHA entered into a formal educational partnership with the purpose of fostering improvement in the management of safety and health issues in health care organizations and minimizing duplication in compliance activities between the two organizations.

Although a complete discussion of the relevant Joint Commission standards is beyond the scope of this book, the astute and well-prepared Environmental Health and Safety director should be as knowledgeable about and conversant in the relevant Joint Commission standards as about the applicable regulations enforced by federal, state, and local governmental agencies.

The Joint Commission's accreditation process focuses on systems critical to the safety and the quality of care, treatment, and services. It represents a shift from a focus survey preparation to a focus on a continuous operational improvement by encouraging health care facilities to incorporate the standards as a guide for routine operations.

Under this accreditation process, the unannounced full survey is the on-site evaluation piece of a continuous process. The accreditation process encourages organizations to embed the standards into routine operations in order to achieve and maintain excellent operational systems on an ongoing basis. Initiatives such as the continuous Periodic Performance Review (PPR) and the sharing of Priority Focus Process (PFP) information facilitate this.

THE ROLE OF THE ENVIRONMENTAL HEALTH AND SAFETY DEPARTMENT

Just as it is not enough to rely on others to keep us safe and healthy in our personal lives, it is not enough to rely solely on the efforts of government agencies and other organizations to ensure the health and safety of employees and patients in health care facilities. It is incumbent on the Environmental Health and Safety Department in a facility to keep current with changes in the rules, regulations, guidelines, recommendations, and other activities of these organizations and agencies. The Environmental Health and Safety Department must also establish and maintain good working relationships with its counterparts in these groups.

References

1. U.S. Congress. Occupational Safety and Health Act of 1970, Public Law 91–596. *U.S. Statutes at Large* 84 (1970), p. 1590. Available at http://www.osha.gov/pls/ oshaweb/owadisp.show_document?p_table=OSHACT&p_id=2743 (accessed 2/9/2006).
2. U.S. Department of Labor. *Ethylene Oxide* (29 CFR 1910.1047). Available at http://www.osha.gov/pls/oshaweb/owadisp.show_document?p_table= STANDARDS&p_id=10070 (accessed 2/17/2006).
3. U.S. Congress. "Section 5: Duties." Occupational Safety and Health Act of 1970, Public Law 91–596. *U.S. Statutes at Large* 84 (1970), p. 1590. Available at http://www.osha.gov/pls/oshaweb/owadisp.show_document?p_table= OSHACT&p_id=3359 (accessed 2/17/2006).
4. U.S. Department of Labor. *OSHA Regulations (Standards, 29 CFR)*. Available at http://www.osha.gov/pls/oshaweb/owasrch.search_form?p_doc_type= STANDARDS&p_toc_level=0&p_keyvalue= (accessed 2/17/2006).
5. U.S. Department of Labor. *All About OSHA: Occupational Safety and Health Administration* (OSHA 2056-07R 2003). Available at http://www.osha.gov/Publications/ osha2056.pdf (accessed 2/17/2006).
6. U.S. Congress. Occupational Safety and Health Act of 1970, Public Law 91–596. *U.S. Statutes at Large* 84 (1970), p. 1590. Available at http://www.osha.gov/ pls/oshaweb/owadisp.show_document?p_table=OSHACT&p_id=2743 (accessed 2/9/2006).

7. U.S. Department of Labor. *Incorporation by Reference* (29 CFR 1910.6). Available at http://www.osha.gov/pls/oshaweb/owadisp.show_document?p_table=STANDARDS&p_id=9702 (accessed 2/17/2006).

8. Joseph J. Lazzara, "Safeguarding: Are ANSI Standards Really Voluntary?" *Occupational Hazards* (December 2004). Available at http://www.occupationalhazards.com/articles/12790 (accessed 2/17/2006).

9. U.S. Department of Labor. *Incorporation by Reference* (29 CFR 1910.6). Available at http://www.osha.gov/pls/oshaweb/owadisp.show_document?p_table=STANDARDS&p_id=9702 (accessed 2/17/2006).

CHAPTER 5

INTEGRATING WORKPLACE AND FAMILY SAFETY AND HEALTH: THE HOLISTIC APPROACH

In the closet, in the corner, there was a bag filled with pieces of cloth. Some of the pieces were brilliant shades of blue, red, and green. Other pieces were muted shades of brown or yellow. A few pieces had prints of flowers or other patterns, and some were textured. The cloth was cotton, silk, and wool.

The pieces were pulled from the bag and sorted by color and texture. They were carefully cut into smaller pieces—some square, some curved. Then the carefully cut pieces were arranged so that they formed a perfect square. A needle and thread worked through the fabric, joining each small piece to another until a square had been made, and the next square was started.

Soon there was a stack of squares all the same size, each with part of a seemingly random design. The squares were taken up and the needle and thread worked up and down, in and out, until two of the squares were joined. A third square was added, and then another, and another, until all the squares had been stitched together.

The finished piece was laid flat. The small pieces had become part of larger pieces, and the larger pieces had become part of a single piece. The once seemingly random design was now apparent. The scraps of cloth that once were a loose collection in a bag in a corner of a closet, and that by themselves made no sense, had now been organized and integrated into a background of solid colors of red and blue and green with rings, partly patterned and partly textured, that appeared to be interlocked. The random shapes and colors had been integrated into a single thing. None of the pieces alone was anything more than a scrap of cloth. None of the squares by themselves was anything more than a square of cloth, but together they had become a quilt that was a thing of its own.

When we were children, our parents always had something to tell us: "Look both ways before crossing the street." "Don't play with matches." "Don't talk to strangers." "Eat your vegetables." "Play nice with the other kids." "Do your homework." Each admonition was seemingly unrelated to the others, but taken together they were intended to keep us safe and healthy and to teach us how to get along in the world.

The rules of safety and health that we are confronted with as adults are far more complex than the simple rules that applied when we were children. We are barraged with rules and regulations from seemingly disjointed agencies. The Food and Drug Administration (FDA) tells us what and how to eat. The Environmental Protection Agency (EPA) tells us how to keep our air and water and our bodies free from contamination. The Occupational Safety and Health Administration (OSHA) has rules for working safely. Health departments require that we receive vaccinations. There are rules for driving and learning, and even for buying and selling. Individually those rules, just like the pieces of cloth, form a small part of the quilt of our lives. Just as the small pieces of the quilt blend into the larger pattern, we often fail to understand that the rules of working safely are as important to the fabric of our daily lives as they are on our jobs.

Disease prevention requires more than childhood vaccinations. Nutrition and exercise are as important to physical well-being as vaccinations. Furthermore, no matter how effective a government regulation may be, the likelihood of suffering a workplace injury or illness is greatly enhanced if a weakened immune system or poor nutrition diminishes an individual's health.

The ability to work safely is also directly related to the stress of our personal lives. Births, deaths, acute or chronic illness in our families, marriage, and divorce—those "small" events in our lives—are all stressful situations. When people are focused on events that have occurred away from the job or are depressed, it is likely that they will be unable to focus on the work tasks before them.

Based on data from the Bureau of Labor Statistics (BLS), each day approximately 800 health care workers incur some type of injury that damages their health or causes them to be unable to work, but work is not the only way in which these workers and their families are hurt. In 2002 more than 80 percent of the 20.4 million disabling injuries and 95 percent of the 99,500 unintentional-injury deaths were unrelated to work. Counting a family member among those injured or made ill is something no one wants to experience. Family members want to believe that their parents, spouse, children, and grandchildren will never be robbed of the gift of health as a result of a senseless accident at work, home, or play. To realize this hope, employees must integrate in their personal lives those practices that are intended to keep them safe and well at work.

Taking Environmental Health and Safety Principles into Employees' Homes

Family safety and health involvement is a key factor in reducing the number of off-the-job injuries and illnesses. As employers and employees experience the benefits of safe and healthy work practices, they will extend those practices to their personal lives to the benefit of themselves and their families. A holistic ap-

Figure 5-1. Examples of Family Safety and Health Programs

- Vacation safety
- Home fire safety
- Educating children who stay home alone
- Seatbelt safety
- Electrical safety
- Ergonomic awareness (e.g., eye rest breaks from computer monitors)
- Chemical hazard safety
- Safeguards for elderly relatives
- Caring values among family members (e.g., handling difficult situations, increasing communication, being aware of how our own behavior affects the way others see us, and respecting others)

proach that integrates traditional workplace safety and health principles with those of family safety and health, stress management, fitness, hygiene, nutrition, and appropriate lifestyle choices forms the quilt of a healthier life. Examples of family safety and health programs that can benefit from the lessons learned in a successful Environmental Health and Safety program are listed in figure 5-1.

Many of these examples of family safety and health are no different from those elements of a successful Environmental Health and Safety program. Home fire safety is no different from fire safety at work. Wearing seatbelts saves lives whether the driver and passengers are traveling as part of their work duties or running errands on a Saturday morning. The principles and practices of working safely with electricity, chemicals, and when lifting are the same at work as they are at home. If basic safety and health principles are properly taught, the course of instruction will show how those principles apply to employees' personal lives as well as their professional environments.

Workers' Family Protection Act

Hazardous chemicals and substances can threaten the health and safety of workers. If they are transported out of the workplace on workers' clothing or bodies, these chemicals and substances can pose an additional threat to the health and welfare of workers and their families.

On October 26, 1992, Congress amended the Occupational Safety and Health Act of 1970 (OSH Act) to grant authority to the director of the National Institute for Occupational Safety and Health (NIOSH) to evaluate and investigate— and, if necessary, for the secretary of labor to regulate—employee-transported releases of hazardous material that result from contamination of an employee's clothing or body and that may adversely affect the health and safety of workers and their families.[1] [CD-ROM 5.1]

THE IMPACT OF OFF-THE-JOB INJURIES AND ILLNESSES

If an injury or illness happens off the job, the employer faces many of the same costs as if it had happened on the job. In addition to medical costs, there are many hidden costs:

- ☐ The sick or injured employee may need to be replaced.
- ☐ Replacement workers may have to be trained, leading to lost productivity and additional payroll expense.
- ☐ Other employees are required to assume additional responsibilities.
- ☐ Benefit costs (insurance rates) may increase.
- ☐ Employee morale may decline.
- ☐ Managers have to devote time to rectifying the situation instead of managing.
- ☐ If the injured employee was a key player on a project, the project could be delayed, costing the facility thousands of dollars.
- ☐ Holidays and vacations may have to be postponed for other employees in order to maintain staffing levels.

In addition, injuries can affect employees and their families in the following ways:

- ☐ Injuries cause pain and suffering to the injured person.
- ☐ Injuries may create stress among people close to the injured worker.
- ☐ Financial difficulties may result.
- ☐ Substance abuse may result.
- ☐ Lowered self-esteem and a sense of worthlessness may result.
- ☐ When an employee has been off work for an extended period, it is often difficult for the employee to return to work.

When someone is seriously injured or killed, everyone close to that person is affected. No event is isolated. A work-related injury affects co-workers and families, and an accident or illness at home has a negative impact on that person's co-workers. Understanding the relationship between family safety and health and workplace safety and health can lead to significant improvements in a person's working life and personal life.

CREATING A NEW DIMENSION IN HEALTH AND SAFETY

Integrating workplace and family safety and health will create a new dimension in health and well-being for health care facilities and for families. This holistic approach:

- ☐ Integrates workplace safety and health principles with those of personal safety and health.

□ Focuses on prevention rather than treatment.

□ Demonstrates how stress management, nutrition, basic hygiene, and physical fitness are essential to reducing injuries and illnesses, no matter where they occur.

□ Addresses caring values that affect safety and health, such as respect and courteous treatment, by enhancing the relationships between employees, patients, families, and the general public.

When employers establish policies and guidelines that teach and enforce the principles and practices of working in a safe and healthy manner, and also show employees how those principles and practices relate to their personal lives, employees begin to focus on prevention rather than treatment. This approach will translate into improved patient care and increased productivity. In a similar fashion, if the facility provides information and training on stress management, personal hygiene, and physical fitness, and shows employees how those lifestyle factors can have a positive effect by helping them to work in a healthier and safer manner, employees will begin to see how easily work practices and personal practices can be integrated to foster a climate of improved patient care and increased productivity while reducing injuries and illnesses. Integrating work practices with personal practices will lead to successful implementation of the health care facility's plan to build broad-based awareness programs using the best elements from around the world while maintaining a focus on caring values, business objectives, and federal and state regulations.

Some examples of work-related health and safety practices that can be translated to employees' personal lives include the following:

Safe Driving

Being a safe driver is an important element of both job safety and personal safety. A number of factors can adversely affect driving ability, including trying to meet deadlines, distraction, anger and aggression, ill health, vision or hearing problems, and drug or alcohol use. By improving defensive driving skills and maintaining a healthy lifestyle, employees will experience fewer accidents both on and off the job.

Hazardous Materials

Employees who have been trained in hazard communication and handling hazardous materials should translate their knowledge and skills to their use of potentially hazardous materials, such as paint, solvents, cleansers, bleach, herbicides, and pesticides, off the job. Hazard communication training at work should provide employees with the tools they need to understand the potential hazards of the chemicals they use at home and to protect themselves and their families.

Personal Security

At work employees are taught how to take control of their personal security by recognizing potentially dangerous situations and taking appropriate measures to avoid them or make them less dangerous. Avoiding poorly lit and isolated areas in our personal lives is just as important as avoiding them at work. Learning how to calm a potentially violent patient will help to mitigate aggressive behaviors encountered when dealing with family members or with strangers while shopping or driving.

Ergonomics

Physical fitness is one of the essential tools in the prevention of musculoskeletal disorders (MSDs). Ergonomic injuries are less likely to occur if employees maintain good physical health.

Learning to lift properly and to avoid tasks that require repetitive motion at work is no different from learning how to lift groceries, children, boxes, or other heavy items at home. Taking short breaks during prolonged computer work in the office and at home will help prevent eyestrain. Using proper posture while typing will help prevent back and leg problems. A wrist rest, whether used with the office computer or the home computer, will help prevent carpal tunnel syndrome.

Slips, Trips, and Falls

Many slips, trips, and falls occur as part of the approximately 18,000 steps each of us takes every day, from walking the dog to going up the stairs at work. The admonition "Don't run in the hall" that we learned in school still applies at work and at home. At home slips, trips, and falls can be prevented by avoiding the use of small rugs at the top of stairs and by applying non-skid backing to them for use in other places. Repairing broken steps, filling cracks and holes in paved surfaces, and keeping walkways free of ice and snow will reduce the likelihood of a slip, trip, or fall, whether at work or at home.

Personal Protective Equipment and Engineering Controls

Personal protective equipment is used to protect employees from chemical exposures, eye injuries, head injuries, and noise. Just as in the workplace, there are dangerous chemicals used in homes. Some paints, furniture strippers, and cleaning agents pose potential health threats at home and should be used only with appropriate personal protective equipment. At work, employees are taught how to use ventilation to help protect them from chemical exposures. At home, fans can be used and windows can be opened to remove fumes. However, consumer fans are not as powerful as industrial ventilation systems, and care should be exercised to ensure that dangerous chemicals are used only in areas with adequate ventilation.

Ladder Safety

At work, approved ladders and step stools are required to reach high places. However, at home people often use chairs, boxes, or other items that are not stable or strong enough to hold their weight. By choosing the correct ladder or step stool for home use, a wide variety of accidents can be avoided. In the work environment, care is taken to ensure that metal ladders are not placed too close to or in contact with power lines. In many work situations, nonconductive ladders made of fiberglass are used to help prevent electrical accidents. The same cautions should be used at home. Fiberglass ladders are readily available for home use, and the cautions concerning placement of ladders near power lines apply equally at home and at work.

Good Housekeeping

In the workplace, efforts are made to replace harsh chemical cleaners with environmentally safer and less toxic products. The same effort should be made in the home. For example, vinegar and water, ammonia and water, and rubbing alcohol may be used as effective and inexpensive cleaning agents.

Many facilities have recycling programs. Those programs are no different from maintaining a personal recycling program at home.

In the health care facility, housekeeping employees are taught to be aware of sharps that have not been disposed of properly. At home, families should learn to avoid sharp objects, such as broken glass and nails, that may be hidden in the trash.

Yard Work

Doing yard work on a weekend requires the same skills and practices that grounds keeping crews use in the health care facility. Grounds keeping and landscape crews can be observed wearing hats to protect them from the sun, drinking lots of water or other liquids to avoid dehydration, applying sunscreen to prevent the harmful effects of ultraviolet radiation, using hearing protection when working with noise-generating power tools, and protecting their hands with gloves and their feet with sturdy work shoes. These same work practices and personal protective equipment will help prevent injuries during yard work at home.

Electrical Safety

At work, electrical equipment is checked to ensure that cords are intact and that the receptacles into which they are plugged are in good condition. Routine inspection of receptacles and electrical cords will also help to prevent electrocutions at home. At work, when an electrical circuit is being worked on, steps are taken to ensure that the circuit is shut off and cannot be turned on until the work is completed; the same precautions should be taken at home.

Tool Safety

At work, the employer makes certain that employees have the correct tools for doing their jobs in order to prevent injuries and to ensure that work is performed properly. The same philosophy should be applied to home repairs. Using the right tool will help ensure that a task is performed safely and correctly. Getting help from a neighbor, family member, or friend with heavy or difficult jobs will help prevent back injuries and crushed fingers or toes.

Fire Safety

In the workplace, fire drills are conducted to make sure that employees know what to do in the event of a fire. Preparing and practicing a family escape plan in case of a fire at home is no different. The health care facility adheres to a fire safety code, as does the builder of new homes. Older homes should be examined to make sure that they comply with existing fire codes. Smoke detectors should be properly located and maintained. Just as the health care facility has fire extinguishers located throughout the building, fire extinguishers placed in the home may prevent property loss and personal injury.

Infection Control

Hand washing is stressed in the health care facility as part of its infection control program. Hand washing needs to be stressed at home for the same reason. Isolation of patients with communicable diseases is no different from isolating family members who have the flu or another easily transmitted disease.

Violence

An ever-increasing problem in the workplace is violence. Sometimes violence is the result of an outsider committing an illegal act in the workplace, or it may be instigated by patients or colleagues. Violence at home is no different. Family violence affects the lives and impacts the safety of employees each day. Stress at work can foster a stressful situation at home, both of which can lead to violence. In addition to workplace violence training, employees should be trained in recognizing signs of family violence, impacts of violence on the workplace, making appropriate referrals, confidentiality, and safety plans. The tools and training provided in the workplace to reduce violence can also be used at home.

BRINGING PERSONAL LIVES INTO THE WORKPLACE

Understanding the relationship between home and work will lead to a new approach to health and safety. For some, this integration is called "common sense." For others, the idea may seem intimidating, and still others readily embrace it. As the partnership between employer and employee progresses, health and well-being in all aspects of their lives benefit. A key step in that progression is understanding how stress, nutrition, and physical fitness are essential to a safe and healthful work experience and personal life.

Stress

A quilt is made of different colors, fabrics, and shapes and is held together by a thread that touches every piece. In life, stress is much like the thread running through the quilt and is a part of virtually every human activity. Stress can be caused by work or life events. Stress is not only work related. Every day we are confronted with situations that make us feel uncertain, afraid, and powerless to make changes. Even joyous events such as weddings, celebrations, and births can be sources of stress. Regardless of the source—work or our personal lives—stress can have a significant impact on how people work, how they feel, and their health.

There are several definitions of stress. The NIOSH definition is specific to work-related stress as is the definition offered by the European Commission, Directorate-General for Employment and Social Affairs. The health and safety executive in the United Kingdom has a more general definition:

> Stress is the reaction people have to excessive pressures or other types of demands placed on them.[2]

Regardless of whether the topic of discussion is work-related stress or general stress, all of the definitions are essentially the same and highlight the fact that stress results in a myriad of mental and physiological reactions.

Studies cited by NIOSH[3] [CD-ROM 5.2] reveal that one-fourth of employees view their jobs as the number one stressor in their lives. In addition, three-fourths of employees believe that the worker today has more on-the-job stress than the worker of a generation ago. The studies also cite data showing that problems at work are more strongly associated with health complaints than are any other life stressor—more so than even financial or family problems.

The NIOSH report lists the following causes of workplace stress:

- *Task design*—Heavy workloads, infrequent rest breaks, long work hours, shift work, work that is hectic, and routine and mundane tasks with little sense of personal control or accomplishment
- *Management style*—Lack of participation by workers in decision making, poor communication in the organization, lack of family-friendly policies
- *Interpersonal relationships*—Poor social environment and lack of support or help from co-workers and supervisors
- *Work roles*—Conflicting or uncertain job expectations, too much responsibility, too many "hats to wear"
- *Career concerns*—Job insecurity; lack of opportunity for growth, advancement, or promotion; rapid changes for which workers are unprepared
- *Environmental conditions*—Unpleasant or dangerous physical conditions, such as crowding, noise, air pollution, or ergonomic problems

Some forms of stress, such as tensions at work or a death in the family, are decidedly negative, while other kinds of stress, such the birth of a baby, are enjoyable experiences. Most often it is the negative stressors that have a deleterious effect on health. According to the NIOSH report, stress has been associated with the following health issues:

- An increased risk of cardiovascular disease, characterized by increased blood pressure, increased heart rate, muscle tension, and headaches
- An increased risk of back and upper-extremity musculoskeletal disease
- Depression and burnout associated with increased anxiety, depression, aggression, and confusion
- An increase in work-related injuries

The NIOSH report also states that there is some evidence of a relationship between stressful working conditions and suicide, cancer, ulcers, and impaired immune function.

Stress can also lead to the behavioral changes listed in figure 5-2.

Figure 5–2. Behavioral Changes That Can Result from Stress

- Increased smoking or drinking
- Irritability
- Obsessive concern with trivial issues
- Poor work performance

In the workplace, these problems can lead to absenteeism, increased accident rates, poor or reduced work output, and worsened interpersonal relations. Employees should be made aware that the range of symptoms they can experience when faced with high levels of stress in the workplace are the same as those that result from stress in their personal lives.

Nutrition and Physical Fitness

Obesity has become a significant health problem in the United States. The Centers for Disease Control and Prevention (CDC) has suggested that obesity may account for as many as 10,000 deaths in the United States. Obesity also affects a person's ability to work by placing undue stress on the body. The surgeon general of the United States reported that in 1999, 61 percent of the adult population was either overweight or obese.[4] Obesity is also related to health problems other than cardiovascular disease, including the following:

- ☐ Hypertension
- ☐ High total cholesterol or high levels of triglycerides
- ☐ Type 2 diabetes
- ☐ Stroke
- ☐ Gallbladder disease
- ☐ Osteoarthritis
- ☐ Sleep apnea and respiratory problems
- ☐ Some cancers (endometrial, breast, and colon)

As an indicator of how obesity is affecting the health of Americans, the prevalence of type 2 diabetes increased 49 percent from 1990 to 2000. Obesity can be reduced through a combination of good nutrition and physical fitness. According to the surgeon general, 40 percent of adults in the United States do not participate in any leisure time physical activity. In addition, less than one-third of adults engage in the recommended amount of physical activity (at least 30 minutes a day most days).

The surgeon general also provides suggestions for a simple exercise program that requires no special skills or training and that can help reverse the trend of increasing obesity in the United States. (See figure 5-3.)

One of the first things that many people learned in grade school was the Food Pyramid. The original Food Pyramid showed how many servings of grains, fruits and vegetables, dairy products, meats, and sweets would make up a healthy diet. However, because of concerns that the Food Pyramid did not consider age, gender, or level of physical activity, the U.S. Department of Agriculture (USDA) revised it in 2005. The new guidance is called "My Pyramid Plan." "My Pyramid Plan" can be used to determine the precise diet that will help an individual maintain a healthy weight. The plan can be obtained from the USDA or can be viewed on a website.[5] The Internet site

Figure 5–3. Suggestions for a Simple Exercise Program

- ☐ Walk. Start slowly and gradually increase the level of activity; start with a 10-minute walk three times a week, and work up to 30 minutes of brisk walking or other form of moderate activity five times a week.
- ☐ Daily exercise can be divided over several short periods (e.g., 10 minutes three times a day) instead of 30 minutes once a day.
- ☐ Select activities that are enjoyable and can fit into your daily life.
- ☐ Do not quit if a day or two is missed, but make exercise a regular part of everyday life.
- ☐ Seek support from friends and family and support the people who are trying to be physically active. Exercise can be a social event that allows interaction with family members or friends or the forming of new relationships.
- ☐ Make fitness a priority.

---

allows people to enter their age, gender, and level of activity to find the mix of foods they need to maintain a healthy weight and diet.

Switching to a healthy diet will make a significant contribution to a person's overall well-being. However, an appropriate level of physical activity is also required to maintain good physical and mental health. The President's Council on Physical Fitness has a website that provides an extensive amount of information to help people of all types to achieve and maintain a healthy lifestyle.[6] [CD-ROM 5.3]

COMPLEMENTARY AND ALTERNATIVE MEDICINE (CAM)

Over the last several decades, there has been a significant change in the public perception and use of nontraditional Western medicine. In recognition of the growing popularity and use of alternative medical practices, the National Institutes of Health (NIH) established the National Center for Complementary and Alternative Medicine (NCCAM).[7] [CD-ROM 5.4] Complementary and alternative medicine (CAM) is defined by NCCAM as:

> A group of diverse medical and health care systems, practices, and products that are not presently considered to be part of conventional medicine—that is, medicine as practiced by holders of M.D. (medical doctor) or D.O. (doctor of osteopathy) degrees and their allied health professionals, such as physical therapists, psychologists, and registered nurses.[8]

The center explains how complementary medicine can be used:

> Complementary medicine is used together with conventional medicine, and alternative medicine is used in place of conventional

medicine. While some scientific evidence exists regarding some CAM therapies, for most there are key questions that are yet to be answered through well-designed scientific studies—questions such as whether these therapies are safe and whether they work for the diseases or medical conditions for which they are used. The list of what is considered to be CAM changes continually, as those therapies that are proven to be safe and effective become adopted into conventional health care and as new approaches to health care emerge.

The NCCAM classifies CAM practices into one of five groups:

Mind-body interventions
Manipulative and body-based methods
Biologically based therapies
Energy therapies
Alternative medical systems

Mind-Body Interventions

Mind-body medicine uses a variety of techniques designed to enhance the mind's capacity to affect bodily function and symptoms. Some techniques that were considered CAM in the past have become mainstream (for example, patient support groups and cognitive-behavioral therapy). Other mind-body techniques are still considered CAM, including meditation, prayer, mental healing, and therapies that use creative outlets such as art, music, or dance.

Manipulative and Body-Based Methods

This category, which includes chiropractic and osteopathic manipulation and massage therapy, focuses on the interactions between the brain, body, and behavior. Chiropractic focuses on the relationship between bodily structure (primarily that of the spine) and function, and how that relationship affects the preservation and restoration of health. Chiropractors use manipulative therapy as an integral treatment tool.

Biologically Based Therapies

Biologically based practices use botanicals, animal-derived extracts, vitamins, minerals, fatty acids, amino acids, proteins, prebiotics and probiotics, whole diets, and functional foods. Botanicals include herbs, which have been used to treat various illnesses for centuries. In some cases botanical preparations have given rise to drugs such as digitalis and quinine. Functional foods include those that have been shown to promote health and well-being, such as foods that have a significant content of anti-oxidants and other vitamins.

Energy Therapies

Energy therapies employ mechanical vibrations (such as sound) and electromagnetic forces such as visible light, magnetism, laser beams, and rays from other parts of the electromagnetic spectrum. They involve the use of specific, measurable wavelengths and frequencies to treat patients. This aspect of CAM also includes the exploitation of what have been termed "biofields." Biofields are thought to be subtle forms of energy that are a part of all life. Practitioners of energy medicine believe that energy flows throughout the body and that they can work with it, see it, and use it to effect changes in the physical body and influence health.

Alternative Medical Systems

Alternative medical systems are complete systems of theory and practice that have evolved independently from or parallel to conventional medicine, and include traditional Chinese medicine and the traditional Eastern Indian practice called Ayurvedic medicine. Major Western whole medical systems include homeopathy and naturopathy. Other systems exist in Native American, African, Middle Eastern, Tibetan, and Central and South American cultures.

USE OF CAM PRACTICES

The National Center for Complementary and Alternative Medicine states that in 1997 Americans spent between $36 billion and $47 billion on CAM.

In May 2004, NCCAM and the National Center for Health Statistics (NCHS), which is a part of the CDC, conducted a survey of 31,044 adult Americans, 18 years of age or older, that explored their use of CAM. At the time of the survey, 36 percent of American adults were using some form of CAM. The principal reasons given for using CAM are listed in figure 5-4.

Figure 5–4. Principal Reasons People Use CAM

□ CAM has the potential to improve a person's health when used in combination with conventional medical treatments: 55 percent.

□ CAM would be interesting to try: 50 percent.

□ Conventional medical treatments would not help: 28 percent.

□ A conventional medical professional suggested trying CAM: 26 percent.

□ Conventional medical treatments are too expensive: 13 percent.

The survey found that most people used CAM as an adjunct to conventional medicine rather than in place of it.

In 1997 the American Medical Association's Council on Scientific Affairs issued a report called *Alternative Medicine* in which they evaluated the current state of scientific evidence supporting complementary and alternative medicine.[9] [CD-ROM 5.5] Their report made the following recommendations:

☐ Maintain an open-minded attitude about all potentially new therapeutic interventions, including those commonly referred to as alternative.

☐ Encourage carefully performed and appropriately controlled studies of these new therapies.

☐ Do not ignore or ridicule the potential of the placebo effect to produce marked therapeutic benefit.

☐ Do not accept all new therapies as efficacious on first acquaintance. Practitioners of quack medicine continue to abound as in all earlier times. Claims of therapeutic efficacy should be rationally examined and tested.

☐ Avoid hubristic and arrogant attitudes toward alternative medical practices because one might be embarrassed by the subsequent demonstrations of their clinical efficacy.

While some believe that complementary and alternative medicine has no place in conventional medicine, others believe that it is superior. Regardless of individual or organizational belief in the value or lack of value of CAM, it is clear that more and more CAM is becoming a square in the quilt of our lives.

THE INFLUENCE OF COMMUNITY RESOURCES ON HEALTH AND SAFETY

The public health community plays an important role in integrating work, environment, and lifestyle health and safety in our lives. One such role is providing information about factors that can contribute to the onset and magnitude of a disease within a population. Employing the resources and expertise of public health officials within communities can result in a cohesive, directed campaign. For example, the U.S. Department of Health and Human Services (HHS) has developed a plan called Healthy People 2010 to improve the quality of life within the United States using numerous resources, including citizens, local government, business organizations, the educational system, public health professionals, and the federal government. By incorporating the assets of the public health community into the employee health and safety programs of the health care facility, employees and their families can receive comprehensive information describing the impact that work, environmental quality, and lifestyle have on specific health outcomes and can benefit from recommendations and guidelines to improve their health status.

Integrating Environmental Health and Safety with personal health and safety will result in a number of positive outcomes. For example, there will be decreases in cancer, cardiovascular disease, and obesity due to reductions in exposures to toxic chemicals, cigarette smoking, dietary fat, and stress. Those health improvements will be achieved through education about and promotion of healthier diets, increased exercise, stress reduction, and spiritual and mental balance.

Some health plans define risky behavior only in terms of sexual practices, rape, and other personal attacks and violations. The definition needs to be expanded to include activities such as driving habits and failure to comply with existing workplace safety standards. For example, between 1992 and 2001, 13,337 civilian workers died in roadway crashes, an average of four deaths each day. Roadway crashes were responsible for 22 percent of workplace deaths, compared with 13 percent from homicide and 10 percent from falls.[10] [CD-ROM 5.6] An inclusive approach to health improvement will encourage state health departments as well as the Department of Transportation (DOT) to actively work with OSHA to develop a combined program to reduce such fatalities. For example, through public service announcements, health departments and other organizations can develop educational campaigns aimed at increasing compliance with OSHA safety and health standards as well as public safety programs designed to reduce vehicle-related injuries and fatalities.

This approach will foster the cooperation and partnership among government, business, and the public that is sought by Healthy People 2010.[11] [CD-ROM 5.7] Healthy People 2010 has identified obesity, diet, and physical activity as priority areas. The plan is based on the strong belief that healthier diets and increased physical activity will lead to decreased obesity as well as reduced morbidity and premature mortality. While this is undoubtedly true, the plan does not explore the significant contribution of occupation on obesity, morbidity, and premature mortality. By the same token, controlling the work environment alone will not achieve the degree of improvement in health status that can be gained by addressing all aspects of an individual's life.

Health screenings have long been a major component of occupational safety and health in the United States and other countries. For example, each OSHA standard that addresses chemical exposure in the workplace includes provisions for periodic medical surveillance as well as pre- and post-employment medical examinations for all potentially exposed workers. Such surveillance or screening programs are the only way to identify the early stages of many diseases. Combining information from workplace surveillance programs with that from county medical screenings will provide a more complete picture of the basis for many health problems.

The principles and recommendations of Healthy People 2010, combined with the principles and practices of Environmental Health and Safety, are analogous to the interlocked rings of the quilt made from the pieces of cloth found in the corner of the closet. By themselves they are nothing more than pieces of cloth, but once they are brought together the pattern is found and the value is clear.

THE ROLE OF THE JOINT COMMISSION IN PROMOTING FAMILY HEALTH AND SAFETY

By understanding the Joint Commission's Environment of Care standards and applying them in their daily work routines, health care workers will discover that many of these standards can also be applied to their non-work life. The Joint Commission standards on safety management (EC.1.10, EC.1.20, EC.1.30), hazardous materials and waste management (EC.3.10), and fire safety (EC.5.10, EC.5.40) all contain elements that can be applied to daily non-work activities. However, just as understanding and complying with OSHA regulations is one part of the total health and safety quilt, so is understanding and applying the Joint Commission's Environment of Care standards.

THE ROLE OF THE ENVIRONMENTAL HEALTH AND SAFETY DEPARTMENT

In addition to serving as a source of knowledge of regulations and other technical responsibilities, the Environmental Health and Safety Department is uniquely suited to help employees and their families integrate workplace health and safety with personal health and safety. The model Environmental Health and Safety Department includes the facility's employee health function along with its wellness program. These two activities, combined with the department's surveillance activities, form a powerful tool for helping employees attain a level of health and fitness that will assist them in being safe at work. Furthermore, the health promotion activities, training, and education expertise of the department can help make employees aware of prevention strategies, including working safely in the facility as well as at home; lifestyle changes that will improve health; and the resources that are available to them in the community.

Chapter 1 presented the philosophy and the scientific evidence to support the establishment of an Environmental Health and Safety Department within each health care facility. The philosophy portion bears repeating:

Carl Sagan once said, "We are, all of us, made of star-stuff,"[12] and John Donne wrote: "No man is an island, entire of itself, every man is a piece of the continent, a part of the main."[13] What were these two men, so separated in time and space, trying to tell us? Their message is clear:

All things are connected.
Quality patient care requires quality employee care and the emphasis on each should be equal.

This book presents many regulations and guidelines. But beyond the "shalls" and "shoulds," it also presents a core philosophy that *all* workers have the right to return from their jobs as healthy as when they arrived at them. But those workers share the responsibility for doing their jobs safely. Employee health and safety is interactive. It is cooperative. It is a joint effort. It is the manifestation of the notion that "no man is an island."

It is not possible for humans to isolate themselves from their friends, families, colleagues, and clients. It is also impossible to compartmentalize safety and health at work separately from that in our personal lives.

References

1. U.S. Congress. Workers' Family Protection Act, Public Law 102–522. *U.S. Statutes at Large* 106 (1992), pp. 3410, 3420. Available at http://www.osha.gov/pls/oshaweb/owadisp.show_document?p_table=OSHACT&p_id=3376 (accessed 2/21/2006).

2. Health and Safety Executive. *Tackling Work Related Stress: A Managers' Guide to Improving and Maintaining Employee Health and Well-being*. Sudbury: HSE Books, 2001. Available at http://www.cipd.co.uk/subjects/health/stress/stress.htm (accessed 3/9/2006).

3. U.S. Department of Health and Human Services. *Stress . . . at Work*. NIOSH Publication No. 99–101. Available at http://www.cdc.gov/niosh/pdfs/stress.pdf (accessed 2/21/2006).

4. U.S. Department of Health and Human Services. www.surgeongeneral.gov (accessed 2/21/2006).

5. U.S. Department of Agriculture. *Steps to a Healthier You*. Available at http://www.mypyramid.gov (accessed 2/21/2006).

6. Executive Office of the President and the Department of Health and Human Services. *HealthierUS.Gov*. Available at www.healthierus.gov (accessed 2/21/2006).

7. National Institutes of Health. *National Center for Complementary and Alternative Medicine*. Available at www.nccam.nih.gov (accessed 2/21/2006).

8. *The Use of Complementary and Alternative Medicine in the United States*. Available at http://nccam.nih.gov/news/camsurvey_fs1.htm (accessed 3/8/2006).

9. American Medical Association. *Alternative Medicine* (Report 12 of the Council on Scientific Affairs (A-97). Available at http://www.ama-assn.org/ama/pub/category/13638.html (accessed 2/21/2006).

10. U.S. Department of Health and Human Services. *Work-Related Roadway Crashes: Prevention Strategies for Employers*. NIOSH Publication No. 2004–136. Available at http://www.cdc.gov/niosh/docs/2004-136/pdfs/2004-136.pdf (accessed 2/21/2006).

11. U.S. Department of Health and Human Services. *Healthy People 2010*. Available at www.healthypeople.gov (accessed 2/21/2006).

12. Sagan, Carl. *Cosmos*. Novel and film series.

13. Donne, John. *The Complete Poetry and Selected Prose of John Donne* (Modern Library Series). New York: Random House, 1994.

CHAPTER 6

INFECTION CONTROL

Ring a ring a roses
A pocket full of posies
Atishoo atishoo
We'll all fall down

Although there has been some wonderfully scholarly discussion about the origin and meaning of this simple nursery rhyme, the most popular interpretation is that it refers to the plague that swept through Europe in the seventeenth or eighteenth century. The populists believe that "Ring a ring a roses" refers to a rash that accompanied the disease and the "pocket full of posies" is a reference to herbs that were believed to ward off the disease. "Atishoo atishoo" is said to mimic the sneezing that occurred just prior to death, when they "all fall down."

The "medicinal" approach to infection control described in this nursery rhyme was bolstered by an engineering solution in the nineteenth century. When London was beset by a cholera epidemic, an astute anesthesiologist, John Snow, carefully mapped the cases and discovered that they centered around a well on Broad Street that served as the local water supply. Dr. Snow removed the handle from the pump, which prevented its use but also prevented the development of new cases of cholera.

Florence Nightingale realized that introducing fresh air into the dank environment of a closed hospital ward improved patient health. The Austrian physician Ignaz Semmelweiss discovered that fatal infections were being spread by doctors who failed to wash their hands between examinations. He introduced a disinfecting procedure that required hand washing with soap and water between patient visits, and in a solution of chloride of lime following autopsies. Semmelweiss also required doctors to change into clean lab coats before examining patients. As a result of these simple procedures, there were dramatic decreases in infectious disease mortality rates and in the incidence of infectious diseases as well.

John Snow mapped cases of cholera in a London neighborhood and removed a pump handle. Today, epidemiology is the primary tool for identifying epidemics of specific diseases, and removing the pump handle has evolved into regulations for locking equipment and tagging it to ensure that it cannot be operated when it is unsafe to do so.

Florence Nightingale believed that fresh air was important to control disease. Her ventilation system was an open window. Today there are complex heating and ventilation systems that heat, cool, regulate humidity, and provide positive and negative pressure to help isolate patients with infectious diseases.

Semmelweiss understood that the spread of infectious disease could be interrupted by personal hygiene. His harsh chemical disinfection procedures have been replaced by germicidal soaps and less aggressive but more effective cleaning solutions, germicidal lamps, and laundering.

Alexander Fleming is credited with discovering penicillin in a common mold, and Jonas Salk ushered in the science of vaccination. Each of these health care providers contributed to the practice of infection control. Modern infection control has certainly advanced well beyond a "pocket full of posies" and the simple removal of a handle from a water pump, but it nonetheless remains a significant problem in society and in hospitals. But there are lessons to be gained from the myth of the nursery rhyme and the thoughtful science practiced by John Snow, Semmelweiss, Nightingale, Fleming, and Salk. Infection control requires a multifaceted approach using epidemiology, medicine, engineering controls, and personal hygiene.

Despite these advances, infectious diseases pose a continuing danger. Although some diseases have been effectively controlled with the help of aggressive surveillance and advances in immunization, new diseases such as severe acute respiratory syndrome (SARS), West Nile virus, avian influenza (bird flu), and HIV/AIDS have appeared over the last 20 years. Others, such as malaria, tuberculosis, and bacterial pneumonias, are now appearing in forms that are resistant to drug treatment. Furthermore, the twenty-first century has been ushered in with concerns about the use of infectious diseases such as smallpox as weapons.

NOSOCOMIAL INFECTIONS

Of particular importance to health care workers are infectious diseases that have their origin in the health care facility. Such infections are called *nosocomial*, which is derived from the Greek phrase *nosus komeion*, which means "disease taking care of," referring to diseases that arise from taking care of people. In recent years, the term "health care–associated infections" has come into vogue as a substitute for the phrase "nosocomial infections." This book uses the two terms interchangeably. Nosocomial infections typically affect those who are immunocompromised because of age, underlying diseases, or medical or surgical treatments. Aging of our population and increasingly aggressive medical and therapeutic interventions, including implanted foreign bodies, organ transplantations, and xenotransplantations, have created a cohort of particularly vulnerable people.

Over the last 30 years, a considerable effort has been made to reduce the incidence of nosocomial infections in U.S. hospitals. In 1976 the Joint Commission on Accreditation of Healthcare Organizations (JCAHO) published accreditation standards for infection control, creating the impetus for hospitals to provide administrative and financial support for infection control programs. In 1985 the Centers for Disease Control and Prevention's (CDC's) *Study on the Efficacy of Nosocomial Infection Control* reported that hospitals with four key infection control components—an effective hospital epidemiologist, one infection control practitioner for every 250 beds, active surveillance mechanisms, and ongoing control efforts—reduced nosocomial infection rates by approximately one-third.[1]

In 1998 the CDC published an update on nosocomial infections that pointed to the need to increase national surveillance, to "risk-adjust" infection rates so that interhospital comparisons are valid, to develop more noninvasive infection-resistant devices, and to work with health care workers on better implementation of existing control measures such as hand washing.[2] [CD-ROM 6.1]

In 1999 the Department of Health and Human Services (HHS) joined other federal agencies to create a federal Interagency Task Force on Antimicrobial Resistance. The task force developed an action plan that provided a comprehensive approach to combat antimicrobial resistance.[3] The plan provides a blueprint with 84 action items divided into four major categories: surveillance, prevention and control, research, and product development. [CD-ROM 6.2]

Every 10 years, the CDC holds a conference on health care–associated infections. The goal of the 2000 conference was to provide the latest scientific information concerning health care–associated infections and set the agenda for research and prevention activities for the coming decade.[4]

At the 2000 conference, it was reported that the nosocomial infection rate among inpatients is between 5 percent and 10 percent, depending on the size of the facility. Assuming 35 million patient admissions each year, the number of nosocomial infections would be between 1.75 million and 3.5 million, and the corresponding mortality between 52,500 and 105,500 deaths due to all nosocomial infections.[5] According to the World Health Organization (WHO), the rate can exceed 25 percent in developing countries.[6]

The World Health Organization also pointed out that understanding the true magnitude of nosocomial infections is hampered for the following reason: "To date, no statistics exist to illustrate the real extent of the problem. Data on health-care-associated infections are not collected in a consistent way. This is one of the main obstacles to fighting them and needs to be addressed."[7]

There appears to be an effort on the part of some states to start collecting data on nosocomial infections. Until there is a uniform nationwide surveillance system, the full extent of health care facility–acquired infections will not be understood.

For this reason, the most recent summary data concerning the incidence of nosocomial infections was obtained in 1975 and between 1990 and 1996, as shown in table 6-1.[8]

Tracking nosocomial infections by site has become difficult in the last few years because of shorter inpatient stays. For example, the average postoperative

Table 6-1. Sites of Nosocomial Infections

Year	Urinary Tract (%)	Surgical Wound (%)	Lower Respiratory Tract (%)	Bloodstream (%)	Other (%)
1975	42	24	10	5	19
1990–1996	34	17	13	14	21

stay, now approximately five days, is usually shorter than the five- to seven-day incubation period for *Staphylococcus aureus* surgical wound infections.[9]

Although the focus of preventive measures to reduce nosocomial infections is on patients, those illnesses also have a direct effect on the health of workers. Of the 73,400 recordable illnesses among hospital workers reported in 2003, more than 13 percent (9,800) were respiratory illnesses.[10] In addition, a major component of hospital worker injuries can be attributable to needlesticks.

INFECTIOUS DISEASES AND HOW THEY SPREAD

Infectious diseases are caused by living organisms, such as bacteria and viruses, and can be spread within a population if the following conditions exist at the right time and place:

- There is a path into the host (body).
- The organism is present in sufficient numbers to overwhelm the host's defense mechanisms.
- The host is susceptible to the organism and its adverse effects.

Exposures may result in colonization or infection:

- *Colonization* means that the organism is present in or on the body but is not causing illness. An employee who has been colonized can become a carrier and spread infection to other individuals, such as other health care workers, patients, and family members.
- *Infection* means that the organism is present and is causing illness.

Organisms can enter a host through several routes:

- Inhalation of small droplets or nuclei from evaporated droplets following a cough or sneeze
- Ingestion by hand-to-mouth transmission or from eating or drinking contaminated food or liquid
- Injection resulting from puncturing the skin with a contaminated object
- Absorption through broken skin or mucous membranes

The most common means for the transmission of infectious disease include:

Aerosolization of infected body fluids

Breathing air contaminated with bacteria, bacterial spores, or virus particles

Contact with contaminated blood, body fluids, food, water, or surfaces

Zoonotic transmission (i.e., bites from infected animals, insects, and other organisms)

Aerosolization

Droplets expelled during coughing, sneezing, or talking may contain bacteria or virus particles. Diseases that are easily spread through aerosolization include tuberculosis, influenza, diphtheria, pertussis, and the common cold, although they are not restricted to this mode of transmission.

Inhalation

Bacterial and other spores can remain airborne and viable for a significant period of time before encountering a host. To a large extent, weather conditions affect the spread of these spores and may play a role in regional outbreaks of the disease. Once an infection occurs, other modes of transfer come into play. Recirculation of air, for example, can facilitate the spread of bacteria, their spores, and virus particles. In addition, improperly maintained heating, ventilation, and air conditioning (HVAC) systems harbor microorganisms and provide a vehicle for their transmission.

Contact with Contaminated Blood, Body Fluids, Food, Water, or Surfaces

Microorganisms thrive in many body fluids, including those found in or on:

☐ Employee and patient restrooms
☐ Patient examination rooms
☐ Patient waiting areas
☐ Employee break and lunchroom facilities, especially refrigerators and food preparation areas
☐ Stethoscopes
☐ Hands
☐ Implanted devices

Some of the situations where employees are most likely to come into contact with patient blood and body fluids are:

☐ Treatment of patients in the Emergency Department
☐ Contact with patients in intensive care units

☐ Handling trash
☐ Contact with soiled stretchers and beds
☐ Handling needles that were not disposed of properly
☐ Security searches of patients or suspects

Zoonotic Transmission

Many insects, mammals, and other animals carry infectious organisms that can be passed on to humans. This transmission can occur as a result of being bitten by or ingesting an infected animal.

It is difficult to know if an employee has been exposed to disease-causing organisms. Laboratory tests identifying the type of organism may take weeks to complete. By the time the laboratory results return, the employee may already have the disease.

EMERGING INFECTIOUS DISEASES AND THE PANDEMIC THREAT

The recent recognition of emerging infectious diseases, such as acquired immunodeficiency syndrome (AIDS), Lyme disease, hantavirus, West Nile virus (WNV), severe acute respiratory syndrome (SARS), avian influenza, and community-acquired methicillin-resistant *Staphylococcus aureus* (MRSA) has both threatened the health and well-being of the population and challenged health care providers, perhaps to a greater extent than ever experienced in the past. The detection, prevention, and treatment of diseases caused by microbes used for bioterrorism purposes has also become an assumed role of individuals working in the field of infectious diseases, particularly since the anthrax attacks of October 2001.

Avian Influenza

In recent years, public health officials around the world have become increasingly concerned that a new or altered virus with enhanced virulence will sweep the globe, killing millions of people. During the last 100 years, there have been three notable influenza pandemics. The first occurred and was called the Spanish flu. The Spanish flu was caused by a virus derived from one known to infect only birds (avian type) that had acquired the ability to infect humans. That pandemic resulted in about 50 million deaths worldwide, 500,000 of which occurred in the United States.

Similar avian influenza–derived pandemics occurred in 1957–1958 (Asian flu) and 1968–1969 (Hong Kong flu). Those strains were also derived from an avian virus. The Asian flu resulted in about 70,000 deaths in the United States, and the Hong Kong flu was deemed responsible for about 34,000 deaths in the United States.[11]

In recent years, a new avian influenza A (designated H5N1) has emerged and resulted in a significant number of avian deaths, prompting a global effort to prepare for a potential outbreak of a highly virulent human form of the H5N1 virus. Although there have been a number of human fatalities attributable to the avian flu, none of the cases appears to be the result of human-to-human transmission.

The World Health Organization (WHO) has developed guidelines for tracking the progress of pandemic development, which define the stages of a pandemic, outline the role of WHO, and make recommendations for national measures before and during a pandemic.[12] [CD-ROM 6.3, 6.4, 6.4a] Figure 6-1 lists the categories.

Figure 6–1. The Stages of a Pandemic

Interpandemic period

Phase 1: No new influenza virus subtypes have been detected in humans. An influenza virus subtype that has caused human infection may be present in animals. If it is present in animals, the risk of human infection or disease is considered to be low.

Phase 2: No new influenza virus subtypes have been detected in humans. However, a circulating animal influenza virus subtype poses a substantial risk of human disease.

Pandemic alert period

Phase 3: Human infection(s) with a new subtype, but no human-to-human spread, or at most rare instances of spread to a close contact.

Phase 4: Small cluster(s) with limited human-to-human transmission, but spread is highly localized, suggesting that the virus is not well adapted to humans.

Phase 5: Larger cluster(s), but human-to-human spread is still localized, suggesting that the virus is becoming increasingly better adapted to humans but may not yet be fully transmissible (substantial pandemic risk).

Pandemic period

Phase 6: Pandemic increased and sustained transmission in general population.

Note: The distinction between phase 1 and phase 2 is based on the risk of human infection or disease resulting from circulating strains in animals. The distinction is based on various factors and their relative importance according to current scientific knowledge. Factors may include pathogenicity in animals and humans, whether occurrence is in domesticated animals and livestock or only in wildlife, whether the virus is enzootic or epizootic, whether the virus is geographically localized or widespread, and other scientific parameters.

The distinction between phase 3, phase 4, and phase 5 is based on an assessment of the risk of a pandemic. Various factors and their relative importance according to current scientific knowledge may be considered. Factors may include rate of transmission, geographical location and spread, severity of illness, presence of genes from human strains (if derived from an animal strain), and other scientific parameters.

These WHO guidelines can be useful for the infection control programs in health care settings to track the emergence and activity of viral and other outbreaks.

Severe Acute Respiratory Syndrome (SARS)

SARS is a respiratory illness that has been reported in Asia, North America, and Europe. SARS appears to spread primarily by close person-to-person contact with symptomatic individuals (e.g., persons with fever or respiratory symptoms). Touching the skin of other people or objects contaminated with infectious droplets and then touching the eyes, nose, or mouth can spread SARS. Contamination occurs when someone with SARS coughs or sneezes droplets onto themselves, other people, or nearby surfaces. It is also possible for SARS to be spread farther through the air by very small particles. This method is called airborne transmission, but investigations to date suggest that this type of transmission is unusual. It is also possible that SARS may be spread in other ways that are currently not known.[13] [CD-ROM 6.5]

Because SARS is spread by close contact with infected individuals, health care workers are among those most commonly infected. As a result, the CDC has issued interim infection control recommendations for health care and other institutional settings. These guidelines recommend that health care workers entering the room of a SARS patient, and medical transport workers transporting a patient with suspected SARS, use the following:

- ☐ Standard precautions (e.g., hand hygiene)
- ☐ Contact precautions (e.g., use of gown and gloves for contact with the patient or their environment)
- ☐ Eye protection for all patient contact (e.g., safety glasses)
- ☐ A respirator that is at least as protective as an N-95 respirator approved by the National Institute for Occupational Safety and Health (NIOSH)

Infectious material deposited on personal protective equipment (PPE) may cause it to become a vehicle for direct or indirect transmission. Therefore, care is needed when removing PPE to avoid contaminating skin, clothing, and mucous membranes. Standard procedures for removal of PPE that minimize the potential for self-contamination should be developed based on the equipment used, and health care employees should be trained in these procedures. Hand hygiene should be performed following the removal of PPE.

Tuberculosis (TB)

Tuberculosis (TB) is not generally considered to be an emerging infectious disease because it has existed for centuries. However, because it is very difficult to remove from the human population and because the bacilli have managed to develop antibiotic-resistant strains, tuberculosis remains a significant public health concern. Tuberculosis is a disease caused by a bacterial infection that is sometimes infectious. [CD-ROM 6.6] It can affect many parts of the body, but is found most commonly in the lungs, where it is called *pulmonary tuberculosis*. The most common symptoms that could indicate TB are a cough that lasts longer than three weeks and a fever that lasts more than one week. Other symptoms include shortness of breath, weight loss, night sweats, loss of appetite, and sometimes lumps in the neck or swelling of joints. Physicians can perform skin tests to determine if someone has TB, and chest x-rays can also provide diagnostic evidence of the disease.

Because some TB patients begin feeling better once they begin taking medication for the disease, they often stop taking it before it has been completely used. Since the organism that causes TB is somewhat difficult to kill, failure to take all of the prescribed medicine can lead to the development of drug-resistant forms of the disease.

Drug resistance is more common in:

- People who have spent time with someone with drug-resistant TB disease
- People who do not take their medicine regularly
- People who do not take all of their prescribed medicine
- People who develop TB again, after having taken TB medicine in the past
- Residents of areas where drug-resistant TB is common

HIERARCHY OF CONTROLS

Both public health and occupational safety and health authorities recommend a hierarchy of controls to prevent the transmission of infectious diseases in health care facilities, with administrative controls being more important than engineering controls, and engineering controls being more important than respirator use. This hierarchy of controls is both cost-effective—since administrative controls can cost very little—and critical for minimizing the exposure of employees to undiagnosed infectious diseases.

Administrative Controls

Administrative controls are intended to enable the early detection of infectious diseases among both patients and employees. Administrative controls include screening mechanisms, such as patient and new-employee questionnaires designed to elicit complete medical histories and to identify risk factors. Administrative controls can also include such things as tuberculin skin testing for new employees and written policies for the referral for evaluation and treatment of those who have positive PPD results.

Administrative controls provide for periodic PPD testing and assessment of symptoms or chest x-rays for both patients and staff. Administrative controls emphasize the importance to both patients and staff of identifying, isolating, and treating active disease at the earliest possible instance. In devising administrative controls, programs must proceed from this clear conviction. The more successful programs will institute policies that require the prompt identification, isolation, evaluation, and treatment of people who pose a threat of transmitting infectious diseases.

Engineering Controls

Engineering controls are more expensive than administrative controls and involve the use of specifically designed areas that meet the engineering standards for respiratory isolation. Such engineering standards are rigidly defined. They include the use of adequate ventilation systems, high-efficiency particulate air (HEPA) filters, and other controls that are intended to reduce the concentration of infectious droplet nuclei in the air, prevent the transmission of such nuclei throughout the facility, or render the nuclei noninfectious.

Health care facilities should develop areas or rooms with such controls only in consultation with environmental engineers from local or state public health departments or from other appropriate agencies or organizations. Once the appropriate engineering controls are in place, the designated area or room can be used as an isolation or holding area for any patient who is suspected of having an infectious disease.

Personal Protective Equipment (PPE)

Although PPE is mentioned last in the hierarchy of prevention, it is essential in protecting health care workers from disease transmission. PPE prevents contact with the infectious agent, or a body fluid that may contain the infectious agent, by creating a barrier between the worker and the infectious material. Gloves protect the hands, gowns or aprons protect the skin and clothing, masks and respirators protect the mouth and nose, goggles protect the eyes, and face shields protect the entire face.

The use of respirators in the health care setting is a relatively new but important step forward in efforts to prevent the transmission of infectious diseases. Air-purifying respirators provide a barrier to prevent health care workers from inhaling airborne particles containing infectious diseases. The level of protection a respirator provides is determined by the efficiency of the filter material and how well the face piece fits or how tightly it seals to the health care worker's face.

A number of studies have shown that surgical masks do not provide adequate protection in filtering out infectious disease particles, such as the TB organism. Additionally, surgical masks are not respirators and, therefore, are not NIOSH certified and do not satisfy Occupational Safety and Health Administration (OSHA) requirements for respiratory protection.[14] [CD-ROM 6.7] The proper use of respirators represents a significant improvement in employee protection against airborne infectious diseases. [CD-ROM 6.8]

INFECTION CONTROL METHODS

The principal defenses against infectious disease are the immune system, antibiotics, vaccines, personal hygiene, and hand hygiene. Those with compromised immune systems or those who do not practice good personal hygiene or who fail to receive appropriate vaccinations have a greater risk of contracting and spreading an infectious disease. This traditional approach to preventing infectious diseases can be greatly enhanced by adherence to principles of personal and family health.[15] People who do not practice good personal health and safety habits off the job bring that same attitude to work.

Effective Immune Systems

Diseases and infections most frequently attack individuals who have an underlying illness or a weakened immune system. However, the immune system can be strengthened in a number of ways, including diet, exercise, and proper rest.

Antibiotics

Antibiotics have been used for decades to treat and prevent the spread of infectious diseases. Unfortunately, the non-judicious use of antibiotics has led to the development of antibiotic-resistant organisms. Each time an antibiotic is taken, bacteria are killed. However, bacteria may be resistant or become resistant. Resistant bacteria do not respond to the antibiotic and continue to cause infection. Each time an antibiotic is taken unnecessarily or improperly, the chances for the development of drug-resistant bacteria increase. Because of such resistant bacteria, some diseases that used to be easy to treat are now becoming nearly impossible to treat. [CD-ROM 6.9]

Taking antibiotics appropriately and becoming immunized will help to prevent the need for more dangerous and costlier medications. The appropriate use of antibiotics will help to prevent the development of drug resistance in bacterial strains. Medicine should be taken exactly as prescribed.

Basically, there are two main types of germs that cause most infections.[16] These are viruses and bacteria. Illnesses caused by each type of agent are listed in figure 6-2.

Figure 6–2. Diseases Caused by Viruses and by Bacteria

Diseases Caused by Viruses	Diseases Caused by Bacteria
□ All colds and flu	□ Most ear infections
□ Most coughs	□ Some sinus infections
□ Most sore throats	□ Strep throat
Antibiotics cannot kill viruses.	Antibiotics do kill specific bacteria.

Vaccines

Many vaccines can prevent infection or mitigate the effect of an infectious disease. Decisions about the use of vaccines can be made by considering the likelihood of exposure to vaccine-preventable diseases and the potential consequences of not vaccinating, the type of contact expected between patients and their environment, and the characteristics of the patient population within the facility.

Personal Hygiene

Apart from the selective and appropriate use of antibiotics, the most fundamental weapon in the disease prevention arsenal is the same one articulated by Semmelweiss more than 100 years ago. Good personal hygiene and aggressive hand washing are the first and foremost methods of preventing the transmission of infectious diseases.

Personal hygiene is essential to good health. Every part of the body demands basic attention on a regular basis, including the hair, skin, teeth, hands, nails, feet, and personal parts of the body.

Proper care of the skin will help prevent a number of dermatological conditions. Poor oral hygiene can lead to infection of the gums and loss of bone and teeth. Infections of the gums often result in halitosis and contribute to sinus infections. Some people are sensitive to highly scented personal care products such as shampoos, perfumes, colognes, and hairsprays. Therefore, personal care products should be used in small quantities. Substituting them with products that are scent free, if possible, should help eliminate the problem.

Hand Hygiene

When Semmelweiss encouraged hand hygiene, his arsenal of cleansers was limited to soap and water and harsh chemicals. In the 100 years since his time, there have been significant advances in the development of soaps and chemical sanitizing agents, presenting the health care worker with a vast and sometimes confusing array of choices. In the evaluation of hand hygiene products for use in health care facilities, product selection should be based on several factors:

- The relative efficacy of antiseptic agents against various pathogens
- Acceptance of the product by personnel
- Characteristics of the product (either soap or alcohol-based hand sanitizers)

Despite the fact that hand hygiene remains the simplest and most effective means of reducing the transmission of germs, many employees do not consistently follow hand hygiene recommendations, such as those issued by the CDC.[17] [CD-ROM 6.10] Prevention is everyone's business—that of health care providers, administrators, and patients. The Joint Commission, together with the Centers for Medicare & Medicaid Services (CMS), launched a national program to encourage patients to take a role in preventing health care errors by becoming active, involved, and informed participants on the health care team. The program features brochures, posters, and buttons on a variety of patient safety topics. The Association for Professionals in Infection Control and Epidemiology (APIC),[18] the CDC, the American Hospital Association (AHA),[19] and other organizations collaborated with the Joint Commission[20] in 2004 to help Americans fight the spread of infections in health care settings and in the community and to avoid contagious diseases such as the common cold, strep throat, and influenza (the flu). The program, *Three Things You Can Do to Prevent Infection*, is designed to encourage patients to play an active role in their health care by asking questions and requesting that their clinicians wash their hands before performing an examination.[21] This program specifies three easy steps to help employees fight the spread of infection:

1. Clean your hands.
2. Cover your mouth and nose.
3. Avoid close contact and stay home if you're sick.

These steps can help prevent the spread of infection from colds, influenza, and diseases such as SARS, TB, and strep throat.

Because many employees frequently wash their hands, there is the possibility of developing dermatitis. This is particularly true if there is an excessive use of products that contain alcohol, which may dry the skin, or products the employee may be allergic to. As the Environmental Health and Safety Department collects and reviews illness data relating to dermatitis, these factors must be taken into consideration. Any dermatological condition that results from hand hygiene must be recorded on OSHA Form 300, Log of Work-Related Injury and Illness.

Guidelines for Employee Infection Control

The CDC and OSHA infection control standards, precautions, and guidelines provide methods for reducing the transmission of infections from patients to health care personnel.

The 1998 *Guideline for Infection Control in Health Care Personnel* by the CDC [CD-ROM 6.11, 6.11a] updates and replaces the CDC *Guideline for Infection Control in Hospital Personnel*, published in 1983. The revised guideline, designed to provide methods for reducing the transmission of infections from patients to health care personnel and from personnel to patients, also provides an overview of the evidence for recommendations considered prudent by consensus of the Hospital Infection Control Practices Advisory Committee members.

The document focuses on the epidemiology of and preventive strategies for infections known to be transmitted in health care settings and for which there are adequate scientific data on which to base recommendations for prevention. The prevention strategies in this document include immunizations for vaccine-preventable diseases, isolation precautions to prevent exposures to infectious agents, management of health care personnel exposure to infected persons (including post-exposure prophylaxis), and work restrictions for exposed or infected health care personnel. In addition, because latex barriers are frequently used to protect personnel against transmission of infectious agents, the guide-line addresses issues related to latex hypersensitivity and provides recommen-dations to prevent sensitization and reactions among health care personnel.

The infection control objectives of the Environmental Health and Safety Department's Employee Health Services function should be an integral part of the facility's general program for infection control. The objectives should include the following:

- Educating employees about the principles of infection control and stressing individual responsibility for infection control
- Collaborating with the Infection Control Department in monitoring and investigating potentially harmful infectious exposures and outbreaks among personnel
- Providing care to personnel for work-related infection risks and instituting appropriate preventive measures
- Containing costs by preventing infectious diseases that result in absenteeism and disability

These objectives cannot be met without the support of the health care facility's administration, medical staff, and other health care personnel.

The CDC guideline also identifies certain elements that are necessary to attain the infection control goals of employee health services:

- Coordination among departments to ensure adequate surveillance and organization of activities, and to ensure that preventive measures are promptly implemented

□ Medical evaluations of new employees to ensure that they are not at undue risk of particular infectious diseases and that their immunization status is current

□ Clearly written policies, guidelines, and procedures to ensure uniform, efficient, and effective coordination of activities

□ Health and safety education appropriate in content and vocabulary

□ Institution of comprehensive immunization and screening programs

□ Encouraging employees to report job-related illnesses or exposures to infectious diseases, including policies for work restrictions for infected or exposed personnel

□ Health counseling about the risk of illness or other adverse outcome from exposures and the potential consequences of exposures or communicable diseases for family members, patients, or other employees

□ Effective recordkeeping in accordance with OSHA's standards 29 CFR 1910.1020, Access to employee exposure and medical records [CD-ROM 6.12]; 29 CFR 1910.1030, Bloodborne pathogens (BBP) [CD-ROM 6.13]; and 29 CFR 1904, Recording and reporting occupational injuries and illnesses [CD-ROM 6.14]

DISPOSABLE ITEMS

Methods for the disinfection and sterilization of health care facility equipment and patient care items were developed more than three decades ago. In recent years, disposable items have been introduced into the health care setting for the purpose of preventing nosocomial infections. Disposable items have the advantage of being pre-sterilized and prepackaged, and they can be discarded rather than sterilized for reuse. In considering the use of disposable items, thought should be given to the impact it will have on the facility's waste stream.

PREVENTING AND CONTROLLING EMERGING INFECTIONS

Approximately one-third of nosocomial infections are preventable. Wenzel and Edmond reported that hand washing could eliminate at least 25 percent of all nosocomial bloodstream infection–related deaths that occur in ICUs. They also suggest that the use of indwelling catheters that have antibiotics bonded to the surface could help prevent septicemia.[22]

To meet and exceed this level of prevention, according to Wenzel and Edmond, several strategies must be pursued simultaneously:

□ Improved national surveillance of nosocomial infections
□ Valid surveillance
□ Improved design of invasive devices
□ Aggressive antibiotic control programs

□ Increased emphasis on newer microbiologic methods through epidemiology

□ Control of TB

Weinstein suggests that, given the choice of improving technology or improving human behavior, technology is the better option, and all infection control measures will need to continue to pass the test of the "four P's"[23] (see figure 6-3).

The last point suggests that technology alone is not the solution. As with all things, technology is only as good as its application and the understanding of the people who apply it. If technology is applied without an understanding of the human aspects, it will fail to solve the problem.

Infection control is an essential component of health care facility operations. Improved infection control will save patient lives and will also reduce the number of hospital-associated illnesses incurred by health care workers. Although infection control among patients and improvements in worker health and safety may appear to be unrelated, they are in fact directly related. A septicemic patient poses a risk to a health care worker who incurs a needle-stick injury, and an unprotected health care worker is at risk of developing a respiratory infection while treating a patient with a bacterial or viral respiratory disease. By the same token, already compromised patients are at further risk if a health care worker who has an infectious disease or does not practice good personal hygiene is treating them.

CONTROL OF INFECTIONS DUE TO NEEDLESTICKS AND OTHER SHARPS INJURIES

Blood and other potentially infectious materials have long been recognized as a potential threat to the health of employees who are exposed to these materials by percutaneous contact (penetration of the skin). Injuries from contaminated needles and other sharps have been associated with an increased risk of disease from more than 20 infectious agents. The primary agents of concern in current occupational settings are the human immunodeficiency virus (HIV), hepatitis B virus (HBV), and hepatitis C virus (HCV).

Figure 6–3. Weinstein's Test of the Four P's

□ Are the recommendations *plausible* biologically (e.g., are they likely to work)?

□ Are they *practical* (e.g., are they affordable)?

□ Are they *politically* acceptable (e.g., will the administration agree)?

□ Will *personnel* follow them (e.g., can they and will they)?

Needlesticks and other percutaneous injuries continue to be of concern due to the high frequency of their occurrence and the severity of the health effects associated with exposure. The CDC has estimated that health care workers in hospital settings sustain 600,000 to 800,000 needlestick and other percutaneous injuries annually. When these injuries involve exposure to infectious agents, the affected workers are at risk of contracting diseases. Workers may also suffer from adverse side effects of drugs used for postexposure prophylaxis and from psychological stress due to the threat of infection following an exposure incident.

To reduce the health risk to workers whose duties involve exposure to blood or other potentially infectious materials, in 1991 OSHA promulgated its Bloodborne pathogens (BBP) standard. [CD-ROM 6.15]

> 29 CFR 1910.1030(a)
> Scope and Application. This section applies to all occupational exposure to blood or other potentially infectious materials as defined by paragraph (b) of this section.

> 29 CFR 1910.1030(b)
> "Blood" means human blood, human blood components, and products made from human blood.
>
> "Other Potentially Infectious Materials" means (1) The following human body fluids: semen, vaginal secretions, cerebrospinal fluid, synovial fluid, pleural fluid, pericardial fluid, peritoneal fluid, amniotic fluid, saliva in dental procedures, any body fluid that is visibly contaminated with blood, and all body fluids in situations where it is difficult or impossible to differentiate between body fluids; (2) Any unfixed tissue or organ (other than intact skin) from a human (living or dead); and (3) HIV-containing cell or tissue cultures, organ cultures, and HIV- or HBV-containing culture medium or other solutions; and blood, organs, or other tissues from experimental animals infected with HIV or HBV.

Although the language describing "Other Potentially Infectious Materials" seems to be focused on HIV, it is clear that OSHA was expressing its concern for any type of infectious disease that may be transferred by blood or other infected human material.

The provisions of the BBP standard were based on OSHA's determination that a combination of engineering and work practice controls, personal protective equipment, training, medical surveillance, hepatitis B vaccination, signs and labels, and other requirements would minimize the risk of disease transmission. A key element of the BBP standard is the requirement to develop an infection control plan.

The term *infection control* is typically used in health care to mean control of nosocomial infections. Although the principles of controlling infection may be similar to those involved with controlling employee exposure, the focus of the BBP standard is on protecting the employee from occupational exposure to bloodborne pathogens. Therefore, in order to most effectively express the intent of this standard, OSHA believes that a clarification of the terms is necessary. The title of paragraph (c) of the final standard is "Exposure Control" and paragraph (c)(1) is titled "Exposure Control Plan."

The exposure control plan required by paragraph (c)(1) is a key provision of the BBP standard because it requires the employer to identify the individuals who will receive the training, protective equipment, vaccination, and other provisions of this standard:

1910.1030(c)(1)(i)
Each employer having an employee(s) with occupational exposure as defined by paragraph (b) of this section shall establish a written Exposure Control Plan designed to eliminate or minimize employee exposure.

1910.1030(c)(1)(ii)
The Exposure Control Plan shall contain at least the following elements:

1910.1030(c)(1)(ii)(A)
The exposure determination required by paragraph (c)(2).

1910.1030(c)(1)(ii)(B)
The schedule and method of implementation for paragraphs (d) Methods of Compliance, (e) HIV and HBV Research Laboratories and Production Facilities, (f) Hepatitis B Vaccination and Post-Exposure Evaluation and Follow-up, (g) Communication of Hazards to Employees, and (h) Recordkeeping, of this standard, and

1910.1030(c)(1)(ii)(C)
The procedure for the evaluation of circumstances surrounding exposure incidents as required by paragraph (f)(3)(i) of this standard.

The BBP standard also requires the following:

1910.1030(c)(1)(iii)
Each employer shall ensure that a copy of the Exposure Control Plan is accessible to employees in accordance with 29 CFR 1910.1020(e).

1910.1030(c)(1)(iv)
The Exposure Control Plan shall be reviewed and updated at least annually and whenever necessary to reflect new or modified tasks and procedures, which affect occupational exposure, and to reflect new or revised employee positions with occupational exposure. The review and update of such plans shall also:

1910.1030(c)(1)(iv)(A)
Reflect changes in technology that eliminate or reduce exposure to bloodborne pathogens; and

1910.1030(c)(1)(iv)(B)
Document annually consideration and implementation of appropriate commercially available and effective safer medical devices designed to eliminate or minimize occupational exposure.

1910.1030(c)(1)(v)

An employer, who is required to establish an Exposure Control Plan, shall solicit input from non-managerial employees responsible for direct patient care who are potentially exposed to injuries from contaminated sharps in the identification, evaluation, and selection of effective engineering and work practice controls and shall document the solicitation in the Exposure Control Plan.

1910.1030(c)(1)(vi)

The Exposure Control Plan shall be made available to the Assistant Secretary and the Director upon request for examination and copying.

(The "Assistant Secretary" means the head of the OSHA, and the "Director" means the director of NIOSH or designated representative.)

Since publication of the BBP standard, a wide variety of medical devices have been developed to reduce the risk of needlesticks and other sharps injuries. These "safer medical devices" replace sharps with non-needle devices or incorporate safety features designed to reduce the likelihood of injury. In a September 9, 1998, Request for Information (RFI), OSHA solicited information on occupational exposure to bloodborne pathogens due to percutaneous injury. Based in part on the responses to the RFI, OSHA has pursued an approach to minimize the risk of occupational exposure to bloodborne pathogens that involves three components, which are listed in figure 6-4.

Needlestick Safety and Prevention Act

Compliance with OSHA's BBP standard significantly reduces the risk of employees contracting a bloodborne disease during work. Nevertheless, occupational exposure to bloodborne pathogens from accidental sharps injuries in health care and other occupational settings continues to be a serious problem. For that reason, Congress felt that a modification to OSHA's BBP standard was appropriate, to set forth in greater detail (and make more specific) OSHA's requirement for employers to identify, evaluate, and implement safer

Figure 6–4. The Occupational Safety and Health Administration's Approach to Minimizing the Risk of Occupational Exposure to BBP

First, OSHA proposed that the revised Standard 29 CFR 1904, Recording and reporting occupational injuries and illness, include a requirement that all percutaneous injuries from contaminated needles and other sharps be recorded on OSHA Form 300.

Second, OSHA issued a revised compliance directive for the BBP standard on November 5, 1999, to reflect advances made in medical technology and treatment. The directive guides OSHA's compliance officers in enforcing the BBP standard and ensures that consistent inspection procedures are followed.

Third, in 2001, OSHA amended the BBP standard to more effectively address sharps injuries.

medical devices. The Needlestick Safety and Prevention Act (NSPA) (Public Law 106-430) was signed into law on November 6, 2000. [CD-ROM 6.16] The NSPA mandated additional requirements for maintaining a sharps injury log and for the involvement of nonmanagerial health care workers in evaluating and choosing devices.

The NSPA made specific revisions to the BBP standard, including the following:

- ☐ Adding and expanding definitions relating to engineering controls
- ☐ Identifying and choosing safer needle devices
- ☐ Revising and expanding the exposure control plan
- ☐ Adding additional recordkeeping requirements
- ☐ Soliciting input from nonmanagerial employees responsible for direct patient care who are potentially exposed to injuries from contaminated sharps

Definitions

The NSPA revised the definitions used in the BBP standard (at 29 CFR 1910. 1030(b)) as follows:

- ☐ The definition of *engineering controls* was expanded to include as additional examples of controls the following: "safer medical devices, such as sharps with engineered sharps injury protections and needleless systems."
- ☐ The term *sharps with engineered sharps injury protections* was added to the definitions and defined as "a nonneedle sharp or a needle device used for withdrawing body fluids, accessing a vein or artery, or administering medications or other fluids, with a built-in safety feature or mechanism that effectively reduces the risk of an exposure incident."
- ☐ The term *needleless systems* was added to the definitions and defined as "a device that does not use needles for: (a) the collection of bodily fluids or withdrawal of body fluids after initial venous or arterial access is established; (b) the administration of medication or fluids; or (c) any other procedure involving the potential for occupational exposure to bloodborne pathogens due to percutaneous injuries from contaminated sharps."

Exposure Control Plan

The NSPA added to the existing requirements concerning exposure control plans described in the BBP standard (at 1910.1030(c)) as follows:

- ☐ Exposure control plans must "reflect changes in technology that eliminate or reduce exposure to bloodborne pathogens."

☐ Exposure control plans must "document annually consideration and implementation of appropriate commercially available and effective safer medical devices designed to eliminate or minimize occupational exposure."

☐ Employers required to establish an exposure control plan must "solicit input from nonmanagerial employees responsible for direct patient care who are potentially exposed to injuries from contaminated sharps, in the identification, evaluation, and selection of effective engineering and work practice controls and shall document the solicitation in the Exposure Control Plan."

Engineering and Work Practice Controls

The NSPA amplified the requirements stated in the BBP standard on the use of safer needle devices. Paragraph (d)(2)(i) of the BBP standard (29 CFR 1910.1030) requires the use of engineering and work practice controls to eliminate or minimize employee exposure to bloodborne pathogens.

Recordkeeping

The NSPA added an additional recordkeeping requirement to the BBP standard (1910.1030(h)(5)). Employers must keep a *sharps injury log* "for the recording of percutaneous injuries from contaminated sharps," and the record must include at a minimum the requirements listed in 1910.1030(h)(5)(i):

☐ The type and brand of device involved in the incident

☐ The department or work area where the exposure incident occurred

☐ An explanation of how the incident occurred

The sharps injury log requirement does not apply to an employer who is not required to maintain a log of occupational injuries and illnesses under 29 CFR 1904. The sharps injury log must be maintained for the period required by 29 CFR 1904.6, Incorporation by reference.

NIOSH Needlestick Prevention Resource

A web-based resource from NIOSH shares information on ways in which some health care facilities have established programs for protecting employees from the risk of job-related needlesticks. The NIOSH website is titled *Safer Medical Device Implementation in Health Care Facilities: Lessons Learned.*[24]

The site describes five essential steps for developing, establishing, and maintaining a needlestick prevention program. It also offers firsthand experiences from hospitals, nursing homes, home health agencies, and dental facilities as to how they put those steps into effect. The firsthand accounts from the facilities discuss barriers they encountered in establishing the programs, how those barriers were overcome, and lessons learned from their experiences.

The five strategic steps for needlestick prevention programs are:

1. Forming a sharps injury prevention team
2. Identifying priorities
3. Identifying and screening safer medical devices
4. Evaluating safer medical devices
5. Instituting and monitoring the use of safer devices

For each step, the NIOSH web page includes links to accounts from health care facilities describing how they put that step into effect. For purposes of confidentiality, the site does not disclose the names or locations of the facilities involved.

CONSTRUCTION AND RENOVATION CONSIDERATIONS

Improper ventilation design or maintenance has been associated with opportunistic infections, including aspergillosis in highly immunocompromised populations such as bone marrow transplant patients. Airborne infections related to ventilation systems, such as tuberculosis, have caused outbreaks among patients, workers, and visitors. Potential terrorist threats related to anthrax, smallpox, and other diseases being introduced through ventilation systems have highlighted the importance of facility design in enhancing the control of infectious agents.

In response to these concerns, professional, accreditation, and oversight agencies have provided guidance for new construction and major renovations in health care facilities that builds infection prevention and safety into the planning process.

Planning for new construction or major renovation requires early consultation and collaboration among infection control professionals (ICPs), epidemiologists, architects, engineers, risk managers, and health and safety professionals to ensure that infection prevention is included in the design. The Environmental Health and Safety director is an essential member of this team.

Infection Control Risk Assessment (ICRA)

A necessary first step in the development of a comprehensive construction and renovation plan is an *infection control risk assessment* (ICRA). The ICRA addresses each phase of the project from concept to completion. An ICRA is a multidisciplinary, organizational, documented process that:

  □ Focuses on the reduction of risk from infection
  □ Acts through the phases of facility planning, design, construction, renovation, and maintenance
  □ Coordinates and weighs knowledge about infectious agents

An ICRA considers the following factors:[25]

- ☐ The facility's patient population
- ☐ The facility's programs
- ☐ The impact of disrupting essential services on patients and employees
- ☐ Patient placement or relocation
- ☐ Placement of effective barriers to protect susceptible patients from airborne contaminants, such as *Aspergillus* spp.
- ☐ Air handling and ventilation needs in surgical services, airborne infection isolation and protective environment rooms, laboratories, local exhaust systems for hazardous agents, and other special areas
- ☐ Determination of the need for additional isolation rooms and other isolated environments
- ☐ Evaluation of the water supply and HVAC system to limit *Legionella* spp. and other waterborne opportunistic pathogens

The *ICRA matrix* is a published assessment tool that is widely accepted by engineers and architects and is one effective method for completing an ICRA. Although the ICRA does not have to be done as a matrix, it does help nonclinical staff understand the management of patient groups without requiring specific diagnoses.

Each facility should categorize patients by group within a specific patient population. The development of the *patient risk groups* is quite relative, and the criteria are dependent on the facility's mix of patients.

The key principle used for categorizing patients considers:

- ☐ Inherent susceptibility to infection (e.g., immunosuppression due to chemotherapy or radiation, such as in bone marrow allograft patients, who as a group remain at greatest risk)
- ☐ Invasiveness (e.g., a healthy patient undergoing surgery is at greatest risk when sterile tissues are exposed to the operating room environment)

The key principle for classifying projects is determining the degree of dust created. The patient groups are matched with project categories to select the level of required precautions. The ICRA takes into consideration preconstruction, demolition, intraconstruction, postconstruction, and cleanup activities, as well as educational and monitoring needs before, during, and after construction/renovation.

The American Institute of Architects (AIA) and the Joint Commission require documentation of the ICRA. One component of the ICRA may be submission of an infection control permit or project approval signature block.

The construction matrix tool includes a sample permit that follows the format of the matrix, assessing patient risk categories and environmental risk groups to determine the appropriate class or level of precautions.

ICRA Key Resources

To assist in planning and conducting an ICRA, a number of resources are available from key agencies. The three main resources are described in the following sections. The CDC also provides other helpful guidelines.[26,27]

The CDC Guidelines for Environmental Infection Control in Health-Care Facilities

Guidelines for Environmental Infection Control in Health-Care Facilities contains the recommendations of the CDC and the Healthcare Infection Control Practices Advisory Committee (HICPAC).[28] [CD-ROM 6.17, 6.17a] These guidelines provide a comprehensive set of recommendations for infection control practitioners, epidemiologists, employee health and safety personnel, engineers, facility managers, information systems professionals, administrators, environmental service professionals, and architects. The report also suggests a series of performance measurements as a means to evaluate infection control efforts. Figure 6-5 lists recommendations relevant to construction and renovation.

Figure 6–5. Recommendations Relevant to Construction and Renovation

- Assess the infection control impact of ventilation system and water system performance.
- Establish a multidisciplinary team to conduct infection control risk assessment.
- Use dust control procedures and barriers during construction, repair, renovation, and demolition.
- Implement environmental infection control measures for special areas with patients who are at high risk.
- Use airborne-particle sampling to monitor the effectiveness of air filtration and dust control measures.
- Implement procedures to prevent airborne contamination in operating rooms where infectious tuberculosis (TB) patients require surgery.
- Dispense guidance on how to recover from water system disruptions, water leaks, and natural disasters (e.g., flooding).
- Implement infection control procedures for equipment using water from the main lines (e.g., water systems for hemodialysis, ice machines, hydrotherapy equipment, dental-unit water lines, and automated endoscope re-processors).
- Implement infection control procedures for the health care facility laundry.

The Guidelines for Design and Construction of Hospital and Health Care Facilities

The Guidelines for Design and Construction of Hospital and Health Care Facilities is a set of guidelines published by the American Institute of Architects and the Facility Guidelines Institute (FGI), with assistance from the Department of Health and Human Services (HHS). These guidelines expand on the ICRA. As a consensus guideline, it relies heavily on input from groups including the American Society of Healthcare Engineering (ASHE), the American Society of Heating, Refrigerating and Air-Conditioning Engineers (ASHRAE), and the CDC. The AIA also maintains files and bibliographies on best practices.

HVAC Design Manual for Hospitals and Clinics

A manual published by ASHRAE, *HVAC Design Manual for Hospitals and Clinics,*[29] provides those involved in the design, installation, and commissioning of HVAC systems for hospitals with a comprehensive reference source for their work. The text covers environmental comfort, infection control, energy conservation, life safety, and operation and maintenance, providing design strategies known to meet applicable standards and guidelines. It also contains information on disaster planning and provides best-practices recommendations.

JOINT COMMISSION INFECTION CONTROL REQUIREMENTS

The Joint Commission has highlighted poor hand hygiene; inadequate staffing levels; sick and immunocompromised patients; technically sophisticated and invasive interventions; poorly cleaned equipment; and ineffective heating, ventilation, and air-conditioning systems as some of the more significant causes of infectious diseases in health care facilities. The Joint Commission's overarching standards for infection control are IC.1.10, IC.2.10, IC.3.10, IC.4.10, IC.5.10, IC.6.10, IC.7.10, IC.8.10, and IC.9.10. These standards focus on the development and implementation of plans to prevent and control infections and are supported by standards in other chapters, such as "Management of the Environment of Care," "Management of Human Resources," "Improving Organization Performance," and "Leadership," to produce a comprehensive approach to infection control.

Some of the specific Joint Commission standards in other chapters that address infection control include medical equipment risks (EC.6.10); maintaining, testing, and inspecting medical equipment (EC.6.20); emergency management (EC.4.10); and managing the design and building of the environment when it is renovated, altered, or newly created (EC.8.30).

THE ROLE OF THE ENVIRONMENTAL HEALTH AND SAFETY DEPARTMENT

The Environmental Health and Safety Department has a crucial role in helping to prevent nosocomial infections. Apart from overseeing the application of OSHA's Bloodborne pathogen and Hazard communication standards, and applicable federal and state medical waste regulations, the department should take an active role in surveillance, housekeeping, and training personnel in the use of appropriate personal protective equipment and clothing. The Environmental Health and Safety Department's goal is to ensure that employees, patients, and the public are provided with a safe and clean environment and that they have the appropriate equipment to protect themselves.

In addition, coordination of efforts with other departments is essential. There should be regular interactions with the Infection Control and Purchasing departments. The Environmental Health and Safety Department should also work closely with the Facilities Department to help identify ventilation and engineering solutions for controlling infectious disease transmission.

The staff of the Environmental Health and Safety Department should also keep abreast of technological advances in respiratory protective devices, ventilation solutions for preventing the spread of airborne infectious diseases, and devices to prevent needlestick injuries.

The Environmental Health and Safety director must be aware of and available to consult on regulations, guidelines, and standards, such as the following:

□ Identifying which employees may have contact with blood and other potentially infectious material (OPIM)

□ Selecting appropriate garb, such as uniforms, shoes, caps, cover-ups, and scrubs apparel

□ Determining the type of personal protective clothing and equipment that is appropriate for each employee

□ Training employees covered by the BBP standard

□ Training employees about the types and use of personal protective equipment for infection control

□ Selecting disposable devices for use in health care facilities

□ Conducting respiratory illness surveillance on employees

□ Administering and conducting the employee TB surveillance program

□ Identifying best practices for reducing the amount of medical waste

□ Improving the accurate reporting of needlestick injuries and nosocomial infections

□ Coordinating with construction project personnel and conducting infection control training for contractors and subcontractors

□ Ensuring that methods for sampling and analysis of airborne microorganisms are implemented

The last item, concerning sampling and analysis, also applies to mold spores that can affect indoor air quality and lead to respiratory illness in employees and patients.

References

1. Haley, R.W., D.H. Culver, J. White, W.M. Morgan, T.G. Amber, V.P. Mann, et al. "The Efficacy of Infection Surveillance and Control Programs in Preventing Nosocomial Infections in U.S. Hospitals," *American Journal of Epidemiology* 121 (1985), pp. 182–205.

2. Weinstein, Robert A. "Nosocomial Infection Update," *Emerging Infectious Diseases* 4, 3 (July–September 1998), Special Issue. Available at http://www.cdc.gov/ncidod/eid/vol4no3/weinstein.htm (accessed 3/17/2006).

3. Interagency Task Force on Antimicrobial Resistance. *A Public Health Action Plan to Combat Antimicrobial Resistance.* Atlanta, GA: Centers for Disease Control, 2001. Available at http://www.cdc.gov/drugresistance/actionplan/aractionplan.pdf (accessed 2/21/2006).

4. Solomon, Steven L. "About the Fourth Decennial International Conference on Nosocomial and Healthcare-Associated Infections," *Emerging Infectious Diseases* 7, 2 (March–April 2001).

5. Wenzel, R.P., and M.B. Edmond. "The Impact of Hospital-Acquired Bloodstream Infections," *Emerging Infectious Diseases* 7, 2 (March–April 2001).

6. *Experts to Tackle Health-Care Associated Infections.* Note to the press. EURO/06/04, Copenhagen, 27 April 2004. Available at http://www.euro.whol.int/Press Room/pressnotes/20050620_11 (accessed 3/13/2006).

7. *Experts to Tackle Health-Care Associated Infections.* Note to the press. EURO/06/04 Copenhagen, 27 April 2004. Available at http://www.euro.whol.int/Press Room/pressnotes/20050620_11 (accessed 3/13/2006).

8. Weinstein, Robert A. "Nosocomial Infection Update," *Emerging Infectious Diseases* 4, 3 (July–September 1998), Special Issue. Available at http://www.cdc.gov/ncidod/eid/vol4no3/Weinstein.htm (accessed 3/17/2006).

9. Weinstein, Robert A. "Nosocomial Infection Update," *Emerging Infectious Diseases* 4, 3 (July–September 1998), Special Issue. Available at http://www.cdc.gov/ncidod/eid/vol4no3/Weinstein.htm (accessed 3/17/2006).

10. U.S. Department of Labor, Bureau of Labor Statistics. *Incidence Rates of Nonfatal Occupational Illness, by Industry and Category of Illness, 2003* (Table SNR08), Available at http://www.stats.bls.gov/iif/oshwc/osh/os/ostb1350.pdf (accessed 2/21/2006).

11. U.S. Department of Health and Human Services, Centers for Disease Control and Prevention. *Key Facts About Pandemic Influenza* (page last modified 1/17/2006).

12. World Health Organization. *WHO Global Influenza Preparedness Plan: The Role of WHO and Recommendations for National Measures before and during Pandemics* (2005). Available at http://www.who.int/csr/resources/publications/influenza/WHO_CDS_CSR_GIP_2005_5.pdf (accessed 2/21/2006).

13. U.S. Department of Health and Human Services, Centers for Disease Control and Prevention, National Institute for Occupational Safety and Health. *Understanding Respiratory Protection against SARS.* Available at http://www.cdc.gov/niosh/npptl/topics/respirators/factsheets/respsars.html (accessed 2/21/2006).

14. U.S. Department of Labor. *Respiratory Protection.* Occupational Safety and Health Administration, 29 CFR 1910.134. Washington, DC: U.S. GPO. Available at www.osha.gov (accessed 2/21/2006).

15. Mulry, Ray. *In the Zone: Making Winning Moments Your Way of Life.* Arlington, VA: Great Ocean Publishers, 1995.

16. U.S. Department of Health and Human Services, Centers for Disease Control and Prevention. *An Ounce of Prevention Keeps the Germs Away: Use Antibiotics Appropriately.* Available at http://www.cdc.gov/ncidod/op/antibiotics.htm (accessed 2/21/2006).

17. U.S. Department of Health and Human Services, Centers for Disease Control and Prevention. "Guideline for Hand Hygiene in Health-Care Settings," *MMWR* 51, RR-16 (October 25, 2002). Available at http://www.cdc.gov/mmwr/preview/mmwrhtml/rr5116a1.htm (accessed 2/21/2006).

18. Association for Professionals in Infection Control and Epidemiology, http://www.apic.org (accessed 2/21/2006).

19. American Hospital Association, http://www.hospitalconnect.com (accessed 2/21/2006).

20. Joint Commission on Accreditation of Healthcare Organizations, http://www.jcaho.org (accessed 2/21/2006).

21. Joint Commission on Accreditation of Healthcare Organizations. *Three Things You Can Do to Prevent Infection: A Speak Up^TM Safety Initiative.* Available at http://www.jcaho.org/general+public/gp+speak+up/infection_control_brochure.pdf (accessed 2/21/2006).

22. Wenzel, R.P., and M.B. Edmond. "The Impact of Hospital-Acquired Bloodstream Infections," *Emerging Infectious Diseases*, Special Issue. Available at http://www.cdc.gov/ncidod/eid/vol7no2/wenzel.htm (accessed 3/13/2006).

23. Weinstein, R.A., "SHEA Consensus Panel Report: A Smooth Takeoff," *Infection Control and Hospital Epidemiology* 19 (1998), pp. 91–93.

24. U.S. Department of Health and Human Services, Centers for Disease Control and Prevention, National Institute for Occupational Safety and Health. *Safer Medical Device Implementation in Health Care Facilities: Lessons Learned.* Available at http://www.cdc.gov/niosh/topics/bbp/safer/ (accessed 2/21/2006).

25. American Institute of Architects and the Facility Guidelines Institute. *The Guidelines for Design and Construction of Hospital and Health Care Facilities.* New York: AIA, 2001. Available from AIA Bookstore, 1735 New York Avenue, NW, Washington DC 20006 and at www.aia.org (accessed 2/21/2006).

26. U.S. Department of Health and Human Services, Centers for Disease Control and Prevention. "Guidelines for Preventing Healthcare-Associated Pneumonia, 2003," *MMWR* 53, RR-3 (2004), pp. 1–36.

27. U.S. Department of Health and Human Services, Centers for Disease Control and Prevention. "Guidelines for Preventing the Transmission of *Mycobacterium* Tuberculosis in Health-Care Settings, 2005," *MMWR*, 54, RR-17 (December 30, 2005), pp. 1–141. Available at www.cdc.gov. Also available on the CD-ROM accompanying this book.

28. Sehulster L., and R.Y.W. Chinn. "Guidelines for Environmental Infection Control in Health-Care Facilities," *MMWR* 52, RR-10 (June 6, 2003). Available at http://www.cdc.gov/mmwr/preview/mmwrhtml/rr5210a1.htm.

29. American Society of Heating, Refrigerating and Air-Conditioning Engineers, *HVAC Design Manual for Hospitals and Clinics.* Atlanta, GA: ASHRAE, 2003. Available from ASHRAE Bookstore, 1791 Tullie Circle, N.E. Atlanta, GA 30329 and at http://www.ashrae.org (accessed 2/21/2006).

CHAPTER 7

CHEMICALS

There seemed to be no use in waiting by the little door, so she went back to the table, half hoping she might find another key on it, or at any rate a book of rules for shutting people up like telescopes: this time she found a little bottle on it ("which certainly was not here before," said Alice), and tied round the neck of the bottle was a paper label, with the words "DRINK ME," beautifully printed on it in large letters.

It was all very well to say, "Drink me," but the wise little Alice was not going to do that in a hurry. "No, I'll look first," she said, "and see whether it's marked 'poison' or not"; . . . she had never forgotten that, if you drink much from a bottle marked "poison," it is almost certain to disagree with you, sooner or later.

However, this bottle was not marked "poison," so Alice ventured to taste it, and finding it very nice (it had, in fact, a sort of mixed flavour of cherry-tart, custard, pine-apple, roast turkey, toffy, and hot buttered toast), she very soon finished it off.

Lewis Carroll, *Alice's Adventures in Wonderland*[1]

Alice had basic information about the hazards of chemicals—very basic. In fact, her knowledge was rudimentary. She knew that if the bottle said "Poison," it was "almost certain to disagree with you sooner or later." But what was the nature of that "disagreement"? Had Alice known it would shrink her to the size of a small cat, would she have drunk from the bottle? What if the same thing would have happened to Alice if she had simply spilled some of the bottle's contents on her arm? How much was too much to drink? Most important, would she be able to return to her normal size any time soon, or would she remain that way forever? Alice's lack of knowledge was bolstered by her faith that unless the bottle had the word "Poison" on it, no harm would come to her.

Had Alice lived in the twenty-first century, the simple, beautifully printed label that said "DRINK ME" would have been a multi-page material safety data sheet (MSDS) that would provide Alice with the name of the enticing liquid and a description of what the contents looked like, smelled like, and perhaps tasted like. It would also explain that if she drank "too much" from the bottle, she would shrink, and it would tell her how much was too much. It would also give her information on treatment, specify whom to call in an emergency, and state whether drinking was the only way the chemical in the bottle could cause her to shrink. In other words, the potential hazards would have been communicated to Alice.

INTRODUCTION TO THE HAZARD COMMUNICATION STANDARD (HCS)

This chapter explores the Occupational Safety and Health Administration's (OSHA's) Standard 29 CFR 1910.1200, Hazard communication [CD-ROM 7.1], and discusses its importance to a workplace health and safety program. The standard is commonly known as the Hazard communication standard (HCS), HAZCOM, or the Right-to-Know Law. The HCS is based on a simple concept—that employees have both a need and a right to know the identities and hazards of the chemicals they are exposed to when working, as well as what protective measures are available to prevent adverse effects from occurring.

Knowledge acquired under the HCS will help employers provide safer workplaces for their employees. When employers have information about the chemicals being used, they can take steps to reduce exposures, substitute less hazardous materials, and establish proper work practices. These efforts help prevent the occurrence of work-related illnesses and injuries caused by chemicals. [CD-ROM 7.2]

The HCS addresses the issues of evaluating and communicating hazards to workers. Evaluation of chemical hazards involves a number of technical concepts; it is a process that requires the professional judgment of experienced experts. That is why the HCS is designed so that employers who simply use chemicals, rather than produce or import them, are not required to evaluate the hazards of those chemicals. Hazard determination is the responsibility of the producers and importers of the materials, who are then required to provide the hazard information to employers that purchase their products.

Employers that do not produce or import chemicals need only focus on those parts of the rule that deal with establishing a workplace program and communicating information to their workers.

Important aspects of the HCS and its implementation include the following:

- It is generic and performance oriented.
- It is criteria based, not limiting coverage to a list that can become outdated—all chemicals are covered.
- It incorporates a downstream flow of information from producers to users.

- ☐ Trade secrets have been addressed to ensure protection of legitimate claims, with disclosure required where necessary for health and safety.
- ☐ It has an impact on interstate commerce and international trade.
- ☐ It interfaces with other federal requirements for classification and labeling.
- ☐ It is designed in part based on communication theory, in addition to technical data and the concept of modifying behavior through transmittal of key information.

OSHA-Approved State Plan States

Some states have their own OSHA-approved plans for regulating occupational safety and health. These are referred to as "OSHA-approved state plan states." The only requirement for states that develop such plans is that their regulations be at least as comprehensive and stringent as the federal OSH Act. Employers in states with OSHA-approved state plans should check with their state OSHA office to determine whether there are hazard communication requirements that differ from those of the federal OSH Act.

Hazardous Drugs

Preparation, administration, and disposal of hazardous drugs (HDs) may expose pharmacists, nurses, physicians, and other health care workers to potentially significant workplace levels of these chemicals. In response to numerous inquiries, OSHA published guidelines for the management of cytotoxic (antineoplastic) drugs in the workplace in 1986. At that time, surveys indicated little standardization in the use of engineering controls and personal protective equipment. Although practices improved in subsequent years, problems still existed.

As a result of the February 21, 1990, Supreme Court decision (see *Dole, Secretary of Labor, et al. v. United Steelworkers of America et al.,* No. 88-1434), all provisions of the HCS are now in effect for all industrial segments. This includes the coverage of drugs and pharmaceuticals in the non-manufacturing sector. On February 9, 1994, OSHA issued a revised Hazard Communication Final Rule with technical clarification regarding drugs and pharmaceutical agents. The HCS requires that drugs posing a health hazard—with the exception of those in solid, final form for direct administration to the patient (i.e., tablets or pills)—be included on lists of hazardous chemicals to which employees are exposed. Appendixes A and B of the HCS outline the criteria used to determine whether an agent is hazardous.

In the past several years, the occupational management of hazardous drugs has been further clarified. These trends, in conjunction with many information requests, prompted OSHA to revise its recommendations for hazardous drug handling. These revisions are incorporated in a new section of OSHA's technical manual. The informational guidance document applies to all settings where employees are occupationally exposed to HDs, such as hospitals, physician's offices, and home health care agencies. Some common drugs that are considered hazardous and are covered under the HCS are listed in OSHA's technical manual *Controlling Occupational Exposure to Hazardous Drugs.*[2] [CD-ROM 7.3]

Purpose of the Hazard Communication Standard (29 CFR 1910.1200(a))

> (1) The purpose of this section is to ensure that the hazards of all chemicals produced or imported are evaluated, and that information concerning their hazards is transmitted to employers and employees. This transmittal of information is to be accomplished by means of comprehensive hazard communication programs, which are to include container labeling and other forms of warning, material safety data sheets, and employee training.

The Hazard communication standard was written in response to a wave of actions by state and local governments that were developing similar legislation on their own. The Occupational Safety and Health Administration realized that commerce would be adversely affected if shippers and manufacturers were required to comply with different regulations in each location in which they did business. With that in mind, the reason for the language in paragraph (a)(2) of the standard becomes clear:

> (2) This occupational safety and health standard is intended to address comprehensively the issue of evaluating the potential hazards of chemicals, and communicating information concerning hazards and appropriate protective measures to employees, and to preempt any legal requirements of a state, or political subdivision of a state, pertaining to this subject. Evaluating the potential hazards of chemicals, and communicating information concerning hazards and appropriate protective measures to employees, may include, for example, but is not limited to, provisions for: developing and maintaining a written hazard communication program for the workplace, including lists of hazardous chemicals present; labeling of containers of chemicals in the workplace, as well as of containers of chemicals being shipped to other workplaces; preparation and distribution of material safety data sheets to employees and downstream employers; and development and implementation of employee training programs regarding hazards of chemicals and protective measures. Under section 18 of the Act, no state or political subdivision of a state may adopt or enforce, through any court or agency, any requirement relating to the issue addressed by this Federal standard, except pursuant to a Federally-approved state plan.

This paragraph presents several concepts and requirements that are intended to give both employers and employees information that they need in order to work safely with chemicals, including evaluating the potential hazards of chemicals, communicating information concerning hazards, and providing information on appropriate protective measures, including personal protective equipment (PPE).

HEALTH HAZARD DEFINITIONS

Learning how to work safely with hazardous chemicals and understanding the potential hazards they pose is the core of the HCS and of this chapter, but first one must know what a health hazard is. Although safety hazards related to the physical characteristics of a chemical can be objectively defined in terms of testing requirements (e.g., flammability), health hazard definitions are less precise and more subjective. In Appendix A of the HCS [CD-ROM 7.4] OSHA defines health hazards:

> Health hazards may cause measurable changes in the body.

What are "measurable changes"? Alice measurably shrunk, but in the real world of chemical exposure it is often difficult to clearly see a measurable change in the body. Bernardino Ramazzini, an eighteenth-century Italian physician who studied the effects of work on humans, wrote that such changes often "steal in on them little by little."[3] The Occupational Safety and Health Act (OSH Act) defines measurable changes in terms of "diminished health, functional capacity, or life expectancy." [CD-ROM 7.5] Some changes in the body are obvious and occur almost instantly, such as a dermatologic condition. Others do not appear for years, such as cancer or pulmonary disease. Still others do not manifest themselves until the next generation is born, such as birth defects.

Some changes are indicated by the occurrence of signs and symptoms in the exposed employees—such as shortness of breath, which is a nonmeasurable, subjective feeling. Employees exposed to such hazards must be told about both the change in body function and the signs and symptoms that may occur to signal that change.

There have been many attempts to categorize effects and to define them in various ways. Generally, the terms *acute* and *chronic* are used to delineate effects on the basis of severity or duration.[4] Acute effects usually occur rapidly as a result of short-term exposures and are of short duration. Chronic effects generally occur as a result of long-term exposure and are of long duration.

Acute Effects

For the purposes of the HCS, OSHA relied on the American National Standards Institute (ANSI)[5] definition of acute effects, which includes irritation, corrosivity, sensitization, and lethal dose. OSHA recognized that this list was not complete. For example, acute effects can also include narcotic effects such

Figure 7–1. Chemicals Commonly Found in Health Care Facilities That Can Cause Acute Health Effects

☐ Xylene found in laboratories

☐ Glutaraldehyde found in x-ray development areas and where cold sterilization is performed

☐ Cleaning chemicals used by housekeeping staff

☐ Paints and solvents used in maintenance jobs

as headache, nausea, and loss of coordination. Some chemicals commonly found in health care facilities that can cause acute health effects are listed in figure 7-1.

Acute effects can also be caused by conditions at the worksite, such as heat and noise. Although heat and noise are not chemicals, they are mentioned here to create awareness that not only chemicals can cause adverse health effects.

Chronic Effects

Most often the term *chronic health effect* is used to refer to cancer, mutagenicity, or teratogenicity. Other long-term debilitating illnesses include chronic bronchitis, blood dyscrasia, and liver disease. Some chemicals commonly found in health care facilities that can cause chronic health effects are listed in figure 7-2.

PHYSICAL HAZARD DEFINITION

Physical hazard refers to a chemical for which there is scientifically valid evidence that it is a combustible liquid, a compressed gas, explosive, flamma-

Figure 7–2. Chemicals Commonly Found in Health Care Facilities That Can Cause Chronic Health Effects

☐ Xylene found in laboratories (peripheral neuropathy)

☐ Ethylene oxide used for sterilization (cancer)

☐ Anesthetic gases (reproductive effects)

☐ Benzene in solvents (blood dyscrasia and leukemia)

☐ Pesticides and herbicides used in groundskeeping (neurological damage)

ble, an organic peroxide, an oxidizer, pyrophoric, unstable (reactive), or water reactive.

CHEMICALS AND CHEMICAL EXPOSURE

This section provides basic information about chemicals, the nature of a chemical exposure, and how exposure information is conveyed by OSHA, the National Institute for Occupational Safety and Health (NIOSH), the American Conference of Governmental Industrial Hygienists (ACGIH), and other organizations. Employees must learn this information in order to understand how to read an MSDS and labels on containers.

Chemicals

Everything is either a chemical or made from chemicals. Chemicals are divided into two main groups:

> **Inorganic.** Inorganic chemicals are typically single elements or relatively simple combinations thereof. For example, mercury (Hg), iron (Fe), and lead (Pb) are inorganic chemicals. So is saline, which is sodium chloride (NaCl) dissolved in water (H_2O). Inorganic chemicals can cause adverse health effects. Mercury and lead, for example, can cause neurological damage. Others, such as some forms of cobalt, are radiation sources. And some metals give off fumes when they are heated that can cause metal fume fever, a disease characterized by flu-like symptoms.
>
> **Organic.** Organic chemicals are relatively large compounds principally comprising various combinations of carbon (C), hydrogen (H), nitrogen (N), oxygen (O), phosphorus (P), and sulfur (S). Organic chemicals occupy a significant position in health care facilities and include glucose, anesthetics, sterilants, pharmaceuticals, cleaning agents, solvents, pesticides, and herbicides. The nature of the health effects attributable to organic chemicals is vast and includes neurological effects, pulmonary damage, sensitization reactions, reproductive effects, kidney damage, and liver damage.

Chemical Names

Chemicals have names, sometimes many. This is particularly true for organic chemicals. The most complicated of these names is the IUPAC (International Union of Pure and Applied Chemists) name.[6] Using the IUPAC rules, each compound has a distinct name that can't be confused with that of another compound. For the average person, this standardized name is much too complicated to use as a general identifier, except for a few of the simplest compounds, so common names are generally used. Common names are much less sophisticated than IUPAC chemical names. They are simpler, easier to remember, and easier to read, pronounce, and write.

Physical States and Properties of Chemicals

Chemicals exist in one of three physical states: solid, liquid, or gas. Adverse health effects can occur from exposure to any hazardous chemical, regardless of its physical state.

Chemicals also have properties, including the following:

- ☐ Volatility (vapor pressure)
- ☐ Flammability (including explosivity)
- ☐ Dielectric constant (ability to conduct electricity)
- ☐ Reactivity (ability to react with other chemicals, sometimes violently)

Chemical Exposure

Routes of Chemical Exposure

Exposure to chemicals can occur in one or more of three ways:

Inhalation
Skin or eye contact
Ingestion

Inhalation Inhalation is the most common route of exposure. All physical states of chemicals can be inhaled—for example, dust generated during construction or when applying solid herbicides or pesticides; gases used for anesthesia, sterilization, and welding; and the vapors of volatile liquid chemicals such as xylene, cleaning solutions, and solvents.

Skin or Eye Contact Many chemicals can have a direct effect on the skin, damaging it by either removing the fat or removing the water in the skin. Chemicals can be absorbed through the skin, resulting in systemic effects, dermatitis (a significant cause of recordable injuries and illnesses in health care facilities), and sensitization. Though rare in the health care setting, systemic effects can occur through skin exposure if some chemicals are used imprudently, such as mercury and certain of its compounds or solvents used routinely and in significant quantities.

Some chemicals may burn or irritate the eye. Occasionally they may be absorbed through the eye and enter the bloodstream. The eyes are easily harmed by chemicals, so any eye contact with chemicals should be considered a serious incident.

Ingestion The least common source of exposure in the workplace is swallowing chemicals, but ingestion can occur if good personal hygiene is not practiced. Chemicals can be ingested if they are left on hands, clothing, or beard, or accidentally contaminate food, drinks, or cigarettes. Eating food with contaminated hands can result in ingestion of a chemical.

Dose

Remember Alice?

> She had never forgotten that, if you drink much from a bottle marked "poison," it is almost certain to disagree with you, sooner or later.

Alice, who was confused by how much of the bottle she should drink and whether or not it was a poison, could have learned a lot if she had only been aware of the sixteenth-century Renaissance Swiss physician, Paracelsus, who wrote:

> All things are poison and nothing is without poison. Solely it is the dose that makes a thing poisonous.[7]

Paracelsus was explaining the concept of dose. It is not enough to simply be exposed to a chemical; unless the exposure is at a high enough concentration in air or enough has been ingested, it may not result in an adverse health effect. For example, ethylene oxide can cause a variety of adverse health effects, but only if it is not properly controlled. Common aspirin can relieve pain and reduce inflammation, but if too much is taken, it can result in gastric ulcerations and problems with blood clotting.

For the purposes of the HCS, exposure dose is expressed in terms of the amount of a chemical in a precise volume of air. Dose can also be expressed as the amount of substance in a known volume of liquid or simply as a total amount. When chemicals are in air, their concentration is typically expressed in terms of parts of the substance per million parts of air (ppm). They may also be expressed in terms of the weight of the chemical in a known volume of air, usually a cubic meter (e.g., mg/cubic meter of air). These two expressions, ppm and mg/m^3, are the typical ways in which OSHA, NIOSH, the ACGIH, and others express occupational exposure limits.

Occupational exposure limits establish the amount of a chemical that workers can be routinely exposed to over their working lifetime without suffering adverse health effects. Although OSHA, NIOSH, and the ACGIH all publish exposure limits, only those of OSHA are legally enforceable. The three types of limits are different:

□ Permissible exposure limit (PEL)—established by OSHA. These limits were established following a public administrative process of information gathering, hearings, and rule making. When establishing PELs, OSHA sometimes relies on NIOSH research, as well as research from other sources.

□ Recommended exposure limit (REL)—established by NIOSH. The National Institute for Occupational Safety and Health is mandated by Congress to conduct scientific research regarding hazardous chemicals and develop criteria for safe exposure limits. This is also a public process involving review and comment by all interested parties from government, industry, labor, and academia.

□ Threshold limit values (TLV)—established by ACGIH, a nongovernmental agency. Each chemical's TLV is established based on information gathered and reviewed by ACGIH's members. The OSHA PELs listed in 29 CFR 1910.1000 table Z-1 were adopted from the ACGIH 1968 TLV list when the OSH Act was passed in 1970.

At the present time, for a variety of reasons, many of the ACGIH TLVs are more current than either OSHA PELs or NIOSH RELs. It is incumbent on the Environmental Health and Safety Department to be aware of the exposure limits for the toxic substances used in the facility and to ensure that even if there is no PEL, the most protective measures are being implemented. Protective measures can be found on the MSDS.

How Exposure Information Is Collected and Conveyed

As a rule, the concentration of a contaminant in air in the workplace varies with time. That variation is due to a number of factors, including ventilation rate, amount of the substance being used or generated, frequency of use, and fluctuations in processes.

In Section 20(a)(3) of the OSH Act,[8] Congress stated that one of the goals was to allow workers to have regular exposure to chemicals and harmful physical agents for their working lifetime without suffering material impairment of health. Regular exposure is generally taken to mean 8 hours per day, 5 days per week, 50 weeks per year for a 40-year working lifetime. Therefore, when studies are conducted on populations to determine whether their exposure has resulted in an adverse health effect, industrial hygienists collect air samples, airborne concentrations are determined, and the results are expressed as if the exposure had occurred over an 8-hour work shift. However, as discussed above, exposure concentrations vary, and even though there may be periods of relatively high exposure during a workday, there may be

Figure 7–3. Relation between Exposure Concentration and Process as a Function of Time

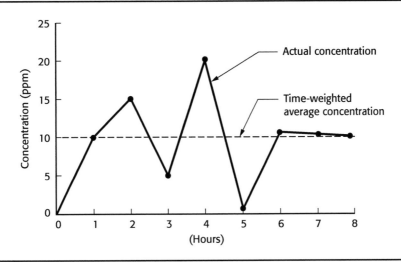

other periods with relatively low or even no exposure. Figure 7-3 demonstrates what that fluctuation in concentration may look like over an 8-hour work shift.

The following terms are used by OSHA, NIOSH, the ACGIH, and professionals in occupational/environmental health and safety:

Time-weighted average (TWA)
Short-term exposure limit (STEL)
Ceiling (C)
Action level

Time-Weighted Average (TWA)   The TWA is the typical method for expressing what the average exposure concentration over an 8-hour work shift is and for protecting workers against chronic health effects. Other time periods of exposure, such as 10 hours or 4 hours, can be expressed as TWA concentrations. For example, xylene has an 8-hour TWA PEL of 100 ppm.

Short-Term Exposure Limit (STEL)   As demonstrated in figure 7-3, there are often short periods of time during which exposure concentrations are great enough to result in acute health effects. To protect against those, OSHA sometimes requires that those short-term exposures be limited. Based on work published by NIOSH and adapted by the ACGIH, the concept of the STEL was developed. A STEL is the maximum concentration of a substance that a worker may be exposed to during any 5-, 10-, or 15-minute period without experiencing acute health effects. Usually only four such periods are allowed in any 8-hour work shift. If a chemical has the potential for causing both chronic and acute health effects, its OSHA PEL may be expressed as a combination of an 8-hour TWA and a STEL. As noted previously, xylene has an 8-hour TWA PEL of 100 ppm. It also has a STEL of 50 ppm.

Ceiling (C)   Sometimes exposure to high concentrations of a chemical over a short period of time can be debilitating or, as in the case of ethylene oxide, can cause permanent damage or cancer. To prevent this scenario, OSHA sometimes includes a concentration that at no time should be exceeded. This is called a ceiling concentration. As is the case with a STEL, an OSHA PEL may be expressed as a combination of an 8-hour TWA and a C. For example, ethylene oxide has an 8-hour TWA REL of 0.1 ppm with a ceiling of 5 ppm over a 10-minute period.

Action Level   Because industrial hygienists know that there are fluctuations in exposure concentration and that sometimes the actual concentration can exceed the 8-hour TWA, they have developed the concept of the action level. OSHA standards for specific chemicals often include an action level. The action level is important because it gives the industrial hygienist information about how the process is working and whether there has been a breakdown in the controls. The action level is generally taken to be one-half of the 8-hour TWA. For example, in the case of xylene, the action level would be an 8-hour TWA concentration of 50 ppm. Because they understand that there are daily fluctuations in airborne concentrations, industrial hygienists know that if the action level is exceeded, it is likely that the TWA has also been exceeded. Thus, the action level serves as a trigger for investigating the source of the exposure and making any necessary corrections.

WRITTEN HAZARD COMMUNICATION PROGRAM (29 CFR 1910.1200(E))

In health care facilities, when employees are exposed to hazardous chemicals, the facility must develop and maintain a written hazard communication program that describes how the HCS will be implemented in the facility (1910.1200(e)(1)). Figure 7-4 lists OSHA's requirements for a written program.

Preparation of a written program is not just a paper exercise; all of the elements must be implemented in the workplace in order to be in compliance with the rule. The plan does not have to be lengthy or complicated. It is intended to be a blueprint for implementation of the facility's program—an assurance that all aspects of the requirements have been addressed.

Figure 7–4. Elements Required for a Written Hazard Communication Program

☐ Lists of hazardous chemicals in the workplace (1910.1200(e)(1)(i))

☐ Labels and other forms of warning (1910.1200(f))

☐ Material safety data sheets (1910.1200(g))

☐ Employee information and training that includes the chemical hazards used in the facility and protective measures employees can take (1910.1200(h))

If OSHA inspects the health care facility for compliance with the HCS, the OSHA compliance officer will ask to see the written plan at the outset of the inspection. The written program must describe how the requirements for labels and other forms of warning, material safety data sheets, and employee information and training are going to be met in the facility.

Identifying Hazardous Chemicals (29 CFR 1910.1200(e)(1)(i))

The HCS requires a list of hazardous chemicals and drugs that are found in the workplace as part of the written hazard communication program. The list will eventually serve as an inventory of everything for which an MSDS must be maintained. Preparing the list will help in completing the rest of the program because it gives an idea of the scope of the program required for compliance in the facility.

The Occupational Safety and Health Administration considers a chemical hazardous if any of the following apply:

☐ It causes cancer.

☐ It is corrosive.

☐ It is toxic or highly toxic based on its median lethal dose (the dose at which 50 percent of animals in an experimental study die).

☐ It is an irritant.

☐ It causes sensitization.

☐ It has an effect on a particular organ such as liver, kidneys, the nervous system, or the hematopoietic system; or it is an agent that damages lungs, skin, eyes, or mucous membranes.

The best way to prepare a comprehensive list is to survey the workplace. Purchasing records may also be useful. Employers should establish procedures to ensure that Purchasing Department procedures result in MSDSs being received before a material is used in the workplace.

The broadest possible perspective should be taken when the survey is conducted. Sometimes people think of chemicals as being only liquids in containers. The HCS covers chemicals in all their physical forms, whether they are contained or not. The hazardous nature of the chemical and the potential for exposure are the factors that determine whether a chemical is covered. If it is not hazardous, it is not covered. If there is no potential for exposure (e.g., the chemical is inextricably bound and cannot be released), the rule does not cover the chemical.

Look around. Identify chemicals in containers, including pipes, but also think about chemicals generated in work operations. For example, welding fumes, dusts, and exhaust fumes are all sources of chemical exposure. Read labels provided by suppliers for hazard information. Make a list of all chemicals in the workplace that are potentially hazardous. For information and planning, note on the list the location(s) of the products within the workplace and an indication of the hazards as found on the label. This step will help in preparing the rest of the program.

Paragraph (b) of the HCS, *Scope and Application,* includes exemptions for various chemicals or workplace situations. After compiling the complete list of chemicals, review paragraph (b) to determine whether any of the items can be eliminated from the list because they are exempted materials. For example, food, drugs, and cosmetics brought into the workplace for employee consumption are exempt.

Once a list of the potentially hazardous chemicals in the workplace is compiled, the next step is to determine whether MSDSs have been received for all of them. Check files against the inventory just compiled. If an MSDS is missing, contact the supplier and request one. It is a good idea to document these requests, by filing either a copy of a letter or a note regarding a telephone conversation. If there are MSDSs for chemicals that are not on the list, figure out why. Perhaps the chemical is no longer used. Or perhaps it was missed in the survey. If suppliers provide MSDSs for products that are not hazardous, they do not have to be maintained.

Employees should not be permitted to use any chemicals for which there is no MSDS. The MSDS provides information needed to ensure that proper protective measures are implemented prior to exposure.

Labels and Other Forms of Warning (29 CFR 1910.1200(f))

Containers of hazardous chemicals must be labeled, tagged, or marked with the identity of the material and appropriate hazard warnings. Chemical manufacturers, importers, and distributors are required to ensure that every container of hazardous chemicals they ship is appropriately labeled with such information and with the name and address of the producer or other responsible party. Employers purchasing chemicals can rely on the labels provided by their suppliers. If the employer subsequently transfers the material from a labeled container to another container, the employer must label that container unless it is subject to the portable container exemption. Paragraphs (6) and (7) of section (f) provide specific exemptions for labeling requirements.

The primary information to be obtained from an OSHA-required label is an identity for the material and appropriate hazard warnings. The identity is any term that appears on the label, the MSDS, and the list of chemicals, and thus links these three sources of information. The identity used by the supplier must include the common name, the trade name, and the formal IUPAC chemical names. The hazard warning is a brief statement of the hazardous effects of the chemical (e.g., "flammable," "causes lung damage"). Labels also include other information, such as safe handling procedures, control measures, and emergency and first aid procedures. Labels must be legible and prominently displayed. There are no specific requirements for size or color or any specified text.

Material Safety Data Sheets (MSDSs) (29 CFR 1910.1200(g))

The HCS establishes uniform requirements to ensure that the hazards of all chemicals imported into, produced by, or used in U.S. workplaces are evaluated, and that the resultant hazard information and associated protective measures are transmitted to employers and potentially exposed employees via container labels and MSDSs. The MSDS is a detailed information sheet prepared by the manufacturer or importer of a chemical that describes the chemical and its potential hazards.

Many suppliers of MSDSs include a disclaimer at the end of the sheet that in essence states that they are not responsible for the information contained in the MSDS. Such disclaimers are contrary to the Hazard communication standard, which makes it clear that the preparer of the MSDS is responsible for its accuracy.[9]

The following requirement for MSDSs is provided in OSHA's HCS:

Material safety data sheets

1910.1200(g)(1)
Chemical manufacturers and importers shall obtain or develop a material safety data sheet for each hazardous chemical they produce or import. Employers shall have a material safety data sheet in the workplace for each hazardous chemical that they use.

1910.1200(g)(2)
Each material safety data sheet shall be in English (although the employer may maintain copies in other languages as well), and shall contain at least the following information:

1910.1200(g)(2)(i)
The identity used on the label, and, except as provided for in paragraph (i) of this section on trade secrets:

1910.1200(g)(2)(i)(A)
If the hazardous chemical is a single substance, its chemical and common name(s)

1910.1200(g)(2)(i)(B)
If the hazardous chemical is a mixture which has been tested as a whole to determine its hazards, the chemical and common name(s) of the ingredients which contribute to these known hazards, and the common name(s) of the mixture itself; or

1910.1200(g)(2)(i)(C)
If the hazardous chemical is a mixture which has not been tested as a whole:

1910.1200(g)(2)(i)(C)(1)
The chemical and common name(s) of all ingredients which have been determined to be health hazards, and which comprise 1% or greater of the composition, except that chemicals identified as carcinogens under paragraph (d) of this section shall be listed if the concentrations are 0.1% or greater; and

1910.1200(g)(2)(i)(C)(2)
The chemical and common name(s) of all ingredients which have been determined to be health hazards, and which comprise less than 1% (0.1% for carcinogens) of the mixture, if there is evidence that the ingredient(s) could be released from the mixture in concentrations which would exceed an established OSHA permissible exposure limit or ACGIH Threshold Limit Value, or could present a health risk to employees; and

1910.1200(g)(2)(i)(C)(3)
The chemical and common name(s) of all ingredients which have been determined to present a physical hazard when present in the mixture

1910.1200(g)(2)(ii)
Physical and chemical characteristics of the hazardous chemical (such as vapor pressure, flash point)

1910.1200(g)(2)(iii)
The physical hazards of the hazardous chemical, including the potential for fire, explosion, and reactivity

1910.1200(g)(2)(iv)
The health hazards of the hazardous chemical, including signs and symptoms of exposure, and any medical conditions which are generally recognized as being aggravated by exposure to the chemical

1910.1200(g)(2)(v)
The primary route(s) of entry

1910.1200(g)(2)(vi)
The OSHA permissible exposure limit, ACGIH Threshold Limit Value, and any other exposure limit used or recommended by the chemical manufacturer, importer, or employer preparing the material safety data sheet, where available

1910.1200(g)(2)(vii)

Whether the hazardous chemical is listed in the National Toxicology Program (NTP) Annual Report on Carcinogens (latest edition) or has been found to be a potential carcinogen in the International Agency for Research on Cancer (IARC) Monographs (latest editions), or by OSHA

1910.1200(g)(2)(viii)

Any generally applicable precautions for safe handling and use which are known to the chemical manufacturer, importer or employer preparing the material safety data sheet, including appropriate hygienic practices, protective measures during repair and maintenance of contaminated equipment, and procedures for cleanup of spills and leaks

1910.1200(g)(2)(ix)

Any generally applicable control measures which are known to the chemical manufacturer, importer or employer preparing the material safety data sheet, such as appropriate engineering controls, work practices, or personal protective equipment

1910.1200(g)(2)(x)

Emergency and first aid procedures

1910.1200(g)(2)(xi)

The date of preparation of the material safety data sheet or the last change to it; and

1910.1200(g)(2)(xii)

The name, address and telephone number of the chemical manufacturer, importer, employer or other responsible party preparing or distributing the material safety data sheet, who can provide additional information on the hazardous chemical and appropriate emergency procedures, if necessary

1910.1200(g)(3)

If no relevant information is found for any given category on the material safety data sheet, the chemical manufacturer, importer or employer preparing the material safety data sheet shall mark it to indicate that no applicable information was found

Employee Information and Training (29 CFR 1910.1200(h))

Robert A. Heinlein, a noted science fiction writer, might have had Alice in mind when he wrote the novel *Stranger in a Strange Land*.[10] Once Alice fell down the rabbit hole, she surely was a stranger in a strange land, with no knowledge of whom she would encounter or of the customs in this new world, and certainly no knowledge of what a beautifully printed label that simply said "DRINK ME" might mean, how to interpret it, or whether other information was available. Alice could have used a guide or a teacher, or perhaps just some good solid training and information, before she drank from the bottle with the beautifully printed label.

Effective training is vital to understanding the information provided on chemical container labels and in MSDSs, and to applying that information in the workplace to protect against chemical hazards.

Training is vital to understanding, integrating, and classifying the many pieces of information that relate to chemical hazard communication. In health care facilities, employees may be confronted with posted hazard warnings, signs, tags, labels, manuals explaining the facility's hazard communication program, lists of chemicals, and information furnished by the union, if there is one. This wide variety of communications will differ in format, content, and reading level. These differences can obscure the important hazard communication messages. Training can reduce background noise by presenting the necessary information in a structured and logical manner.

Training sessions serve another important purpose—they provide a forum for employees to share their health and safety concerns and to obtain answers from managers, department liaisons, and Environmental Health and Safety professionals. Employees can also share their ideas and job experiences; they have often acquired real expertise in dealing with potentially hazardous situations.

The Occupational Safety and Health Administration is concerned about how training should be delivered. Although OSHA recognizes that there are many computer- and video-based training courses available that may serve as useful tools during training, the agency has published the following statement:

> Use of computer-based training by itself would not be sufficient to meet the intent of most of OSHA's training requirements. Our position on this matter is essentially the same as our policy on the use of training videos, since the two approaches have similar shortcomings. OSHA urges employers to be wary of relying solely on generic "packaged" programs in meeting their training requirements. [CD-ROM 7.6]

OSHA's Specific Training Requirements

1910.1200(h) Employee Information and Training

(1) Employers shall provide employees with effective information and training on hazardous chemicals in their work area at the time of their initial assignment, and whenever a new physical or health hazard the employees have not previously been trained about is introduced into their work area. Information and training may be designed to cover categories of hazards (e.g., flammability, carcinogenicity) or specific chemicals. Chemical-specific information must always be available through labels and material safety data sheets.

Simply knowing that an MSDS is available is not enough to be informed. The Occupational Safety and Health Administration requires that all employees be given certain information about the HCS and substances they may encounter in their work areas. That information includes the following:

1910.1200(h)(2)(i–iii)

The requirements of this section.

Any operations in their work area where hazardous chemicals are present.

The location and availability of the written hazard communication program, including the required list(s) of hazardous chemicals, and material safety data sheets required by this section.

The Occupational Safety and Health Administration also specifies the content of the training that employees must have:

1910.1200(h)(3)(i–iv)

☐ Methods and observations that may be used to detect the presence or release of a hazardous chemical in the work area (such as monitoring conducted by the employer, continuous monitoring devices, visual appearance or odor of hazardous chemicals when being released).

☐ The physical and health hazards of the chemicals in the work area.

☐ The measures employees can take to protect themselves from these hazards, including specific procedures the employer has implemented to protect employees from exposure to hazardous chemicals, such as appropriate work practices, emergency procedures, and personal protective equipment to be used.

☐ The details of the hazard communication program developed by the employer, including an explanation of the labeling system and the material safety data sheet, and how employees can obtain and use the appropriate hazard information.

Translating the Meaning of OSHA's Training Requirements

What do all these information and training requirements mean? The following definitions are from OSHA's *Draft Model Training Program for Hazard Communication:*[11] [CD-ROM 7.7]

☐ *Effective* means that the information and training program must work. Employees must carry the knowledge from the training into their daily jobs. For example, if asked, they should know where hazardous chemicals are present in their work area and should know how to protect themselves.

☐ *In their work area* means just what it says. The information and training must be specific to each work area. The facility cannot stop at training about general hazards found in work areas. The potential hazards that employees are actually going to encounter must be addressed.

☐ *Time of initial assignment.* This means that new employees must be informed and trained before going on the job so they are not faced with unknown hazards.

☐ *New physical or health hazard.* Sometimes new hazardous chemicals are introduced into the workplace, and sometimes employees are assigned to new jobs that involve potential exposure to new hazards. Either way, no employee should be in the position of encountering unfamiliar or unknown hazards.

☐ *Categories of hazards.* OSHA is aware that many workplaces contain so many different chemicals that it would be difficult and confusing to attempt to train employees about each one separately. Fortunately, many chemicals fall into categories, such as flammables or acids and bases. In these instances, it is not only acceptable but also more effective to discuss the hazards of the category as a whole. If individual chemicals within a category present a special safety or health hazard, these unique properties must be pointed out.

☐ *Specific chemicals* are those that don't belong in a category or should be singled out for some other reason. For example, they may present a special hazard or be represented in great quantity in the workplace.

☐ *Chemical-specific information must always be available through labels and material safety data sheets.* Whether categories or any other training method is selected, labels and MSDSs must always be available and accessible to employees at all times.

☐ *Informed.* Providing information is not quite the same as training but both terms are included under the general term "training" in OSHA's model training program. It means that employees must know what the standard means and where things are kept. Information can be furnished with the help of signs, notices, handouts, or other means. Whatever information measures are chosen, however, they must be effective. For example, employees should be able to tell someone where the written program is housed and also how to locate the material safety data sheet collection.

☐ *Requirements of this section* are simply the requirements of the HCS. It is a good idea to inform the employees about the rights and responsibilities of the employer as well as the employee.

☐ *Operations in their work area.* This phrase points again to the need to be specific in the information and training program. Generalities about operations that have no relevance to these specific employees are not sufficient.

☐ *Location and availability* must again be specific. For example, the written hazard communication program may be kept in Building A or in the supervisor's office, where it must be available at all times. Employees should know exactly where it is and how to gain access.

□ *Training.* This term covers anything that is done to impart new knowledge or skills or to refresh employees' memories on previously learned knowledge or skills. It can best be imagined as bridging the gap between what employees know now and what they have to know to identify hazards and protect themselves against them. Many different training methods and media can be used to achieve this goal.

□ *Methods and observations* mean any active or passive means that can be used to detect the presence or release of a hazardous chemical. For example, some chemicals such as chlorine can be detected by their odor, color or other unique properties.

□ *Physical and health hazards.* These terms apply only to the physical and health hazards of chemicals. A physical hazard is associated with a chemical that is a combustible liquid, a compressed gas, explosive, flammable, an organic peroxide, an oxidizer, pyrophoric, unstable or water-reactive. All these can harm as a result of physical reaction. Health hazard means that exposure to the chemical can cause acute or chronic health effects. Examples are carcinogens and eye irritants.

□ *Measures employees can take to protect themselves.* These can include any control, including everything from learning the meaning of emergency signals to observing "No Entry" areas or selecting the correct personal protective equipment.

□ *Details of the hazard communication program.* This allows employees to learn what label statements mean, what information can be found in the material safety data sheet, and how to find out if a chemical presents a potential hazard.

Prioritizing Hazard Communication Training

What should be done first? It is often necessary to prioritize hazard communication information and training needs. Health care facilities often use many different chemicals and frequently hire new employees or transfer existing employees to new jobs. In these situations, it is necessary to prioritize training activities. As this text from OSHA's *Draft Model Training Program* illustrates, prioritizing is easier when planning is done first:

1. Use existing facility records to define groups potentially exposed to hazardous chemicals:
   □ Inventory of chemicals used, stored, or otherwise present in the workplace.
   □ Index of MSDSs for hazardous materials.
   □ Description of job tasks—gives information on potential exposures.
   □ Further definitions of exposure groups obtained from industrial hygiene monitoring data.

2. Review previous training history:
   - ☐ Have all new employees been trained?
   - ☐ Have all employees assigned to new tasks, with potential new exposures, been trained?
   - ☐ What training has been conducted?
     - How often? How recently?
     - What was the content of training?
     - How effective was it? Do employees have the knowledge and/or skills to protect themselves against possible harm?

The Occupational Safety and Health Administration's *Voluntary Training Guidelines* (OSHA 2254)[12] [CD-ROM 7.8] suggest that employees can assist in this process by providing, "in writing, and in their own words, descriptions of their jobs. These should include the tasks performed, and the tools, materials and equipment used." It is also helpful to observe employees at the worksite as they perform tasks, asking about the work and recording the employees' answers.

OSHA's Model Training Program and How It Helps Health Care Facilities

The Occupational Safety and Health Administration's *Draft Model Training Program* is designed to help health care and other industries provide effective hazard communication training.

Section II addresses the issue of effective and site-specific training. A section titled "Guidance for Site-Specific Training" expands on guidance provided in OSHA's *Voluntary Training Guidelines*. Included are the steps that lead to an effective program, as well as a discussion about how to assist employees who lack basic skills. Using the guidance, facilities can develop and administer hazard communication training programs that are specific to their workplace.

Section III identifies training components that are not site specific and apply to all employees. These topics are portable and can stay with employees when they go from one worksite to another. The topics are made into training "modules" that are self-contained lesson plans. The lesson plans include visual aids that can be modified to reflect the facility's site-specific hazard communication program. The visual aids can be printed as handouts, made into overhead transparencies, or projected digitally on a computer screen. Also included at the end of each lesson plan is a quiz that can be printed for distribution. The lesson plans, called *general elements*, can be incorporated into the facility's overall program.

There are two kinds of general elements in the OSHA model. The first group covers topics that help employees understand the HCS and the information that is communicated by MSDSs and labels. The second group covers four common chemical categories.

The *Draft Model Training Program* includes appendixes that contain a glossary of terms and a section on where to go for further help.

GUIDELINES FOR EMPLOYER COMPLIANCE (ADVISORY) (29 CFR 1910.1200, APPENDIX E)

Appendix E of the HCS is a general guide for health care and other industries to help them determine what is required under the rule. [CD-ROM 7.9] It does not supplant or substitute for the regulatory provisions, but provides a simplified outline of the steps an average employer would follow to meet OSHA's requirements.

The HCS is long, and some parts of it are technical, but the basic concepts are simple. One difference between this rule and many others adopted by OSHA is that this one is performance oriented. This means that health care facilities have the flexibility to adapt the rule to the needs of the workplace, rather than having to follow specific, rigid requirements. It also means that the facility will have to exercise more judgment to implement an appropriate and effective program.

OCCUPATIONAL EXPOSURE TO HAZARDOUS CHEMICALS IN LABORATORIES (29 CFR 1910.1450)

Standard 29 CFR 1910.1450, Occupational exposure to hazardous chemicals in laboratories, covers all workers who use hazardous chemicals in laboratories. [CD-ROM 7.10] *Laboratory use* means performing chemical procedures using small quantities of hazardous chemicals on a laboratory scale and not as part of a production process in an environment where protective laboratory practices and equipment are in common use. This standard requires employers to comply with employee exposure limits (PELs) specified in the standard on air contaminants (29 CFR 1910.1000, table Z-2, Toxic and Hazardous Substances) [CD-ROM 7.11] and in other substance-specific health standards. As with the requirements in OSHA's Hazard communication standard, if engineering, administrative, and work practice controls fail to maintain exposures below PELs, workers must use respirators to achieve that end. Employers must provide appropriate respiratory protection at no cost to workers, provide appropriate training and education regarding its use, and ensure that workers use it properly in accordance with OSHA Standard 29 CFR 1910.134, Respiratory protection. [CD-ROM 7.12] The employer must establish and maintain for each employee an accurate record of any measurements taken to monitor employee exposure and any medical consultation or examination, including tests or written opinions.

If laboratory employees use hazardous chemicals, the facility must develop and implement a written chemical hygiene plan to protect them. In addition to appropriate safety and health procedures and hygiene practices for hazardous chemicals in laboratories, the plan must include the following:

- Criteria for reducing employee exposure to hazardous chemicals
- Requirements for the use of personal protective equipment
- Requirements ensuring that fume hoods and other protective equipment are functioning properly
- Provisions for employee training
- Circumstances requiring employer approval of certain laboratory operations, procedures, or activities before implementation
- Provisions for medical consultation
- Measures to protect employees from particularly hazardous substances
- Assignment of a chemical hygiene officer, a qualified employee who by training or experience can provide technical guidance in developing and implementing the chemical hygiene plan

ADDITIONAL RESOURCES

The Chemical Reactivity Worksheet is a free program that health care facilities can use to find out about the reactivity of substances or mixtures of substances (reactivity is the tendency of a substance to undergo chemical change). It includes a database of reactivity information for more than 6,000 common hazardous chemicals. The program also includes an option to virtually mix chemicals to find out what dangers could arise from accidental mixing.

The database includes information about the intrinsic hazards of each chemical and about whether a chemical reacts with air, water, or other materials. It also includes case histories on specific chemical incidents.

The Chemical Reactivity Team at the Office of Response and Restoration, National Ocean Service, National Oceanic and Atmospheric Administration (NOAA), developed the Chemical Reactivity Worksheet.[13]

JOINT COMMISSION STANDARDS FOR THE SAFE USE AND HANDLING OF CHEMICALS

The Joint Commission addresses the safe use and handling of chemicals under the broad rubric of Clinically Related Risks in their publication *Protecting Those Who Serve: Health Care Worker Safety.*[14] Published in conjunction with OSHA, *Health Care Worker Safety* presents a good general discussion of chemicals in the health care setting and devotes particular attention to ethylene oxide, formaldehyde, and glutaraldehyde.

The overarching Joint Commission standard for chemical safety is EC.1.10, safety management. A specific Joint Commission standard (EC.3.10) states that the facility manages its hazardous materials and waste risks, which requires health care facilities to identify materials they use that need special handling and to implement processes to minimize the risks of their unsafe use. Standard EC.3.10, EP2 explicitly requires health care facilities to create and maintain an inventory that identifies hazardous materials using criteria consistent with applicable laws and regulations (e.g., OSHA).

Other standards that are important in the overall approach to worker safety include monitoring and environmental conditions (EC.9.10), analyzing environmental issues (EC.9.20), and improving the environment (EC.9.30). Additional pertinent standards include initial job training (HR.2.10), roles and responsibilities (HR.2.20), and ongoing education (HR.2.30).

THE ROLE OF THE ENVIRONMENTAL HEALTH AND SAFETY DEPARTMENT

Development of and compliance with an effective hazard communication program is not a one-shot deal. It must be a continuing program in each health care facility. The Environmental Health and Safety Department should assume leadership and responsibility for both the initial and ongoing activities that are required for compliance with the rule.

The principal functions of the Environmental Health and Safety Department include:

- ☐ Training employees about the HCS
- ☐ Assisting in establishing and maintaining the inventory of hazardous chemicals in each department
- ☐ Maintaining copies of all MSDSs and reviewing them for accuracy and completeness and correcting errors
- ☐ Working with other departments to find ways in which inventories of hazardous chemicals can be reduced

In the model Environmental Health and Safety Department presented in this book, each department within the organization has a liaison who works with the Environmental Health and Safety Department. The role of the department liaison is critical to the success of the hazard communication program. Just imagine the aggravation Alice might have saved herself if Wonderland had had a liaison who could have told her that, no matter how beautifully printed the label on the bottle was, drinking its contents was probably not a very good idea. The department liaisons are in the best position to help develop the inventory of hazardous chemicals in their departments and to identify training needs and ensure compliance with the HCS. For example, the facility's hazardous drug officer is ideally suited to serve as a liaison to the Environmental Health and Safety Department, as are the facility's chemical hygiene officer, biological safety officer, and radiation safety officer.

References

1. Carroll, Lewis. *Alice's Adventures in Wonderland* (facsimile ed.). New York, 1941, pp. 9–11.

2. U.S. Department of Labor. *Controlling Occupational Exposure to Hazardous Drugs.* OSHA Technical Manual. Section VI, Chapter 2, Appendix VI: 2-1. Available at http://www.osha.gov/dts/osta/otm/otm_vi/otm_vi_2.html (accessed 2/22/2006).

3. Ramazzini, Bernardino. *Diseases of Workers* (trans. from the Latin text *DeMorbis Articum* (1713) by Wilmer Cave Wright). Thunder Bay, Canada: OH&S Press, 1993, p. 233.

4. U.S. Department of Labor. *Hazard Communication Standard* (29 CFR 1910.1200) (August 14, 1987), Appendix A, *Health Hazard Definitions (Mandatory).* Available at www.osha.gov/1910_1200_APP_A.html (accessed 2/20/2006).

5. American National Standards Institute. *Hazardous Industrial Chemicals— Precautionary Labeling* (Z129.1-2000). Available at www.ansi.org.

6. International Union of Pure and Applied Chemists (IUPAC). IUPAC Secretariat, P.O. Box 13757, Research Triangle Park, NC 27709-3757, USA.

7. Paracelsus. *Selected Writings* (J. Jacobi, ed.; N. Guterman, trans.). New York: Pantheon, 1951.

8. U.S. Congress. Occupational Safety and Health Act of 1970, Public Law 91-596, Section 20(a)(3), Research and Related Activities. *U.S. Statutes at Large* 84 (1970), p. 1590. Available at http://www.osha.gov/pls/oshaweb/owadisp.show_document?p_table=OSHACT&p_id=2743 (accessed 2/9/2006).

9. U.S. Department of Labor. OSHA Hazard Communication Standard (29 CFR 1910.1200), Appendix B, *Hazard Determination (Mandatory).* Available at www.osha.gov/1910_1200_APP_B.html (accessed 2/20/2006).

10. Heinlein, Robert A. *Stranger in a Strange Land.* New York: Ace Books, 1995.

11. U.S. Department of Labor. *Draft Model Training Program for Hazard Communication.* Available at http://www.osha.gov/dsg/hazcom/ MTP101703.html (accessed 3/10/2006).

12. U.S. Department of Labor. *Training Requirements in OSHA Standards and Training Guidelines.* OSHA 2254 1998 (Revised). Available at http://www.osha.gov/dsg/hazcom/MTP101703.html (accessed 3/10/2006).

13. Office of Response and Restoration, National Ocean Service, National Oceanic and Atmospheric Administration. *The Chemical Reactivity Worksheet.* Available at http://response.restoration.noaa.gov/type_subtopic_entry.php?RECORD_KEY%28entry_subtopic_type%29=entry_id,subtopic_id,type_id&entry_id(entry_subtopic_type)=328&subtopic_id(entry_subtopic_type)=3&type_id(entry_subtopic_type)=3 (accessed 3/10/2006).

14. *Protecting Those Who Serve: Health Care Worker Safety.* Oakbrook Terrace, IL: Joint Commission on Accreditation of Healthcare Organizations, 2005.

CHAPTER 8

WASTE MANAGEMENT

Sarah Cynthia Sylvia Stout
Would not take the garbage out.
She'd wash the dishes and scrub the pans
Cook the yams and spice the hams,
And though her parents would scream and shout,
She simply would not take the garbage out.
And so it piled up to the ceiling . . .
It filled the can, it covered the floor,
It cracked the windows and blocked the door,
Prune pits, peach pits, orange peels . . .
The garbage rolled on down the halls,
It raised the roof, it broke the walls . . .
. . . finally it touched the sky,
And none of her friends would come to play,
And all of her neighbors moved away;
And finally, Sarah Cynthia Stout
Said, "Okay, I'll take the garbage out!"
But then, of course it was too late,
The garbage reached across the state,
From New York to the Golden Gate;
Remember Sarah Stout,
And always take the garbage out.

Shel Silverstein, *Where the Sidewalk Ends*[1]

Whether at home or at work, there is always garbage, and someone needs to take it out. Sarah obviously resented the job, and when she finally realized it had become a problem, it was too late. If Sarah owned a restaurant, the local health department would have closed its doors. If Sarah was a business owner, the Occupational Safety and Health Administration (OSHA) could have cited her for failing to "provide a place of employment free from recognized hazards," the fire department would have cited her for garbage blocking the door, and once the garbage spilled out of the door, the Environmental Protection Agency (EPA) could have fined her for operating an unlicensed hazardous waste site. If Sarah happened to run a hospital, it is highly likely that in addition to the local health department, the fire department, OSHA, the EPA, the U.S. Food and Drug Administration (FDA), and the Joint Commission would also want to have a little chat with her about the disposal of her pharmaceuticals and radiation sources. Sarah's neighbors simply moved to get away from her mess. But in the real world of commerce and industry, it is likely that Sarah would have had to have tea with the local citizens' environmental group and one or two of their lawyers.

Sarah's job really was very simple—bag the garbage and take it to the garbage can. However, the disposal of waste in health care facilities is far more complex. Sarah didn't have to separate the orange peels from the prune pits. She didn't need to make any decisions about which parts of the waste might be hazardous and need special handling, and she obviously was not concerned about being a good neighbor.

Sarah should have been cognizant of the effect that her disregard for her neighbors was having on them, but she was not—nor was she concerned about the ultimate cost of disposing of all her waste. On the other hand, health care facilities must demonstrate a responsible approach to handling their waste and understand the environmental, economic, and social impacts it can have. By implementing an aggressive health care waste management program, facilities can help achieve a healthy and safe environment for their employees, patients, and community and reduce both procurement and disposal costs.

HEALTH CARE FACILITY WASTE

It has been estimated that health care facilities generate more than 4 million tons of nonhazardous waste each year, costing the industry millions of dollars. Between 75 and 90 percent of the waste produced by health care providers is nonrisk or "general" health care waste. In many ways, general waste is comparable to domestic waste and is primarily derived from the administrative, housekeeping, engineering, and food service functions of the facility. The remaining 10 to 25 percent of health care waste is regarded as hazardous waste that may create a variety of health risks, thus requiring costly special handling or incineration.[2] [CD-ROM 8.1] Failing to comply with state and federal waste handling regulations can also be costly. In 2003 various violations among 10 New York state hospitals for improper waste handling ranged from $2,000 up to $500,000.[3]

Health care facilities are institutions of healing, centers for wellness, and are viewed by the public within that framework. However, health care

Table 8–1. Classification of Health Care Waste

Waste Category	Description
Chemical	Waste containing chemical substances
Pharmaceutical	Waste containing pharmaceuticals
Genotoxic	Waste containing substances with genotoxic properties
Infectious (medical)	Waste suspected to contain pathogens, human tissues, or fluids
Pathologic (medical)	Waste containing human tissues or fluids
Sharps	Sharp waste
Radioactive	Waste containing radioactive substances
General	Common waste

facilities have complex waste problems. Not only must they deal with an enormous amount of solid waste, but they must segregate that waste into hazardous chemical waste, medical waste, radioactive waste, and common waste, and dispose of each component accordingly.

Health care facilities have a "duty of care" for the environment and for public health, and this carries particular responsibilities in relation to the waste they produce. The burden is on health care facilities to ensure that there are no adverse health and environmental consequences of their waste handling, treatment, and disposal activities.

WASTE CATEGORIES AND DESCRIPTIONS

Classification of health care wastes is summarized in table 8-1.

HEALTH IMPACTS OF HAZARDOUS TYPES OF HEALTH CARE WASTE

Exposure to hazardous types of health care waste can result in disease or injury. The hazardous nature of health care waste may be due to one or more of the following characteristics:

- ☐ It contains toxic or hazardous chemicals or pharmaceuticals.
- ☐ It is genotoxic.
- ☐ It contains infectious agents.
- ☐ It contains sharps.
- ☐ It is radioactive.

All individuals exposed to hazardous types of health care waste are potentially at risk, including those within health care establishments that generate hazardous types of waste and those outside these sources who either handle such waste or are exposed to it as a consequence of careless management. The main groups at risk are the following:

- ☐ Employees in support services such as environmental services, laundries, waste handling, maintenance, and transportation
- ☐ Medical doctors, nurses, and volunteers
- ☐ Patients
- ☐ Visitors to the facility

HAZARDOUS WASTE

In the mid-1970s, it became clear to Congress and the American people that action had to be taken to ensure that wastes were managed properly. This realization began the process that resulted in the passage of the Resource Conservation and Recovery Act (RCRA). The goals set by RCRA are:

- ☐ To protect human health and the environment from the hazards posed by waste disposal
- ☐ To conserve energy and natural resources through waste recycling and recovery
- ☐ To reduce or eliminate, as expeditiously as possible, the amount of waste generated, including hazardous waste
- ☐ To ensure that wastes are managed in a manner that is protective of human health and the environment

To achieve these goals, RCRA established three distinct yet interrelated programs (see figure 8-1).

RCRA Subtitle C, the hazardous waste program, establishes a system for controlling hazardous waste from the time it is generated until its ultimate disposal—in effect, from cradle to grave.[4]

A hazardous waste is a waste with properties that make it dangerous or capable of having a harmful effect on human health or the environment. Unfortunately, to develop a regulatory framework that ensures adequate protection, this simple narrative definition is not enough. Determining what is a hazardous waste is paramount, because only wastes with specific attributes are subject to Subtitle C regulation.

Figure 8–1. RCRA Programs

Subtitle D	Subtitle C	Subtitle I
Solid waste program	Hazardous waste program	Underground storage tank program

RCRA is the primary federal legislation that governs the identification and disposal of both nonhazardous and hazardous wastes. Just as Congress stated its purpose and intent when it crafted the Occupational Safety and Health Act of 1970 (OSH Act) [CD-ROM 8.2], it also stated its purpose and intent for dealing with the ever-increasing burden of waste and waste disposal when it crafted RCRA.

US Code Collection, Title 42, Chapter 82, Subchapter 1
Sec. 6902. Objectives and national policy

b) National policy

The Congress hereby declares it to be the national policy of the United States that, wherever feasible, the generation of hazardous waste is to be reduced or eliminated as expeditiously as possible. Waste that is nevertheless generated should be treated, stored, or disposed of so as to minimize the present and future threat to human health and the environment.

How Does a Material Become a Hazardous Waste?

There are two primary ways in which a waste material can become classified as a hazardous waste, subject to the RCRA requirements:

1. *Listed wastes:* Wastes from certain industrial processes are automatically classified as hazardous. Each waste of this type is given a code number. The full list of hazardous waste codes appears in the Code of Federal Regulations (40 CFR 261). [CD-ROM 8.3]
2. *Characteristic wastes:* Wastes that do not appear on the CFR lists may nevertheless be classified as hazardous if they have one of four properties:

   □ Ignitability (readily burns)
   □ Corrosiveness ($pH < 2$ or $pH > 12$, i.e., a strong acid or a strong base)
   □ Reactivity (reacts readily with other substances and can be explosive)
   □ Toxicity

In addition, materials can acquire hazardous waste status if they are mixed with, contaminated with, or derived from other wastes that are themselves hazardous. An example of mixing waste would be putting nonhazardous cleaning agents in a container of used hazardous solvents.

The generator of the waste is responsible for determining if the waste is hazardous. The rules can get complicated. In addition to determining whether a waste is hazardous, health care facilities must know how each particular waste is classified. The rules that apply to each facility depend on how much waste and what type of waste the facility generates. Misclassifications can (and do) lead to citations and penalties.

The EPA Healthcare Environmental Resource Center website provides additional information regarding hazardous waste regulations and management.[5]

Types of Hazardous Waste and Potential Health Hazards

Hazardous waste consists of discarded solid, liquid, and gaseous chemicals from laboratories, medical and research equipment, housekeeping, and maintenance. Some of the hazardous chemicals used most commonly in health care facilities are discussed next.

Formaldehyde

Formaldehyde, once used to clean and disinfect heat-labile equipment (e.g., hemodialysis or surgical equipment), is now primarily used to preserve specimens and disinfect liquid infectious waste, and in pathology, autopsy, dialysis, embalming, and nursing units. Formaldehyde causes upper respiratory, eye, and mucous membrane irritation and has been associated with cancer in long-term studies using rodents.

Mercury

As a reproductive toxin and a potent neurotoxin, mercury affects the brain and the central nervous system. Pregnant women, women of childbearing age, and small children are at greatest risk. Mercury can cross the placenta and cause irreparable neurological damage to the fetus. Mercury poses a special problem in the health care facility waste stream. [CD-ROM 8.4] Mercury can be found in many common health care devices:

- ☐ Fever thermometers
- ☐ Blood pressure cuffs
- ☐ Sphygmomanometers
- ☐ Some gastrointestinal tubes
- ☐ Dental amalgams
- ☐ Some laboratory chemicals
- ☐ Pharmaceutical products: ophthalmic and contact lens products, nasal sprays, and vaccines
- ☐ Cleaners and degreasers
- ☐ Mercuric oxide batteries and button batteries
- ☐ Fluorescent light ballasts, high-density discharge lamps, and ultraviolet lamps
- ☐ Electrical equipment: tilt switches, float switches, thermostats, reed relays, plunger or displacement relays, and thermostat probes

- Thermostat probes in gas-fired appliances with pilot lights, such as ranges, ovens, clothes dryers, water heaters, and furnaces
- Industrial thermometers: air and water heating and cooling systems
- Pressure gauges: laboratory manometers and barometers
- Plumbing

Ethylene Oxide

Ethylene oxide is used for the sterilization of heat-labile material and has been associated with ocular damage, respiratory irritation, and cancer in long-term studies using rodents.

Glutaraldehyde

The most commonly used chemical for high-level cold disinfection is glutaraldehyde. Use of glutaraldehyde in health care facilities has revealed serious and wide-ranging health risks to workers, including dermatitis, rhinitis, conjunctivitis, and respiratory sensitization. In the United Kingdom, the National Health Service (NHS), as of May 2002, has banned the use of glutaraldehyde in hospitals.

Photographic Chemicals

Photographic fixing and developing solutions are used in x-ray departments. The fixer usually contains 5 to 10 percent hydroquinone, 1 to 5 percent potassium hydroxide (both of which can cause eye and skin irritation), and less than 1 percent silver. The developer contains approximately 45 percent glutaraldehyde, which can cause respiratory sensitization. Acetic acid, which can cause mucous membrane irritation, is used in both stop baths and fixer solutions.

Solvents and Waste Organic Chemicals

Solvents and waste organic chemicals generated in health care facilities include:

- Solvents used in pathology and histology laboratories and engineering departments such as methylene chloride, chloroform, trichloroethylene, refrigerants, and non-halogenated compounds such as xylene, methanol, acetone, isopropanol, toluene, ethyl acetate, and acetonitrile
- Disinfecting and cleaning solutions, such as phenol-based chemicals used for scrubbing floors and perchlorethylene used in workshops and laundries

□ Oils such as vacuum pump oils and used engine oil from vehicles (particularly if there is a vehicle service station on the facility premises)
□ Insecticides and rodenticides

Inorganic Chemicals

Apart from silver and mercury, waste inorganic chemicals consist mainly of acids and alkalis (e.g., sulfuric, hydrochloric, nitric, and chromic acids, and sodium hydroxide and ammonia solutions).

Pharmaceutical and Genotoxic Materials

Pharmaceutical and genotoxic materials are a special class of hazardous waste and include pharmaceuticals that have expired, are unused, or are split, and contaminated pharmaceutical products, drugs, vaccines, and sera that are no longer required. [CD-ROM 8.5] This category also includes discarded items used in the handling of pharmaceuticals, such as bottles or boxes with residues, gloves, masks, connecting tubing, and drug vials.

Genotoxics are highly hazardous and may have mutagenic, teratogenic, or carcinogenic properties. Such waste raises serious safety problems both inside health care facilities and after disposal. Genotoxic waste may include certain cytotoxic drugs, vomit, urine, or feces from patients treated with cytostatic drugs, chemicals, and radioactive material.

The cytotoxicity of many antineoplastic drugs is cell cycle–specific, targeted at specific intracellular processes such as DNA synthesis and mitosis. Other antineoplastics, such as alkylating agents, are not phase specific but are cytotoxic at any point in the cell cycle. Experimental studies have shown that many antineoplastic drugs are carcinogenic and mutagenic; secondary neoplasia (occurring after the original cancer has been eradicated) is known to be associated with some forms of chemotherapy.

Many cytotoxic drugs are extremely irritating and have harmful local effects after direct contact with skin or eyes. They may also cause dizziness, nausea, headache, or dermatitis. Additional information on health hazards from cytotoxic drugs may be obtained on request from the International Agency for Research on Cancer (IARC).[6] Of particular concern are the numerous published studies describing the potential health hazard associated with the handling of antineoplastic drugs. Many of those studies found increased urinary levels of mutagenic compounds in exposed workers. Those increased urinary concentrations were associated with an increased risk of spontaneous abortions. Another study demonstrated that exposure of personnel cleaning hospital urinals exceeded that of nurses and pharmacists. Unfortunately, because of a lack of training about the potential hazards, those individuals were less aware of the danger and took fewer precautions.[7]

Figure 8–2. Federally Regulated Universal Wastes

    □ Spent batteries
    □ Waste pesticides
    □ Used fluorescent lamps
    □ Used mercury-containing thermostats

UNIVERSAL WASTES

Universal wastes are hazardous wastes that are more common and pose a lower risk to people and the environment than do other hazardous wastes. Federal (40 CFR part 273) [CD-ROM 8.6] and state-specific regulations identify universal wastes and provide simple rules for their handling, recycling, and disposal. Specific information for each state can be found on the EPA's website.[8] Federally regulated universal wastes are listed in figure 8-2.

The lists of universal wastes in various states may include these same items along with different wastes.

All universal wastes are hazardous wastes and, without the new rules, would have to be managed under the same stringent standards as other hazardous wastes. Also, universal wastes are generated by a wide variety of sources, in contrast to the industrial businesses that are primarily responsible for the generation of other hazardous wastes.

Additional information about universal wastes can be found on the EPA's Healthcare Environmental Resource Center website.[9]

MEDICAL WASTE

Different federal agencies refer to waste derived from humans and animals variously as *medical waste, regulated waste, regulated medical waste, biohazardous waste,* or *infectious medical waste.* For example, OSHA Standard 29 CFR 1910.1030, Bloodborne pathogens [CD-ROM 8.7], uses the term *regulated waste* and the EPA uses the term *regulated medical waste.* These seemingly different designations refer to the same materials. In addition to this confusion at the federal level, most states have their own regulations and definitions. In this chapter, these wastes are referred to as *medical waste.*

Medical waste is the portion of the waste stream that may be contaminated by blood, body fluids, or other potentially infectious materials, thus posing a significant risk of transmitting infection.

Although not specifically regulated by the EPA, medical waste requires special handling. Its treatment and disposal are subject to state regulations, which require the medical waste to be rendered noninfectious before it can be disposed of as solid waste. These wastes are also referred to as *red-bag* or *infectious* wastes, and it is estimated they cost about $800 per ton to dispose of; general waste, in comparison, costs about $60 per ton.[10]

Medical waste is unique to the health care sector and presents a number of compliance challenges. Unlike many regulations that apply to health care, most regulations governing medical waste are defined at the state rather than the federal level. Compounding the complexity, the authority for medical waste rules often lies with multiple agencies at the state level.

Who Regulates What?

The state agencies involved in medical waste regulation generally include:

- ☐ State health departments, which are typically responsible for defining what categories of waste are regulated and delineating the acceptable treatment/disinfection methods
- ☐ State environmental agencies, which are typically responsible for outlining requirements related to the labeling, storage, transportation, and end disposal of medical waste

The specific division of responsibilities can vary from state to state. Although state agencies typically assume primary responsibility for developing and enforcing the regulations that apply to most health care facilities, federal agencies can also play a role in overseeing medical waste management:

- ☐ The Centers for Disease Control and Prevention (CDC) issues guidelines for infection control.
- ☐ The Occupational Safety and Health Administration (OSHA) issues and enforces rules protecting workers who handle medical waste.
- ☐ The U.S. Department of Transportation (DOT) regulates issues such as packaging and labeling medical waste for shipment.

The defined categories of medical waste and the methods used to treat and process medical waste provide a quantitative system for its general handling. The revisions resulting from the Medical Waste Tracking Act are intended to protect the health and safety of the public, as well as those individuals within and outside health care facilities who must manage medical waste. The quantity, as well as the quality, of the waste must be considered in determining if it should be designated as medical waste.

Types of Medical Waste

Six categories exist within the general classification of medical waste:[11]

Pathology and anatomy wastes
Bulk human blood, blood products, bulk body fluids, or other potentially infectious material

Microbiological waste
Sharps
Wastes from highly communicable diseases
Animal wastes

Pathology and Anatomy Wastes

Definition: All human anatomical wastes and all wastes that consist of human tissues, organs, or body parts removed by trauma or during surgery, autopsy, studies, or another hospital procedure and that is intended for disposal.

It is important to understand the distinction between anatomical and pathological waste. While both are wastes derived from the human body, pathological wastes are unique in that these are typically samples of tissues that are examined in a laboratory setting to understand the nature of the disease or affliction from which a patient suffers. For the most part, pathological waste refers to very small tissue sections and body materials derived from biopsies or surgical procedures that are then examined in the laboratory. Anatomical wastes are typically distinguished as recognizable human organs, tissue, and body parts, and may require special treatment under state regulations.

Some states do not consider hair, teeth, and nails to be pathological/anatomical waste.

Bulk Human Blood, Blood Products, Bulk Body Fluids, or Other Potentially Infectious Material (OPIM, as defined by OSHA)

Definition: Bulk waste human blood, human blood components, products derived from blood (including serum, plasma, and other blood components), or bulk human body fluids as defined by OSHA to include semen, vaginal secretions, cerebrospinal fluid, synovial fluid, pleural fluid, pericardial fluid, peritoneal fluid, amniotic fluid, saliva in dental procedures, any body fluid that is visually contaminated with blood, and all body fluids in a situation where it is difficult or impossible to differentiate between body fluids.

This category includes samples of these fluids taken in hematology laboratories, as well as drainage from surgery, and urine or feces when visibly contaminated by blood.

Microbiological Waste

Definition: Cultures and stocks of infectious agents, and associated microorganisms and biologicals; discarded cultures, culture dishes, and devices used to transfer, inoculate, and mix cultures, stocks, specimens, live and attenuated vaccines, and associated items if they are suspected to contain organisms likely to be pathogenic to healthy humans; discarded etiologic agents and wastes from the production of biologicals and antibiotics that may have been contaminated by organisms likely to be pathogenic to healthy humans; and waste originating from clinical or research laboratory procedures involving communicable infectious agents.

Note: Microbiological waste that is also considered a *sharp,* as defined next, should be managed first and foremost as a "sharp." It is also important to note what materials the facility's laboratory is working with, as there are special guidelines from the CDC on how to handle infectious microorganisms at biosafety level (BSL) 3 and BSL 4. Recent federal regulations require health care facility laboratories to maintain the capability of destroying discarded cultures and stocks on-site if these laboratories isolate from a clinical specimen any microorganism or toxin identified as a *select agent* from a clinical specimen.[12,13]

Sharps

Definition: Items that can induce subdermal inoculation of infectious agents or that can easily penetrate the skin or puncture waste bags and cardboard boxes; objects capable of penetrating the skin that have been used or are intended to be used in human or animal care, medical research, or industrial laboratories, including hypodermic needles, syringes, Pasteur pipettes, capillary tubes, and broken glass from the laboratory, including slides and slide covers, razor blades, and scalpel blades.

Sharps require special handling and packaging under both OSHA and DOT specifications. To avoid confusion, the state's guidelines should be consulted in identifying which items are classified as sharps.

Wastes from Highly Communicable Diseases

Definition: Biological waste and discarded materials contaminated with blood, excretion, exudates, or secretion from humans or animals isolated to protect others from highly communicable diseases (Lassa fever virus, Marburg virus, monkey pox virus, Ebola virus, and others).

Animal Waste

Definition: Animal carcasses, body parts, bedding, and related wastes that may have been exposed to infectious agents during research, production of biologicals, or testing of pharmaceuticals.

Managing Medical Waste through Universal Precautions

According to the CDC and OSHA, *universal precautions* refers to an infection control system based on the assumption that any direct contact with a patient, particularly with body fluids, has the potential for transmitting disease. This type of system resulted from the heightened awareness and concern over the potential risk of transmitting human immunodeficiency virus (HIV) and hepatitis B (HBV) and other bloodborne pathogens to health care providers. Thus, "universal precautions" denotes a qualitative system designed to ensure the safety of the individual health care provider. Contact with any body fluid, regardless of the quantity, is considered a potential source of infectious agents.

The following description provides clarification of the application of universal precautions in relation to the handling and disposal of tubing used in patient care:

> The critical factors for determining if the tubing used in patient care should be considered as medical waste are: (1) direct contact with any of the fluids identified by OSHA as being possible sources of transmission of infectious agents, and (2) the quantities of these fluids. OSHA has defined human body fluids as semen, vaginal secretions, pleural fluid, cerebrospinal fluid, synovial fluid, pericardial fluid, amniotic fluid, saliva in dental procedures, any body fluid visibly contaminated with blood, and all body fluids in situations where it is difficult or impossible to differentiate between body fluids.[14]

Conversely, feces, urine, and vomitus are not included unless they contain visible blood. For tubing to be designated as medical waste, it would have to have been in contact with those fluids listed by OSHA. For example, tubing used in gastrointestinal procedures that is visibly coated with body fluids should be discarded as medical waste.

OSHA Standard for Bloodborne Pathogens

In 1991 OSHA promulgated Standard 29 CFR 1910.1030, Bloodborne pathogens (BBP). This standard is designed to protect approximately 5.6 million workers in health care and related occupations from the risk of exposure to bloodborne pathogens such as HIV and HBV.

The BBP standard has numerous requirements, including the development of an exposure control plan. The standard also includes rules specific to medical waste. EPA's Healthcare Environmental Resource Center provides the following summary of OSHA's BBP standard relating to medical waste.[15]

Definitions

Exposure Control Plan   The exposure control plan is the employer's written program that outlines the protective measures an employer will take to eliminate or minimize employee exposure to contaminated blood and other potentially infectious materials (OPIM).

The exposure control plan must contain at a minimum:

□ An exposure determination that identifies job classifications and, in some cases, tasks and procedures to be followed when there is occupational exposure to blood and OPIM

□ Procedures for evaluating the circumstances surrounding an exposure incident

□ A schedule of how and when other provisions of the standard will be implemented, including methods of compliance, communication of hazards to employees, and recordkeeping

OSHA's Meaning of "Regulated Waste" The BBP standard uses the term *regulated waste* to refer to the following categories of waste:

□ Liquid or semi-liquid blood or other potentially infectious materials (OPIM)

□ Items contaminated with blood or OPIM and that would release these substances in a liquid or semi-liquid state if compressed

□ Items that are caked with dried blood or OPIM and are capable of releasing these materials during handling

□ Contaminated sharps

□ Pathological and microbiological wastes containing blood or OPIM

This chapter refers to these wastes as "medical waste."

It is the employer's responsibility to determine the existence of medical waste. This determination should not be based on the actual volume of blood, but rather on the potential to release blood (e.g., when compacted in the waste container). If an OSHA inspector determines that sufficient evidence of medical waste exists, either through observation (e.g., a pool of liquid in the bottom of a container, dried blood flaking off during handling) or based on employee interviews, citations may be issued.

OSHA has provided some additional guidance for the determination of medical waste. Bandages that are not saturated to the point of releasing blood or OPIM if compressed would not be considered medical waste. Similarly, discarded feminine hygiene products do not normally meet the criteria for medical waste as defined by the standard. Beyond these guidelines, it is the employer's responsibility to determine the existence of medical waste.

Management of Sharps Containers

1. *How should sharps containers be handled?*

Each sharps container must either be labeled with the universal biohazard symbol and the word *biohazard* or be color-coded red. Sharps containers must be maintained upright throughout their use, be replaced routinely, and not be allowed to overfill. Also, the containers:

□ Must be closed immediately before removal or replacement to prevent spillage or protrusion of contents during handling, storage, transport, or shipping.
□ Must be placed in a secondary container, if leakage is possible. The second container:
  ▪ Must be closable.
  ▪ Must be constructed to contain all contents and prevent leakage during handling, storage, transport, or shipping.
□ Must be labeled or color-coded according to the standard.
□ Must not be opened, emptied, or cleaned manually or in any other manner that would expose employees to the risk of percutaneous injury, if containers are reusable.
□ Must be closed with an impenetrable lid that is securely sealed (e.g., with duct tape).

2. *Where should sharps containers be located?*

Sharps containers must be easily accessible to employees and located as closely as possible to the immediate area where sharps are used (e.g., patient care areas).

In areas such as psychiatric units, there may be a problem with placing sharps containers in the immediate use area. If a mobile cart is used in these areas, an alternative would be to lock the sharps container inside the cart.

3. *What type of container should be purchased for the disposal of sharps?*

Sharps containers are made of a variety of products, from cardboard to plastic. As long as they meet the definition of a sharps container (i.e., must be closable, puncture resistant, leak proof on sides and bottom, and labeled or color-coded), OSHA would consider them to be of an acceptable composition.

Disposal Requirements

1. *How should disposal of medical waste be handled?*

Disposal of all medical waste must be in accordance with applicable state regulations. State environmental agencies and/or state departments of health typically publish these rules.

In addition to state rules for disposal of medical waste, there are basic OSHA requirements that protect workers. Medical waste must be placed in containers that are:

- □ Closable
- □ Constructed to contain all contents and prevent leakage of fluids during handling, storage, transport, or shipping
- □ Labeled or color-coded in accordance with the standard
- □ Closed before removal to prevent spillage or protrusion of contents during handling, storage, transport, or shipping
- □ Placed in a second container meeting the OSHA requirements, if outside contamination of the medical waste container has occurred

OSHA has no specific requirement for hospitals or other health care facilities to treat (e.g., autoclave) waste before disposal. Such rules are usually published by state agencies.

Communication of Hazard to Employees

1. When are labels required?

A warning label that includes the universal biohazard symbol, followed by the term *biohazard*, must be included on bags or containers of medical waste, on bags or containers of contaminated laundry, on refrigerators and freezers that are used to store blood or OPIM, and on bags or containers used to store, dispose of, transport, or ship blood or OPIM (e.g., specimen containers). In addition, contaminated equipment that is to be serviced or shipped must have a readily observable label that uses the biohazard symbol and the word *biohazard* along with a statement detailing what portions of the equipment remain contaminated.

2. What are the required colors for the labels?

The background of the label must be fluorescent orange or orange-red, or predominantly so, with symbols and lettering in a contrasting color. The label must be either an integral part of the container or affixed as close as feasible to the container by a string, wire, adhesive, or other method to prevent its loss or unintentional removal.

3. Can there be substitutes for the labels?

Yes. Red bags or red containers may be substituted for the biohazard labels.

4. What are the exceptions to the labeling requirement?

Labeling is not required for:

☐ Medical waste that has been decontaminated.
☐ Containers of blood, blood components, and blood products bearing an FDA-required label that have been released for transfusion or other clinical uses.
☐ Individual containers of blood or OPIM that are placed in secondary labeled containers during storage, transport, shipment, or disposal.
☐ Specimen containers, if the facility uses universal precautions when handling all specimens, the containers are recognizable as holding specimens, and the containers remain within the facility (see the following discussion concerning specimen bags).
☐ Laundry bags or containers containing contaminated laundry, which may be marked with an alternative label or color-coded, provided the facility uses universal precautions for handling all soiled laundry and the alternative marking permits all employees to recognize the containers as requiring compliance with universal precautions. If contaminated laundry is sent off-site to a facility that does not use universal precautions in the handling of all soiled laundry, it must be placed in a bag or container that is red in color or identified by the biohazard label described above.

5. What special procedures are required for specimen bags?

Some health care facilities use plastic bags to transport specimen containers from patient care areas to in-house laboratories. The facilities label the plastic bag "biohazard" and dispose of the plastic bag as infectious waste.

If not contaminated, the plastic transport bags are not considered infectious waste and may be disposed of as solid waste. However, if the bags are labeled "biohazard," there is the risk that the solid waste hauler will refuse to transport the waste because of the belief that the bags contain materials that are infectious.

Biohazard-labeled plastic bags used as secondary containment for internal transport of specimens are not required by OSHA. The labeling exemption, listed in OSHA's Bloodborne pathogens standard (29 CFR 1910. 1030(d)(2)(xii)(A)), applies to facilities that handle all specimens with universal precautions, provided the containers are recognizable as holding specimens. The exemption applies only while these specimens remain within the facility. If the specimens leave the facility, a label or red color coding is required. In addition, secondary containers or bags are required only if the primary container is contaminated on the outside.

6. *Does OSHA accept the DOT labels for waste and specimens to be shipped or transported?*

OSHA's labeling requirements do not preempt either the U.S. Postal Service labeling requirements (39 CFR Part III) or the DOT Hazardous Materials Regulations (49 CFR Parts 171–181).

DOT labeling is required on some transport containers (i.e., those containing "known infectious substances"). It is not required on all containers for which the BBP standard requires the biohazard label. Where there is an overlap between the OSHA-mandated label and the DOT-required label, the DOT label will be considered acceptable on the outside of the transport container provided the OSHA-mandated label appears on any internal containers that may be present. Containers serving as collection receptacles within a facility must bear the OSHA label, since these are not covered by the DOT requirements.

How Medical Waste Can Harm Humans

Pathogens in medical waste may enter the human body by a number of routes, including:

- ☐ Punctures, abrasions, or cuts in the skin
- ☐ Mucous membranes
- ☐ Inhalation
- ☐ Ingestion

There is particular concern about infection with HIV, HBV, or HCV (hepatitis C virus), for which there is strong evidence of transmission via health care waste. These viruses are generally transmitted through injuries from syringe needles contaminated by human blood.

The existence in health care facilities of bacteria resistant to antibiotics and chemical disinfectants may also contribute to the hazards created by poorly managed health care waste. It has been demonstrated, for example, that plasmids from laboratory strains contained in health care waste have been transferred to indigenous bacteria via the waste disposal system. Moreover, antibiotic-resistant *Escherichia coli* were shown to have survived in an activated sludge plant, although there seems to be no significant transfer of this organism under normal conditions of wastewater disposal and treatment.

Concentrated cultures of pathogens and contaminated sharps (particularly hypodermic needles) are probably the waste items that represent the most acute potential hazards to health.

Sharps may not only cause cuts and punctures but also infect these wounds if the sharps are contaminated with pathogens. Sharps carry a double risk of injury and disease transmission. The principal concern is with infections that may be transmitted by subcutaneous introduction of the causative agent (e.g., viral blood infections). Hypodermic needles constitute an important part of the sharps waste category and are particularly hazardous because they are often contaminated with patients' blood.

RADIOACTIVE WASTE

Radiopharmaceuticals—therapeutic drugs that contain radioactive material—are important in the diagnosis and treatment of many diseases. They can be injected into the body, inhaled, or taken orally as medicines or to enable the imaging of internal organs and bodily processes.

Radioactive (radionuclide) waste includes solid, liquid, and gaseous materials contaminated with radionuclides. It is produced as a result of procedures such as in vitro analysis of body tissue and fluid, in vivo organ imaging and tumor localization, and various other investigative and therapeutic practices.

Radionuclides continuously undergo spontaneous disintegration (known as radioactive decay), a process in which energy is liberated. The emissions resulting from radioactive decay are classified according to the energy associated with their release and include alpha, beta, and gamma radiation. Depending on the energy level of the radioactive waste, it can cause transformation of intracellular material. For example, DNA can be altered as a result of such radiation, which is therefore considered to be genotoxic (i.e., harmful to genetic material). X-ray, used for imaging of bones, is a high-energy radiation that does not produce radioactive waste. The decay of radioactive material may occur in fractions of a second or may take millions of years. The time it takes for the amount of radioactivity to decrease by one-half is called the *half-life.* Radionuclides with long half-lives, such as those used in therapeutic procedures, are a particular problem in the health care facility waste stream. However, some radionuclides with long half-lives in solid form can be sterilized and reused.

The majority of radioactive waste generated in hospitals is considered low-level radioactive waste (LLRW) and is treated as such by the Nuclear Regulatory Commission (NRC), which regulates about 4,900 licenses for their possession and use of radioactive materials. [CD-ROM 8.8] The NRC also has agreements with 32 states that have accepted responsibility for licensing. The NRC Office of Nuclear Material Safety and Safeguards (ONMSS) has overall responsibility for the NRC radioactive waste regulation program. The ONMSS has four regional offices (Region 1—Northeast, Region II—Southeast, Region III—Midwest, and Region IV—West/Southwest).

The NRC and the agreement states manage the disposal of radioactive waste. The NRC considers the contaminated items listed in figure 8-3 to be low-level radioactive waste.[16] [CD-ROM 8.9]

Hospitals typically keep their waste stored in special containers or separate rooms that have been posted to identify them as radioactive waste storage areas. Low-level radioactive waste may be stored safely for short periods

Figure 8–3. NRC Items Designated as Low-Level Radioactive Waste

---

   □ Protective shoe covers and clothing
   □ Wiping rags, mops, and filters
   □ Luminous dials
   □ Medical tubes
   □ Swabs
   □ Injection needles and syringes
   □ Laboratory animal carcasses
   □ Tissues

---

while it decays, before its disposal in the common waste stream. However, the NRC prefers that it be disposed immediately rather than stored.

Low-level waste may be stored to allow short-lived radionuclides to decay to innocuous levels and for safekeeping when access to disposal sites is not available. The NRC believes storage can be safe over the short term as an interim measure but favors disposal rather than storage over the long term. Radioactive waste must be transported in containers approved by the DOT.

Types of radioactive waste produced by health care facilities include:

   □ Sealed sources
   □ Spent radionuclide generators
   □ Low-level solid waste (e.g., absorbent paper, swabs, glassware, syringes, and vials)
   □ Residues from shipments of radioactive material and unwanted solutions of radionuclides intended for diagnostic or therapeutic use
   □ Liquids immiscible with water, such as liquid scintillation-counting residues used in radioimmunoassay, and contaminated pump oil
   □ Waste from spills and from decontamination of radioactive spills
   □ Excreta from patients treated or tested with unsealed radionuclides
   □ Low-level liquid waste (e.g., from washing apparatus)
   □ Gases and exhausts from stores and fume cupboards

WASTE MANAGEMENT PLANNING

An effective waste management campaign requires administrative commitment, careful planning, and the cooperation of all employees. Formulation of objectives and planning for their achievement are important for improving waste management in health care facilities. Planning requires the definition of a strategy that will facilitate careful implementation of the necessary measures and the appropriate allocation of resources to achieve program goals. By implementing a waste management program, health care facilities move toward the achievement of a healthy and safe environment for their employees and communities. At a minimum, the waste management plan should include:

> Administrative commitment
> A survey of current waste practices
> Policy and guidelines development
> Adoption of "best practices"
> Training
> Periodic program review

Administrative Commitment

As is the case with all organizational initiatives, unless the administration is committed to the goals and policy, the program cannot achieve complete success. Policy commitment must be reflected in appropriate budgetary allocation.

Survey of Current Waste Practices

A comprehensive survey is essential for planning an effective waste management program. [CD-ROM 8.10] The Environmental Health and Safety Department should complete a wide-ranging questionnaire for the facility, to establish the following:

- □ Number of beds and bed occupancy rate
- □ Types and quantities of waste generated
- □ Personnel involved in the management of waste
- □ Current disposal practices, including segregation, collection, transportation, storage, and disposal methods
- □ Cost associated with the segregation, collection, transportation, storage, and disposal methods
- □ Management and employee responsibilities
- □ Recordkeeping and documentation
- □ Training requirements
- □ State and federal regulations that affect the handling of waste

Policy and Guidelines Development

Guidelines are based on the results of the survey and must be supported by regulations. Their content should provide the technical foundation on which the facility can build its waste management program. A program with specific and realistic goals should be developed, endorsed by the administration, and circulated to all employees. The policy document and guidelines should include the following:

- □ Descriptions of health and safety risks that result from mismanagement of health care waste
- □ Objectives of the program
- □ Rules governing the protection of employees, patients, and visitors
- □ Listing of the facility's approved methods of treatment and disposal for each waste category
- □ Warnings against unsafe practices, such as disposing of hazardous waste in municipal landfills
- □ Management and employee responsibilities
- □ Assessment of the costs of health care waste management in the facility
- □ Key steps of the facility's program, such as identification, handling, separation, treatment, disposal, and minimization
- □ Methods of recordkeeping and documentation
- □ Training requirements

Adoption of "Best Practices"

There are several organizations and cooperative programs that are actively involved in health care waste management, including:

- □ Hospitals for a Healthy Environment (H2E)[17]
- □ Healthcare Environmental Resource Center (HERC)[18]
- □ Sustainable Hospitals[19]
- □ Health Care Without Harm[20]
- □ Kentucky Pollution Prevention Center[21]

These organizations offer a great deal of information, including results of recent research that can help health care facilities reduce their waste streams and save money.

Training

To achieve acceptable practices in health care waste management and compliance with regulations, department heads, Environmental Health and Safety department liaisons, and other involved personnel must receive the appropriate training.

Periodic Program Review

The program should be viewed as a continuous process and thus requires periodic monitoring and assessment. In addition, recommendations on disposal and treatment methods should be updated regularly to keep pace with new developments.

The assessment should be based on Health and Safety Committee reports on the level of success in implementing the plan. It should include a review of reports submitted by departments and random audits of the waste management system. Any deficiencies should be identified in writing, together with recommendations for corrective measures. The time limit for implementation of corrective measures should be specified and the report summary should be included in the annual report to the administration.

Periodic review of the facility's waste management practices should result in improved protection of employees, patients, and the public and in enhanced cost-effectiveness of waste disposal.

WASTE MINIMIZATION

In recent years, many health care facilities have joined in a cooperative program called Hospitals for a Healthy Environment (H2E). H2E is an outgrowth of a 1998 Memorandum of Understanding (MOU) between the American Hospital Association (AHA) (joined by Health Care Without Harm) and the EPA. The MOU listed 11 action items, among which were "Virtual Elimination of Mercury Waste" and "Total Waste Volume Reduction." The latter action item called for a 33 percent reduction in total waste by 2005 and the goal of a 50 percent reduction by 2010. The H2E website[22] contains a significant amount of information about successful waste minimization practices that have saved hospitals thousands of dollars annually.

Careful management of departments will prevent the accumulation of large quantities of outdated chemicals or pharmaceuticals and limit waste to the packaging (i.e., boxes and bottles) plus residues of the products remaining in the containers. These small amounts of chemical or pharmaceutical waste can be disposed of easily and relatively cheaply, whereas disposing of larger amounts requires costly and specialized treatment—emphasizing the importance of waste minimization.[23] [CD-ROM 8.11]

Waste minimization benefits the health care facility. Costs both for the purchase of goods and for waste treatment and disposal are reduced and the liabilities associated with the disposal of hazardous waste are lessened. All employees have a role to play in this process and should be trained in waste minimization.

Suppliers of chemicals and pharmaceuticals can also become responsible partners in waste minimization programs. The facility can encourage this by ordering only from suppliers who provide rapid delivery of small orders and who accept the return of unopened stock.

Reducing the toxicity of waste also reduces the problems associated with its treatment or disposal. For example, in some cases polyvinyl chloride (PVC)–free plastics can be purchased that may be recycled, and goods can be supplied without unnecessary packaging.

Significant reduction of the waste generated in health care facilities may be encouraged by the implementation of certain policies and practices, including the following:

> Source reduction
> Recycling
> Waste segregation
> Secure and safe storage
> Waste conversion
> Pollution prevention

Source Reduction

Source reduction includes buying products that use less packaging and thereby eliminate the use of unnecessary items, working with vendors to reduce packaging, and obtaining items in bulk packages with minimal packaging or in returnable packages. Other measures include utilizing reusable items instead of disposable ones, such as cloth gowns rather than disposable paper gowns. One hospital saved a substantial amount of money by switching from powdered laundry detergent to liquid, which could be metered.

Recycling

A recycling campaign will effectively reduce the amount of waste sent to landfills. Paper products can be recycled, as can aluminum cans and nonhazardous glass containers. Medical and other equipment used in the facility may be reused, provided it has been designed for that purpose. Reusable items may include certain sharps, such as scalpels and hypodermic needles, syringes, glass bottles, and containers. After use, these items should be segregated from non-reusable items, carefully washed, and sterilized. Long-term radionuclides conditioned as pins, needles, or seeds and used for radiotherapy may also be reused after sterilization. Plastic syringes and catheters should be discarded.

Other, nonroutine methods of recycling that can result in savings for the facility include the recovery of silver from fixing baths used in processing x-ray films. Purchasing stills for recovering formalin and alcohols has been shown to result in significant savings by reducing the amount spent on purchasing new chemicals and on their disposal. For example, a hospital in Michigan has saved more than $45,000 a year in its Pathology Department by recycling formalin. In determining the economic viability of recycling, consider the costs of alternative disposal methods and not just the cost of the recycling process and the value of the reclaimed material.

Waste Segregation

Waste segregation is a major component of any waste minimization effort in the health care facility. Appropriate handling, treatment, and disposal of waste by type reduces costs and protects public health. Combining nonhazardous with hazardous waste may increase the amount of hazardous waste subject to regulation, as it can cause the whole batch to become hazardous. Mixing waste can also make recycling difficult, if not impossible. One successful method of waste segregation requires identifying the categories of waste and then properly sorting waste into color-coded bins, plastic bags, or containers. Although this method requires a significant training effort, it will reduce "red-bag" waste and thus the overall cost of disposal. In addition to the color coding of waste containers, the following practices are recommended:

- ☐ Appropriate containers or bag holders should be placed in all locations where particular categories of waste may be generated.
- ☐ Instructions on waste separation and identification should be posted at each waste collection point to remind staff of the procedures.
- ☐ Staff should never attempt to correct errors of segregation by removing items from a bag or container after disposal or by placing one bag inside another bag of a different color.

Secure and Safe Storage

Expensive cleanup costs can be avoided by preventing spills or leaks. Hazardous products and waste containers should be stored in secure areas and inspected frequently for leaks. When leaks or spills occur, the materials used to clean them up also become hazardous.

Waste Conversion

Waste conversionis the process of converting some medical waste to general waste to avoid incineration. Several methods have been introduced in recent years, including autoclaving, shredding with autoclaving, and microwave treatment.

Pollution Prevention

Health care waste management policies have come under increasing scrutiny as facilities have become bigger contributors of pollution to the environment. Among the pollution problems facing health care facilities are the growing use of disposable products and the quality of wastewater and incinerator emissions. By implementing pollution prevention techniques, health care facilities can save money and reduce liability.

Benefits of Pollution Prevention

There are many benefits to pollution prevention, including the following, presented by the Kentucky Pollution Prevention Center:[24]

- ☐ Protection of human health and wildlife through reduction of occupational exposures and releases of hazardous materials to the air, water, and land from wastewater discharges, spills, landfilling, or incineration
- ☐ Avoidance of the costs associated with the use of hazardous materials, such as disposal or recycling, collection and storage prior to disposal, paperwork for tracking hazardous waste disposal, training and equipment for spill response, training for hospital employees who handle hazardous materials, and liability for environmental problems or worker exposure
- ☐ Avoidance of increased regulation in the future
- ☐ Increased public awareness of the dangers of hazardous materials through publicity about the facility's program
- ☐ Enhancement of the positive public image of the health care facility due to publicity about success stories

Pollution Prevention Techniques

In addition to other measures outlined in this section, the following activities will reduce the volume of waste generated by the health care facility, which in turn will reduce disposal costs. Creativity and effort can lead to impressive reductions in waste generation. The Kentucky Pollution Prevention Center provides examples of ideas in figure 8-4.[25]

Products found in health care facilities that contain PVC include intravenous tubing, ID bracelets, blood bags, IV bags, vinyl gloves, and sharps containers. Products found in health care facilities that contain latex include adhesive bandages, disposable syringes, catheters, surgical gloves, and blood pressure cuff and tubing. Mercury can also be released into wastewater and into the atmosphere by spills and improper disposal techniques. In addition, sensitivity to latex is a growing problem, and severe reactions can induce shock. Although products containing mercury are recyclable, those containing PVC and latex are not. Therefore, to eliminate or minimize these problems, facilities can purchase products that contain no mercury, PVC, or latex. Some products have no alternatives that are free of these materials, but there may be alternatives that contain less of the material. For example, all fluorescent lamps contain mercury, but manufacturers are now producing lamps that contain less mercury and work just as well. Vendors can be consulted for specific information.

Figure 8–4. Examples of Pollution Prevention Techniques

☐ Reduce the amount of waste being generated. The less trash sent to the landfill or incinerator, the less the facility pays for disposal. Additionally, less effort is required for preventing pollution in the facility when less waste is being produced.

☐ Make certain that only pathological waste (tissues and organs) are being incinerated. Health care facilities must incinerate pathological wastes to prevent the spread of pathogens, but alternative forms of treatment are available for other infectious wastes. Also, make certain that no products containing mercury or PVC are incinerated. When incinerated, PVC can form dioxins and mercury-containing products release mercury vapor to the atmosphere.

☐ Recycle. Recycling diverts waste materials from the landfill and is a possible source of income. Recycling is not limited to items such as aluminum cans and plastic bottles from vending machines. Mercury-containing products are recyclable, and by recycling them the possibility of releasing mercury to the environment is diminished.

☐ Sort wastes properly. If a patient does not finish a meal or if a tongue depressor falls on the floor, place the waste in the general trash, not in a red biohazardous waste bag. If a recycling program is started, make certain all containers for the recyclables are marked correctly and that employees are told what materials are and are not being recycled.

☐ Eliminate the use of unnecessary items. If any materials or supplies are not necessary, eliminate the use of those products.

☐ Work with vendors to reduce packaging. Try to obtain items in bulk packages with minimal packaging or in returnable packages to reduce the amount of waste being landfilled or recycled.

☐ Choose reusable items instead of disposable ones whenever possible. While disposable syringes are a must in any modern health care facility, disposable paper gowns are not. Use cloth gowns instead.

☐ Reuse items whenever possible. Cardboard, foam peanuts, pallets, solvents, and other items can be reused several times before disposal is needed.

☐ Use and maintain durable equipment and supplies. Less expensive items may be more attractive initially, but quality, durability, and the costs associated with maintenance, disposal, and replacement should be considered.

☐ Find suitable alternatives for products containing mercury, PVC, and latex. Mercury vapor and dioxins can be generated by incinerating mercury-containing products and PVC products, respectively.

☐ Switch to double-sided copying. Less paper and less storage area will be needed, and less packaging waste will be generated.

THE JOINT COMMISSION'S WASTE MANAGEMENT REQUIREMENTS

The Joint Commission standard on hazardous materials and waste management (EC.3.10) requires that health care facilities manage their hazardous materials and waste risks by identifying the materials that require special handling and implementing processes to minimize the risks associated with their unsafe use and improper disposal. Though federal and state agencies distinguish between hazardous waste and medical waste, the Joint Commission makes no such distinction. The Joint Commission requires health care facilities to create and maintain an inventory that identifies hazardous materials and waste using criteria that are consistent with applicable laws and regulations.

Joint Commission standards on safety management (EC.1.10), monitoring environmental conditions (EC.9.10), initial job training (HR.2.10), and ongoing education (HR.2.30) all contain elements that can be applied to managing hazardous health care waste.

THE ROLE OF THE ENVIRONMENTAL HEALTH AND SAFETY DEPARTMENT

Our young friend, Sarah, created a terrible problem for herself, her family, and her neighbors because she "simply would not take the garbage out." Once she had decided that it was time, she was confronted with a terrible dilemma. First, there was just too much for one little girl to handle. Second, there was a tremendous mix of food, paper, cans, glass, and all the other things left over from the process of living that needed to be sorted. Some of Sarah's waste could go directly to the local dump, but some of it most certainly could have been recycled, and perhaps some of her waste may have required special handling. Sarah also might have spent some time thinking about how to reduce the amount of waste that she was producing.

The health care facility is also confronted with a significant waste problem that should not be addressed by just one department. In the model program presented in this book, the Environmental Health and Safety Department directs responsibilities for Subtitle C. The Environmental Health and Safety Department also serves as the coordinating organizational component for the handling of medical waste. However, the proper handling of waste in the health care facility requires the participation of every department. The Environmental Health and Safety department liaisons are in the best position to understand the waste activities in their particular department and to work with the Environmental Health and Safety Department to develop a waste management plan that includes:

> ☐ Conducting a waste audit to evaluate the facility's purchasing and waste management practices. This evaluation should include a survey of current practices and suggest improvements. Follow-up audits should be performed to ensure that changes are implemented.

The process should gain support of employees and identify how the survey will be conducted, and a report must be written.

☐ Consulting state and federal regulatory agencies, such as the EPA and OSHA, to determine the appropriate regulations regarding disposal and employee health and safety issues.

☐ Evaluating the awareness and knowledge of employees regarding such matters as the hazards of handling various types of waste and handling of toxic substances.

☐ Soliciting input from employees for improving waste handling.

Currently, there are many organizations that are working to find solutions to handling health care waste, to prevent the inappropriate mixing of the various types of waste, and to reduce the amount of waste that is produced. The Environmental Health and Safety Department, in coordination with the Purchasing, Housekeeping, and Engineering departments, should take the lead in identifying innovative practices for reducing and recycling waste that will cut the health care facility's waste handling expenses.

References

1. Silverstein, Shel. *Where the Sidewalk Ends: The Poems and Drawings of Shel Silverstein.* New York: HarperCollins Children's Books.

2. Who International. *Safe Management of Wastes from Health Care Activities.* Available at http://www.who.int/water_sanitation_health/medicalwaste/wastemanag/en/ (accessed 3/14/2006).

3. Veit, Lori. "A Closer Look at Waste Management," *Housekeeping Solutions* (March 2004). Available at http://www.cleanlink.com/hs/article.asp?id=1156 (accessed 3/14/2006).

4. United States Environmental Protection Agency. Resource Conservation and Recovery Act of 1976 (40 CFR Parts 260–290). Available at http://www.epa.gov/region5/defs/html/rcra.htm (accessed 3/14/2006).

5. Hospitals for a Healthy Environment (H2E). www.h2e-online.org.

6. Allwood, M., and P. Wright, eds. *The Cytotoxic Handbook.* Oxford: Radcliffe Medical Press, 1993.

7. "Safe Management of Wastes from Health Care Activities." Chapter 3 in *Health Impacts of Health-Care Waste.* Geneva: World Health Organization, 1999. Available at http://www.who.int/water_sanitation_health/medicalwaste/wastemanag/en/(accessed 3/14/2006).

8. www.epa.gov.

9. Healthcare Environmental Resource Center. www.hercenter.org.

10. Veit, Lori. "A Closer Look at Waste Management," *Housekeeping Solutions* (March 2004). Available at http://www.cleanlink.com/hs/article.asp?id=1156 (accessed 3/14/2006).

11. Healthcare Environmental Resource Center. www.hercenter.org.

12. U.S. Department of Health and Human Services, Office of Inspector General. Possession, Use, and Transfer of Select Agents and Toxins, Interim Final Rule

(42 CFR Part 73), *Federal Register* (December 13, 2002) 67 (240), pp. 76885–76905.

13. U.S. Department of Agriculture, Animal and Plant Health Inspection Service. Agricultural Bioterrorism Protection Act of 2002; Possession, Use, and Transfer of Biological Agents and Toxins, Interim Final Rule (9 CFR Part 121), *Federal Register* (December 13, 2002) 667 (2240), pp. 76907–76938.

14. OSHA. Standard 1910.1030 (1910.1030[b]): *Bloodborne Pathogens.* Available at http://www.osha.gov/pls/oshaweb/owadisp.show_document?p_table=STANDARDS&p_id=10051 (accessed 3/14/2006).

15. Healthcare Environmental Resource Center. www.hercenter.org.

16. U.S. Nuclear Regulatory Commission. *Radioactive Waste: Production, Storage, Disposal.* Available at http://www.nrc.gov/reading-rm/doc-collections/nuregs/brochures/br0216/r2/index.html (accessed 3/14/2006).

17. Hospitals for a Healthy Environment (H2E). www.h2e-online.org.

18. Healthcare Environmental Resource Center. www.hercenter.org.

19. Sustainable Hospitals. www.sustainablehospitals.org.

20. Health Care Without Harm. www.noharm.org.

21. Kentucky Pollution Prevention Center. www.kppc.org.

22. Hospitals for a Healthy Environment (H2E). www.h2e.org.

23. "Waste Minimization, Recycling, and Reuse." Chapter 6 in *Health Impacts of Health-Care Waste.* Geneva: World Health Organization, 1999. Available at http://www.who.int/water_sanitation_health/medicalwaste/058to060.pdf (accessed 3/14/2006).

24. Kentucky Pollution Prevention Center. *Healthcare Pollution Prevention: Benefits of Hospital Pollution Prevention.* Available at http://www.kppc.org/about/services/healthcare.cfm#3 (accessed 3/14/2006).

25. Kentucky Pollution Prevention Center. *Pollution Prevention Techniques.* Available at http://www.kppc.org/about/services/healthcare.cfm#3 (accessed 3/14/2006).

CHAPTER 9

PERSONAL PROTECTIVE EQUIPMENT

Sec. (6)(b)(7) Where appropriate, such standard shall also prescribe suitable protective equipment and control or technological procedures to be used in connection with such hazards. (Occupational Safety and Health Act of 1970)

Sec. (5)(b) Each employee shall comply with occupational safety and health standards and all rules, regulations, and orders issued pursuant to this Act which are applicable to his own actions and conduct. (Occupational Safety and Health Act of 1970)

Imagine a hockey goalie preparing for a game. He slips into hip pads, thigh pads, shoulder pads, shin guards, helmet and face mask, and the thick heavy gloves to protect his hands from the impact of skates, hockey sticks, and, of course, the hard rubber disk flying toward him at bone-crushing speed.

Now imagine that one day he decides it's all too bulky, too uncomfortable, and it just doesn't look good, so he enters the goal wearing only his uniform and skates. In the ideal world of the foolish goalie, an impenetrable barrier between the puck and himself would perpetually protect him. But then there would be no point to the game.

In the workplace, such a barrier would be called an "engineering control." Engineering controls are the preferred method for preventing workers from facing hazardous situations. For example, a laboratory worker who uses solvents on a regular basis most likely uses them in a hood with a dedicated ventilation system that removes the fumes so that the worker has no opportunity to inhale them. Another example is the retractable needle, which eliminates the possibility of a needlestick. Unfortunately, like the barrier between the goalie and the rest of the hockey game, engineering controls are sometimes neither feasible nor practical, so the potentially exposed worker needs to use what is called "personal protective equipment (PPE)." The pads, helmet, gloves, and face mask that the goalie wears are PPE.

Another way to prevent goalie injuries is to simply not have a goalie—but then, once again, there would be no point in playing the game. Removing a person from a potentially hazardous situation is called an "administrative control." For example, a robotic device that takes the place of one or more employees is both an engineering and an administrative control. But just as not having a goalie will prevent injury but also make the game impossible, administrative controls are sometimes not possible.

In health care facilities, if there is no human contact, there is no health care delivery. Humans are needed to draw blood, load trucks, work near hot ovens and grills, and use hazardous chemicals in a variety of locations, including laboratories, surgical suites, and areas where medical equipment is being sterilized. For most of these activities, neither engineering controls nor administrative controls are possible.

Drawing blood without protective gloves, working on a loading dock without safety shoes, being in a room with a highly infectious patient without wearing a respirator, and handling dangerous chemicals without appropriate ventilation and respiratory protection are all equivalent to the hockey player more concerned with comfort and style than with his own personal health and safety.

The Occupational Safety and Health Administration (OSHA) requires that employers protect their employees from workplace hazards that can cause injury through the use of engineering controls, work practice controls, administrative controls, or PPE. This order of controls is referred to as the "hierarchy of control."

When engineering, work practice, and administrative controls are not feasible or do not provide sufficient protection, health care facilities must provide PPE to their employees and make sure they use it. Examples of PPE in health care facilities include gloves, foot and eye protection, hearing protection, hard hats, and respirators. [CD-ROM 9.1]

PPE must not be used as a substitute for engineering, work practice, or administrative controls. To do so would place the burden for protection on the employee and runs contrary to the concept of the hierarchy of controls. Under certain circumstances, PPE can be used in conjunction with these controls to provide the employee with the maximum protection in the workplace.

Department managers must be aware of the hazards in their departments and held accountable for their employees' use of PPE. Departments should use ongoing safety discussions and reminders to motivate employees to wear the PPE required for their jobs. Teaming the correct PPE with a good training program can afford the employee a large measure of safety. PPE can be effective only if the equipment is selected based on its intended use, employees are trained in its use, and the equipment is properly tested, maintained, and worn. Employees share accountability for their protection by wearing the proper PPE for the job and ensuring that it is properly worn. In the final analysis, the best protection comes from an engaged management and workforce committed to sound work practices.

The goal of OSHA-required training is that workers be able to demonstrate proficiency in the proper use of PPE. Although OSHA prescribes in detail the requirements for selecting and wearing PPE and the content of training, they do allow employers to decide how to conduct that training. Regardless of how employers decide to conduct the training, OSHA requires written certification that the training has been successfully completed and that employees have gained proficiency in the use and maintenance of PPE.

American National Standards Institute (ANSI) Standards

When the Occupational Safety and Health Act (OSH Act) was passed, it adopted certain standards from other organizations.

> 29 CFR 1910.6
> Incorporation by reference.
> 1910.6(a)(1)
> The standards of agencies of the U.S. Government, and organizations which are not agencies of the U.S. Government which are incorporated by reference in this part, have the same force and effect as other standards in this part. Only the mandatory provisions (i.e., provisions containing the word "shall" or other mandatory language) of standards incorporated by reference are adopted as standards under the Occupational Safety and Health Act.

OSHA requires that workplaces comply with several ANSI standards involving PPE, which are incorporated by reference as specified in Section 1910.6 or shall be demonstrated by the employer to be equally effective. [CD-ROM 9.2]

OSHA Standards for Personal Protective Equipment

There are several OSHA standards that address PPE. [CD-ROM 9.3] Further, there are several standards for chemicals that require specific PPE and designate when and how it should be used. Figure 9-1 lists examples of OSHA standards that address PPE.

All Environmental Health and Safety staff, as well as affected employees and managers, should become familiar with these standards, their intent, and their PPE requirements.

Figure 9–1. Examples of OSHA Standards Addressing PPE

- 29 CFR 1910.95, Noise exposure
- 29 CFR 1910.120, Hazardous waste operations and emergency response
- 29 CFR 1910 Subpart Q, Welding, cutting, and brazing
- 29 CFR 1910 Subpart Z, Toxic and hazardous substances

General Requirements for PPE (29 CFR 1910.132)

> Protective equipment, including personal protective equipment for eyes, face, head, and extremities, protective clothing, respiratory devices, and protective shields and barriers, shall be provided, used, and maintained in a sanitary and reliable condition wherever it is necessary by reason of hazards of processes or environment, chemical hazards, radiological hazards, or mechanical irritants encountered in a manner capable of causing injury or impairment in the function of any part of the body through absorption, inhalation or physical contact.[1] [CD-ROM 9.4]

OSHA requires employers to ensure that PPE be "provided, used, and maintained in a sanitary and reliable condition wherever it is necessary" to prevent injury. This requirement includes protection of any part of the body from hazards through absorption, inhalation, or physical contact. This standard requires that health care facilities be responsible for the following:

☐ Performing a hazard assessment through written certification of work areas or jobs where hazards are likely to be present.

☐ Providing PPE when the hazard assessment determines there is sufficient cause to require it (see the following note).

☐ Training employees on how to don (put on), doff (remove), adjust, and wear PPE; the limitations of PPE; and how to maintain PPE, including replacing worn or damaged PPE.

☐ Periodically reviewing, updating, and evaluating the effectiveness of the PPE program.

☐ Retraining employees when necessary.

☐ Certifying in writing that training has been carried out and that employees understand it. Each written certification must contain the name of each employee trained and the date(s) of training, and must identify the subject certified.

The standard also requires that employees be responsible for:

☐ Properly wearing PPE
☐ Attending training sessions on PPE
☐ Caring for, cleaning, and maintaining PPE
☐ Informing a supervisor of the need to repair or replace PPE

Note: In most cases, the employer must provide and pay for employee PPE required by the facility and for compliance with the OSHA standards. If the equipment is very personal in nature and is usable by the employees off the job, the matter of payment may be left to the facility or labor-management negotiations, as appropriate. If employees provide their own PPE, it is the employer's responsibility to be certain it is adequate and properly maintained. Figure 9-2

Figure 9–2. OSHA General Industry Standards Requiring the Use of PPE

Standards that Require the Employer to Provide PPE:

1910.28	Safety requirements for scaffolds
1910.66	Powered platforms for building maintenance
1910.67	Vehicle-mounted elevating and rotating work platforms
1910.94	Ventilation
1910.119	Process safety management of highly hazardous chemicals
1910.120	Hazardous waste operations and emergency response
1910.132	General requirements (personal protective equipment)
1910.133	Eye and face protection
1910.135	Occupational foot protection
1910.136	Occupational foot protection
1910.137	Electrical protective devices
1910.138	Hand protection
1910.139	Respiratory protection for *M. tuberculosis*
1910.157	Portable fire extinguishers
1910.160	Fixed extinguishing systems, general
1910.183	Helicopters
1910.218	Forging machines
1910.242	Hand and portable powered tools and equipment, general
1910.243	Guarding of portable power tools
1910.252	General requirements (welding, cutting and brazing)
1910.261	Pulp, paper, and paperboard mills
1910.262	Textiles
1910.268	Telecommunications
1910.269	Electric power generation, transmission and distribution
1910.333	Selection and use of work practices
1910.335	Safeguards for personnel protection
1910.1000	Air contaminants
1910.1003	13 carcinogens, etc.
1910.1017	Vinyl chloride
1910.1029	Coke oven emissions
1910.1043	Cotton dust
1910.1096	Ionizing radiation

Standards that Require the Employer to Provide PPE at No Cost to the Employee:

1910.95	Occupational noise exposure
1910.134	Respiratory protection
1910.146	Permit-required confined spaces
1910.156	Fire brigades
1910.266	Logging operations
1910.1001	Asbestos
1910.1018	Inorganic-Arsenic
1910.1025	Lead
1910.1027	Cadmium
1910.1028	Benzene
1910.1030	Bloodborne pathogens
1910.1044	1,2-Dibromo-3-chloropropane
1910.1045	Acrylonitrile
1910.1047	Ethylene oxide
1910.1048	Formaldehyde
1910.1050	Methylenedianiline
1910.1051	1,3-Butadiene
1910.1052	Methylene chloride
1910.1450	Occupational exposure to chemicals in laboratories

Courtesy U.S. Department of Labor, Occupational Safety and Health Administration. *Personal Protective Equipment*. OSHA 3151-12R. 2003. Available at www.osha.gov.

lists OSHA's general industry standards that require the employer to provide PPE and those that require the employer to provide PPE at no cost to the employee.

Protective Clothing

Health care facilities are required to ensure that their employees wear PPE only for the parts of the body exposed to possible injury. Examples of protective clothing are laboratory coats, coveralls, jackets, aprons, and surgical gowns.

Impermeable or low-permeability gowns should be worn to prevent contact with antineoplastic drugs, ribavirin, and blood or body fluids. Contaminated gowns should be properly stored in the area of use until disposal or until they have been laundered.

Lead aprons are used in health care facilities to protect employees and patients from unnecessary radiation exposure from diagnostic radiology procedures.

In the laboratory, lab coats can be used to protect street clothing against biological or chemical spills, as well as to provide some additional bodily protection. They should be removed before employees leave the work area.

The Centers for Disease Control and Prevention/National Institutes of Health (CDC/NIH) *Biosafety in Microbiological and Biomedical Laboratories* (BMBL) guidelines for biocontainment practices recommend the use of a lab coat, gown, smock, or uniform during work in BSL2 laboratories. They further recommend solid-front or wrap-around gowns, scrub suits, or coveralls.[2]

Eye and Face Protection (29 CFR 1910.133)

> The employer shall ensure that each affected employee uses appropriate eye or face protection when exposed to eye or face hazards from flying particles, molten metal, liquid chemicals, acids or caustic liquids, chemical gases or vapors, or potentially injurious light radiation. (1910.133(a)(1)) [CD-ROM 9.5]

Employees can be exposed to a large number of hazards that pose danger to their eyes and face, such as the following:

□ Flying particles in maintenance or repair shops and construction areas
□ Chemicals in either the liquid or gas phase
□ Potentially infected body fluids
□ Potentially harmful light radiation

This standard requires health care facilities to furnish eye and face protection as appropriate to the hazard to all of the facility's personnel and visitors while they are in hazardous areas.

As is the case with many OSHA PPE standards, an eye protection program includes the following:

- Selection
- Fit testing
- Training
- Inspection
- Maintenance

Someone familiar with the standard and skilled in fitting goggles and safety glasses should perform these tasks. Only qualified optical personnel should fit prescription safety eyewear.

Eye protection must meet the following minimum requirements:

- Provide adequate protection against the particular hazard
- Be reasonably comfortable when worn under the designated conditions
- Fit snugly without interfering with the movements or vision of the wearer
- Be durable
- Be capable of being disinfected
- Be easily cleanable and kept clean and in good repair

Over the years, many types and styles of eye and face wear have been developed to protect against a variety of hazards. These include the following:

- Goggles, which should be worn in situations where there is potential for chemical fumes, splashes, mists, sprays, or dust exposure to the eyes. Chemical goggles form a liquid-proof seal around the eyes, protecting them from splashes.
- Safety glasses with or without side shields. Safety glasses effectively protect the eye from solid materials (dust, chips, and flying objects) but are less effective at protecting the eyes from chemical splashes.
- Full-face shields. Face shields should be worn for highest-impact, full-face protection for spraying, chipping, grinding, and critical chemical hazards or biohazards. Goggles with a face shield are required for handling highly reactive substances or large quantities of hazardous chemicals, corrosives, or radiant energy. Face shields are not a substitute for eye protection. Safety glasses should always be worn with goggles under a face shield.

The lenses of eye protectors must be kept clean. Continuous vision through dirty lenses can cause eyestrain—often an excuse for not wearing the eye protection. Employees should inspect and clean their eye protectors daily with soap and hot water or with a cleaning solution and tissue.

Filtered Lenses

Eye and face protection with filtered lenses is required where there is a potential exposure to injurious light radiation, such as during welding and work with lasers.

ANSI Standards   The design, construction, tests, and use of eye and face protection must be in accordance with ANSI Z87.1-1989 USA, Practice for Occupational and Educational Eye and Face Protection.[3]

Emergency Eyewash Stations

Emergency eyewash stations are also considered vital to a sight protection program and must be provided in all areas where the eyes of an employee may be exposed to corrosive materials. First-aid instructions must be posted in areas where potential eye hazards exist, since any delay in providing immediate aid or an early mistake in dealing with an eye injury can result in lasting damage. The instruction sign must comply with OSHA Standard 29 CFR 1910.145, Specifications for accident prevention signs and tags. [CD-ROM 9.6]

Several OSHA regulations refer to the use of emergency eyewash and shower equipment. The primary regulation is contained in 29 CFR 1910.151, Medical services and first aid, which requires that "where the eyes or body of any person may be exposed to injurious corrosive materials, suitable facilities for quick drenching or flushing of the eyes and body shall be provided within the work area for immediate emergency use." [CD-ROM 9.7]

ANSI Standards   ANSI also has a standard for emergency eyewash and equipment, Z358.1, Emergency Eye Wash and Shower Equipment, but it is not incorporated by reference into OSHA standards. The ANSI standard is intended to serve as a guideline for the proper design, performance, installation, use, and maintenance of emergency equipment.

Respiratory Protection (29 CFR 1910.134)

Respirators are a special class of personal protective equipment and are not governed by OSHA's General requirements for PPE (i.e., 1910.132).

> Respirators shall be provided by the employer when such equipment is necessary to protect the health of the employee. The employer shall provide the respirators, which are applicable and suitable for the purpose intended. The employer shall be responsible for the

establishment and maintenance of a respiratory protection program. (1910.134(a)(2)) [CD-ROM 9.8]

A respirator is a protective device that covers the nose and mouth or the entire face or head to guard the wearer against hazardous atmospheres. When health care employees must work in environments with insufficient oxygen or where harmful dusts, fogs, smokes, mists, fumes, gases, vapors, or sprays are present, they need respirators. These health hazards may cause cancer, lung impairment, other diseases, or death. The need for participation in a respiratory protection program is established through industrial hygiene monitoring.

Respirators have their limitations and are not a substitute for effective engineering and work practice controls. Employees should use respirators for protection from air contaminants only if the use of other hazard control methods is not practical or possible, as in the following situations:

□ Engineering or work practice controls are not technically feasible.
□ Engineering controls are being installed or repaired.
□ In emergencies or other temporary situations.

When it is not possible to use controls to reduce airborne contaminants below their occupational exposure limits, respirator use may be the best or only way to reduce employee exposure. In cases where work practices and engineering controls alone cannot keep exposure concentrations below the occupational exposure limit, respirator use is essential.[4] [CD-ROM 9.9]

Before choosing respirators, health care facilities must have a written respirator program that describes the proper procedures for their selection, use, and maintenance. Without a complete respiratory protection program, employees are not likely to receive the best protection from a respirator even if it is the correct choice for a specific job. A respiratory protection program has several elements, including the following:

□ A qualified program administrator
□ Hazard identification and control
□ Exposure assessment
□ Selection of an appropriate respirator approved by the National Institute for Occupational Safety and Health (NIOSH)[5] [CD-ROM 9.10]
□ Respirator fit testing
□ Training, which is essential for correct respirator use
□ Inspection, cleaning, maintenance, and storage
□ Recordkeeping, which must comply with OSHA Standard 29 CFR 1910.1020, Access to employee exposure and medical records[6] [CD-ROM-9.11]
□ Medical evaluations
□ Work area surveillance
□ Written worksite-specific procedures

□ Program evaluation
□ Air quality standards

Employees assigned to tasks that require respirator use must be physically able to perform the work while using the respirator. They must also be psychologically comfortable (e.g., not claustrophobic) about wearing respirators. A physician or licensed health care professional (LHCP) will determine what health and physical conditions are pertinent. Licensed health care professionals may include occupational health nurses, nurse practitioners, or physician assistants, provided they are licensed in the state in which they practice.

The medical evaluation can be performed by a physician or other LHCP by using a medical questionnaire or a medical examination that provides the same information as the questionnaire provided in Appendix C of the OSHA Respiratory protection standard, 29 CFR 1910.134.[7] [CD-ROM 9.12] This evaluation must be done before the employee is fit tested and uses the respirator in the workplace.

The employer must obtain a written recommendation from the physician or LHCP for each employee's ability to wear a respirator. Additional medical evaluations must be provided whenever health care professionals deem them appropriate.

Employees with beards, long sideburns, or even a two-day stubble may not wear respirators, since facial hair prevents the formation of an adequate seal between the skin and the respirator mask and thus allows contaminated air into the wearer's breathing zone. Wearing eyeglasses in some cases will also prevent an adequate seal, as will some facial scars or acne problems.

Different Classes of Respirators

The two main types of respirators are air-purifying respirators (APRs) and supplied-air respirators (SARs).

Air-purifying respirators can remove contaminants in the air that employees breathe by filtering out particulates (e.g., dusts, metal fumes, mists, and microorganisms). Other APRs purify air by adsorbing gases or vapors on an adsorbing material in a cartridge or canister. They are available in several forms and include the following:

□ Particulate respirators (previously called dust, fume, and mist respirators or masks).
□ Chemical cartridge respirators, which can use a combination of chemical cartridges along with a dust prefilter. Properly chosen, this combination can provide protection against multiple air contaminants at the same time.
□ Gas masks (which contain more adsorbent than cartridge-type respirators and can provide a higher level of protection than chemical cartridge respirators).

□ Powered air-purifying respirators (PAPRs), which have a battery-operated pump that draws air through the filter and across the wearer's breathing zone.

Supplied-air respirators supply clean air from a compressed-air tank or through an air line. The air supplied in tanks or from compressors must meet certain standards for purity and moisture content. Examples of SARs include the following:

□ Self-contained breathing apparatus (SCBA)
□ Air line supplied-air respirators

Depending on the level of protection required, SCBAs are sometimes worn with a fully encapsulating suit that is impervious to the contaminant.

Respirator Selection

Choosing a respirator is complex. Experienced health and safety professionals who are familiar with the workplace environment should select the proper respirator after they have evaluated all relevant factors, including the following:

□ The nature of the hazard
□ The extent of the hazard
□ Whether engineering controls are feasible

The typical surgical mask provides little or no protection against small particles including viruses, chemicals, and fumes.

The following questions represent part of a decision logic that a health and safety professional can use when selecting a respirator:

1. What is the nature of the hazard (e.g., chemical properties, concentration in the air, warning properties)?
2. Is the airborne contaminant a gas, a vapor, or a particulate (e.g., fume, mist, or dust)?
3. Are the airborne concentrations below or above the exposure limit, or are they at or above concentrations considered to be immediately dangerous to life or health?
4. What are the health effects of the airborne contaminant (e.g., carcinogenic, potentially lethal, irritating to eyes, or absorbed through the skin)?
5. What activities will the employee be performing while wearing the respirator (e.g., strenuous work)?
6. How long will the employee need to wear the respirator?

7. Does the selected respirator fit the employee properly?
8. Where is the nearest safe area that has respirable air?

Health care facilities must be aware that only National Institute for Occupational Safety and Health (NIOSH)–certified respirators are approved for use under OSHA 1910.134. All respirators must be chosen and used according to the limitations of the NIOSH certification, which appear on the NIOSH certification label.[8] Health care facilities should familiarize themselves with the certification process, noting that any changes or modifications to the respirator can be made only according to NIOSH regulations.

NIOSH provides several documents to help health care facilities select appropriate respirators, one of which is the *NIOSH Respirator Selection Logic (RSL)*. This document provides guidance to respiratory program administrators on respirator selection that incorporates the changes necessitated by the revisions to the respirator use and certification regulations and changes in NIOSH policy. This RSL is not intended to be used for the selection of respirators for protection against infectious agents or against chemical, biological, radiological, or nuclear (CBRN) agents of terrorism. [CD-ROM 9.13] Other resources that should be consulted include *Understanding Respiratory Protection Against SARS* [CD-ROM 9.14], *TB Respiratory Protection Program in Health Care Facilities: Administrator's Guide* [CD-ROM 9.15], *Respirator Fact Sheet: What You Should Know in Deciding Whether to Buy Escape Hoods, Gas Masks, or Other Respirators for Preparedness at Home and Work* [CD-ROM 9.16], *CBRN APR NIOSH Approved Respirators* [CD-ROM 9.17], and *NIOSH-Approved Disposable Particulate Respirators (Filtering Facepieces)* [CD-ROM 9.18].

Head Protection (29 CFR 1910.135)

> The employer shall ensure that each affected employee wears a protective helmet when working in areas where there is a potential for injury to the head from falling objects. (1910.135(a)(1))
>
> The employer shall ensure that a protective helmet designed to reduce electrical shock hazard is worn by each such affected employee when near exposed electrical conductors which could contact the head. (1910.135(a)(2)) [CD-ROM 9.19]

Prevention of head injuries is an important part of every health and safety program. Head injuries are caused by falling or flying objects, or by bumping the head against a fixed object. A survey by the Bureau of Labor Statistics (BLS) noted that most employees who suffered impact injuries to the head were not wearing head protection at the time of the injury and that they were injured while performing their normal jobs at their regular worksite.[9]

The BLS survey found that in most head injury cases, employers had not required their employees to wear head protection (hard hats). Among those employees wearing hard hats, all but 5 percent indicated that they were required to wear them by their employers.

Functions of Head Protection

Head protection, in the form of protective hats, must do two things—resist penetration and absorb the shock of a blow. Protective hats are also used to guard against electrical shock. The type of hard hat needed is dependent on the hazards identified during the assessment.

In health care facilities, head protection should be worn in several areas, including construction areas, confined spaces, and below scaffolding. Bump caps are not acceptable in areas where hard hats are required. Bump caps are lightweight and durable but provide protection only from minor bumps and abrasions.

Care and Maintenance

Care and maintenance of hard hats require inspections for dents and other damage and regular cleaning. In addition, hard hats must be protected from temperature extremes, chemicals, and rough treatment. Hard hats must not be placed where they may be exposed to direct sunlight. Any hat subjected to a heavy blow should be replaced.

ANSI Standards As is the case for certain other personal protective equipment, OSHA relied on ANSI for its head protection requirements. The standards for protective helmets are contained in ANSI's Personnel Protection—Protective Headwear for Industrial Workers: Requirements, Z89.1-1986. Later editions of ANSI Z89 are available and acceptable for use.

Foot Protection (29 CFR 1910.136)

> The employer shall ensure that each affected employee uses protective footwear when working in areas where there is a danger of foot injuries due to falling or rolling objects, or objects piercing the sole, and where such employee's feet are exposed to electrical hazards. (1910.136(a)) [CD-ROM 9.20]

There are many types and styles of protective footwear. Employees must wear protective footwear when working in areas where the feet are exposed to electrical hazards, dangers due to falling or rolling objects, or objects capable of piercing the sole. Rubber-soled shoes can act as insulation against electrical shock. Appropriate footwear with good traction should be worn in wet or slippery areas. In areas where injuries can be caused by crushing, steel-toed shoes must be worn.

Safety shoes should be sturdy and have an impact-resistant toe. In some shoes, metal insoles protect against puncture wounds. Additional protection, such as metatarsal guards, are found in some types of footwear. Safety shoes come in a variety of styles and materials, such as leather or rubber boots and oxfords.

In delivery rooms and surgical areas, nonconducting disposable shoe covers (booties) must be available to not only protect the surgery from contamination but also to protect the employee against exposure to blood and body fluids and to prevent the discharge of static electricity.

Categories of Injuries

There are two major categories of work-related foot injuries: punctures, crushing, sprains, and lacerations, which account for 10 percent of all reported disabling injuries; and those resulting from slips, trips, or falls, which account for 15 percent of all reported disabling injuries. These two categories of foot injuries, however, do not exhaust the range of foot problems that may be work related.

There are other foot conditions, such as calluses, ingrown toenails, or simply tired feet, that are common among employees. Although these may not be considered occupational injuries, they can have serious consequences for health and safety at the workplace. They cause discomfort, pain, and fatigue. Fatigue sets up the employee for further injuries affecting the muscles and joints. Also, an employee who is tired and suffering pain is less alert and more likely to act unsafely. An accident of any kind may result.

Common foot problems occur both on and off the job. Still, there is no doubt that some work-related factors can lead to foot problems, especially in jobs that require long periods of standing. Since the human foot is designed for mobility, maintaining an upright stance is extremely tiring. Standing for hours, day after day, not only tires the employee's feet but can also cause permanent damage. Continuous standing can cause the joints of the bones of the feet to become misaligned (e.g., cause flat feet) and can cause inflammation that can lead to rheumatism or arthritis.

ANSI Standards Safety footwear is classified according to its ability to meet minimum requirements for both compression and impact. As is the case for some other personal protective equipment, OSHA relied on ANSI for its foot protection requirements. The standards for foot protection, which include testing procedures, are contained in ANSI's American National Standard for Personal Protection—Protective Footwear, Z41.1-1991.

Hand Protection (29 CFR 1910.138)

Employers shall select and require employees to use appropriate hand protection when employees' hands are exposed to hazards such as those from skin absorption of harmful substances; severe cuts or lacerations; severe abrasions; punctures; chemical burns; thermal burns; and harmful temperature extremes. (1910.138(a))

Employers shall base the selection of the appropriate hand protection on an evaluation of the performance characteristics of the hand protection relative to the task(s) to be performed, conditions present, duration of use, and the hazards and potential hazards identified. (1910.138(b)) [CD-ROM 9.21]

The determination of the type of hand protection to be used by health care workers must be based on an evaluation of the work that is being performed and the potential exposures that may be encountered.

Types of gloves that health care facilities use include:

- □ Cotton/fabric gloves, which are general work gloves, for parts handling and general maintenance. Cotton/fabric gloves also insulate hands from mild heat or cold.
- □ Leather/cut-resistant gloves, which are best for handling sharp objects that might cause lacerations, such as blades, knives, glass, or sheet metal. Leather/cut-resistant gloves also guard against injuries from heat, sparks, or rough surfaces.
- □ Disposable (latex) gloves, which are widely used in laboratories, housekeeping, and patient care areas.
- □ Chemical-resistant gloves, which are made of rubber, neoprene, polyvinyl, alcohol, or nitrile. Chemical-resistant gloves provide protection against chemicals, such as corrosives, oils, and solvents.

Latex Allergies

As with many products that contain natural latex rubber, employees who frequently use latex gloves are at risk for developing latex allergy. Also, atopic individuals (those with multiple allergic conditions) are at increased risk for developing latex allergy. Latex allergy is also associated with allergies to certain foods, especially the avocado, potato, banana, tomato, chestnut, kiwi fruit, and papaya.

In recent years, employees with frequent exposure to latex in the workplace have begun to develop sensitivity to latex. The most common reaction to latex products such as gloves is contact dermatitis—dry, itchy, irritated areas on the skin, usually the hands. Contact dermatitis can also be caused by exposure to other products and chemicals or hand washing practices.

A true latex allergy (immediate hypersensitivity) can be a serious reaction and may be caused by certain proteins in the latex that cause sensitization. Although the amount of exposure needed to cause sensitization or symptoms is not known, exposures even at very low levels can trigger allergic reactions in sensitized individuals.

When gloves are being selected, the potential for allergic reactions among employees must be considered. Every effort should be made to avoid gloves that have the potential for exposing workers to latex.

Latex allergies can be diagnosed by means of a thorough medical history, skin testing, blood tests, and breathing tests.

There are no ANSI standards for gloves. However, selection must be based on the performance characteristics of the glove in relation to the tasks to be performed.

OCCUPATIONAL NOISE EXPOSURE (29 CFR 1910.95)

The Occupational noise exposure standard (1910.95) has its own PPE requirements that are not controlled by OSHA's General requirements for PPE (1910.132).

> Protection against the effects of noise exposure shall be provided when the sound levels exceed those shown in table G-16. (1910.95 (a)) [CD-ROM 9.22]

Exposure to high noise levels can cause temporary or permanent hearing loss.[10] [CD-ROM 9.23] Excessive noise can also lead to physical and psychological stress. There is no cure for noise-induced hearing loss, so avoidance of excessive noise exposure is the only way to prevent hearing damage. This standard is often referred to as the "hearing conservation standard." The need for participation in a hearing protection program is established through industrial hygiene monitoring.

Depending on the type of noise encountered, specially designed protection is required to prevent noise-induced hearing loss. Some forms of hearing protection, such as preformed or molded earplugs, should be individually fit by a professional. Waxed cotton, foam, or fiberglass wool earplugs are self-forming. When properly inserted, they work as well as most molded earplugs.

Some earplugs are disposable, to be used one time and then thrown away. The nondisposable type should be cleaned after each use for proper protection. Plain cotton is ineffective as protection against hazardous noise.

Earmuff-type hearing protectors are also used and, depending on the source of the noise and its intensity, will provide more adequate protection than earplugs. Earmuffs need to form a perfect seal around the ear to be effective. Glasses, long sideburns, long hair, and facial movements such as chewing can reduce protection.

When hearing protection is required, health care facilities must also develop a comprehensive hearing protection program.

DESIGNING A PPE PROGRAM

A PPE program must be comprehensive. It requires commitment and active participation at the planning, development, and implementation stages from all levels: senior management, supervisors, and employees. [CD-ROM 9.24]

PPE programs must have, and must be seen as having, equal importance with all other organizational policies, procedures, and programs. When new PPE is introduced into the facility, modifications to the program must be planned carefully, developed fully, and implemented methodically. It should be introduced gradually and in phases. Any PPE program must comply with the appropriate OSHA standard.

The greater the employees' involvement in all stages of the program, the smoother the program's implementation and operation will be. Employees must be told why the PPE is to be worn and must be trained in its proper use. The method of implementation affects the acceptance and effectiveness of the whole program.

The protection provided will be dramatically reduced if employees remove the PPE for even short periods of time in the presence of a hazard. The loss of protection during periods when the PPE is not worn can easily outweigh the protection afforded when it is used. For example, to provide full benefit, hearing protectors must be worn at all times during noisy work. If they are removed even for a short period, the protection is substantially reduced.

Flexibility in the choice of protective equipment is important (e.g., the choice between types of glove), provided that the item conforms to safety standards.

An effective PPE program consists of the following elements:

> Hazard assessment
> Selection of PPE
> Fit testing
> Training
> Recordkeeping
> Maintenance
> Program auditing

Hazard Assessment

PPE selection relies on a complete and thorough hazard assessment, and health care facilities are required to assess the workplace to identify hazards. Potential hazards may be physical or health related, and a comprehensive hazard assessment should identify hazards in both categories. In health care facilities, physical hazards include sources of electricity; unguarded machinery; fluctuating temperatures; and sharp objects. Health hazards in health care facilities include chemicals used in the workplace; harmful dusts; sources of light radiation, such as welding, brazing, and thermal cutting; loud noises; and biological hazards such as blood or other potentially infected material.

If the assessment uncovers hazards or the likelihood of hazards, health care facilities must select and direct affected employees to use properly fitted PPE suitable for protection from these hazards.

The workplace should be periodically reassessed for any changes in conditions, equipment, or operating procedures that could affect the potential for occupational hazards. This periodic reassessment should include a review of injury and illness records to spot any trends or areas of concern and follow up with appropriate corrective action. An evaluation of the suitability of existing PPE, including its condition and age, should be included in the reassessment.

A PPE hazard assessment is similar to OSHA's Hazard communication standard (HCS), 29 CFR 1910.1200. (*Note:* 29 CFR 1926.59 is specific to the construction industry and may apply under certain circumstances.) Under the HCS, employees must be told about any hazardous conditions they may encounter so that they can protect themselves.

Health care facilities must document by written certification that a hazard assessment has been performed. Documentation must include the identification of the workplace evaluated, name of the person conducting the assessment, date of the assessment, and identification of the document verifying completion of the hazard assessment. Figure 9-3 is a sample hazard assessment form. A hazard assessment should involve the Environmental Health and Safety Committee as an integral part of the survey team.

Selection of PPE

Selection of PPE must be based on the nature of the hazard. The following are guidelines for selection:

> *Match PPE to the hazard.* On some jobs the same task is performed throughout the entire job cycle, so it is easy to select proper PPE. In other instances, employees may be exposed to two or more different hazards. For example, a nurse may have exposure to blood and other body fluids, as well as anesthetic gases during surgery, glutaraldehyde for sterilization of medical equipment and devices, and needles following surgery. Each of these situations will require different protective equipment. Consideration may also be given to whether disposable items will perform satisfactorily for the task.
>
> The material safety data sheet (MSDS) should be consulted for the proper PPE for chemical hazards.
>
> *Obtain advice.* Advice on proper PPE selection can be obtained from a number of sources, including the manufacturers of PPE. In addition, NIOSH is responsible for the testing and certification of respirators, and OSHA requires specific types of respirators in specific situations under specific standards.
>
> *Involve employees in evaluations.* Not all employees will be able to wear the same PPE from a particular manufacturer. Therefore, it is reasonable to have an assortment of PPE from a variety of manufacturers during the fitting process. The selection of protective equipment and

Figure 9–3. Hazard Assessment Certification Form

Date:	Location:
Assessment Conducted by:	
Specific Tasks Performed at This Location:	

Hazard Assessment and Selection of Personal Protective Equipment
(This form does not include respiratory protection or hearing protection.)

I. Overhead Hazards

Examples of hazards to consider include:
- Suspended loads that could fall
- Overhead beams or loads that could be hit against
- Energized wires or equipment that could be hit against
- Employees working at an elevated site who could drop objects on others below
- Sharp objects or corners at head level

Hazards Identified:

Head Protection

Hard Hat:	Yes	No
If yes, type: • **Type A** (impact and penetration resistance, plus low-voltage electrical insulation) • **Type B** (impact and penetration resistance, plus high-voltage electrical insulation) • **Type C** (impact and penetration resistance)		

II. Eye and Face Hazards

Examples of hazards to consider include:
- Chemical splashes
- Dust
- Smoke and fumes
- Welding operations
- Lasers/optical radiation
- Bio-aerosols

Hazards Identified:

Eye Protection

Safety glasses or goggles	Yes	No
Face shield	Yes	No

(Continued on next page)

III. Hand Hazards

Examples of hazards to consider include:
- Chemicals
- Sharp edges, splinters, etc.
- Temperature extremes
- Biological agents
- Exposed electrical wires
- Sharp tools, machine parts, etc.
- Material handling

Hazards Identified:

Hand Protection

Gloves	Yes	No
• Chemical-resistant • Temperature-resistant • Cut-resistant • Disposable (latex) • Other (explain)		

IV. Foot Hazards

Examples of hazards to consider include:
- Heavy materials handled by employees
- Sharp edges or points (puncture risk)
- Exposed electrical wires
- Unusually slippery conditions
- Wet conditions
- Construction/demolition

Hazards Identified:

Foot Protection

Safety shoes	Yes	No
Types: • Toe protection • Metatarsal protection • Puncture-resistant • Electrical insulation • Other (explain)		

V. Other Identified Safety and/or Health Hazards

Hazard	Recommended Protection

(Continued on next page)

I certify that the above inspection was performed to the best of my knowledge and ability, based on the hazards present on ————————————.

————————————
(Signature)

Courtesy of Office of Health and Safety, Centers for Disease Control and Prevention, 1600 Clifton Road N.E., Mail Stop F05, Atlanta, Georgia 30333, USA. Last Modified:1/2/97

clothing should incorporate input from the employees who will use it. If employees know that PPE was selected with their comfort in mind, it will help to ensure acceptance.

Review standards. All standards must be reviewed to ensure that their PPE requirements are met and that the PPE that was selected complies with those requirements.

Fit Testing

Only qualified personnel should conduct fit testing.

Appendixes A and B of the Respiratory protection standard (1910.134) provide guidance on the proper methods for fit testing respirators. [CD-ROM 9.25, 9.26] In addition, if prescription safety or eye protection is needed, it should be obtained only from a qualified optometrist or ophthalmologist.

Training

Training is vital to a successful PPE program. Training is distinguished from orientation in that training requires a demonstration of proficiency through specialized instruction and practice, while orientation is intended to provide for adaptation to a new environment, situation, or set of ideas. Although OSHA does not prescribe the precise way in which training should be conducted, the agency is specific in its requirements for training and for an objective demonstration that employees have acquired proficiency. The agency also requires that employers provide written certification of the successful completion of each employee's training.[11] Employees must be trained to understand:

- ☐ When PPE is necessary
- ☐ What PPE is necessary
- ☐ How to properly don, doff, adjust, and wear the PPE to achieve the necessary level of protection
- ☐ The limitations of the PPE
- ☐ How to care for the PPE
- ☐ The useful life of PPE
- ☐ Proper disposal of contaminated PPE

Training can be done on an individual basis or in group meetings. Training programs should reemphasize the major goals of the program and reinforce the point that engineering controls have been considered as the primary prevention strategy. It is not good enough to tell someone to wear a respirator just because management or legislation requires it. If a respirator is intended to prevent lung disorders, the employees should be informed of the hazards.

The employees to be trained include those who may be exposed to a hazard on a regular basis and those who might be exposed on an occasional basis. Examples of occasional exposures are emergencies and performance of temporary work in dangerous areas. PPE may be needed to treat a person who has been injured in an automobile accident or an industrial accident or as the victim of a chemical, biological, or nuclear weapon.

After the training, the employees must demonstrate that they understand the components of the PPE program and how to use PPE properly, or they must be retrained. If a previously trained employee is not demonstrating the proper understanding and skill in the use of PPE, that employee should receive retraining. Other situations that require additional training or retraining of employees include changes in the workplace or in the type of required PPE that make prior training obsolete.

Recordkeeping

Health care facilities must document in writing that training has been performed and that employees understand it. Documentation must contain the name of each employee trained, the date(s) of training, and clear identification of the subject of the training.

Maintenance

The effectiveness of PPE cannot be ensured without proper maintenance. Maintenance should include inspection, care, cleaning, repair, and proper storage. A key to proper maintenance is the regular inspection of the equipment for cleanliness and defects. If carefully performed, inspections will identify damaged or malfunctioning PPE before it is used. Equipment that is not performing up to manufacturers' specifications, such as safety glasses with scratched lenses that have lost their ability to withstand impact, should be discarded. Respiratory protection devices require an elaborate program of repair, cleaning, storage, and periodic testing.

Defective or damaged PPE must not be used. Wearing poorly maintained or malfunctioning PPE could be more dangerous than not wearing any protection at all. OSHA Standard 29 CFR 1910.134, Respiratory protection, requires that respirators be regularly inspected and properly maintained.

Program Auditing

Once the PPE program has been put in place, its effectiveness should be monitored in several areas. Program auditing will be effective only if it requires an objective assessment of how the program elements are working. In some cases, this can be obtained by data collection. In other cases, those who are performing the audit may observe employee compliance with standards and in-house policies. Regardless of how the audit is conducted, it must focus on the employees' understanding of the requirements for wearing PPE and a demonstration of their proficiency in wearing it. At a minimum, the program audit must focus on:

□ Employer compliance, including training records
□ Employee compliance with the program
□ Areas that need to be improved to increase compliance
□ Areas in which the program is failing to meet anticipated improvements in rates of injuries and illnesses

PRECAUTIONS IN USING PPE

Using several types of protection at the same time, such as hard hats, earmuffs, and goggles, must not increase the danger or decrease the employee's ability to do the assigned job. Wearing PPE should not in itself create a greater danger. Gloves prevent skin damage but can create an entanglement hazard around machinery that has moving parts in which the glove or other protective clothing can be caught.

According to OSHA requirements, PPE must not be used unless the employer has exhausted the use of engineering controls, work practices, and administrative controls to contain the hazard. The use of PPE does not prevent an accident from happening. It does not eliminate the hazard. It only minimizes the exposure or limits the severity of injury or illness.

JOINT COMMISSION REQUIREMENTS FOR THE USE OF PERSONAL PROTECTIVE EQUIPMENT

The Joint Commission standard on safety management (EC.1.10) provides overarching guidance in Element of Performance (EP) 5, which requires health care facilities to implement procedures and controls to achieve the lowest potential for adverse impact on the safety and health of patients, staff, and other people coming to the health care facility. Standard EC.1.10, EP4 requires that the health care facility conduct comprehensive, proactive risk assessments. Conducting a risk assessment to identify where PPE should be used would fall under this requirement.

According to EC.3.10, EP9, "The hospital identifies and implements emergency procedures that include the specific precautions, procedures, and protective equipment used during hazardous materials and waste spills or exposures"; this language requires health care facilities to develop a written plan for handling wastes that includes personal protective equipment used during hazardous materials and waste spills or exposures.

Other Joint Commission standards that address personal protective equipment include medical equipment management (EC.6.10), utilities management (EC.7.10), initial job training (HR.2.10), roles and responsibilities (HR.2.20), and ongoing education (HR.2.30).

As is the case with other Joint Commission standards, compliance with these standards is not equivalent to compliance with local, state, or federal regulations.

THE ROLE OF THE ENVIRONMENTAL HEALTH AND SAFETY DEPARTMENT

The Environmental Health and Safety Department has responsibility for coordinating the facility's PPE program, as required by OSHA. These duties will most likely be shared by the Safety and Environmental Monitoring functions within the department. The Environmental Health and Safety Department is also responsible for assisting other departments in maintaining PPE and ensuring that it complies with standards and regulations. The latter responsibility is particularly important with respect to OSHA's Respiratory protection standard, 29 CFR 1910.134, since failure to comply with this standard is one of the OSHA citations most frequently issued to health care facilities.

Department managers must be held accountable for their employees' use of PPE. Department liaisons should participate in motivating employees to continue to use protective equipment.

References

1. *OSHA. Personal Protective Equipment.* 29 CFR 1932. Available at http://www.osha.gov/pls/oshaweb/owadisp.show_document?p_table=STANDARDS&p_id=9777 (accessed 3/21/2006).

2. U.S. Department of Health and Human Services. Public Health Service, Centers for Disease Control and Prevention and National Institutes of Health. *Biosafety in Microbiological and Biomedical Laboratories,* 4th ed. Available at http://www.cdc.gov/od/ohs/pdffiles/4th%20BMBL.pdf (accessed 4/27/2006).

3. American National Standards Institute. *Practice for Occupational and Educational Eye and Face Protection.* ANSI Z87.1-1989 USA. New York: ANSI, 1989.

4. OSHA. *Respiratory Protection.* Technical Manual, Section VIII, Chapter 2. Available at http://www.osha.gov/dts/osta/otm/otm_viii/otm_viii_2.html (accessed 3/20/2006).

5. Department of Health and Human Services, Public Health Service. *Respiratory Protective Devices: Final Rules and Notice.* 42 CFR Part 84. Available at http://www.cdc.gov/niosh/pt84abs2.html (accessed 3/20/2006).

6. OSHA. *Access to Employee Exposure and Medical Records.* 29 CFR 1910.1020. Available at http://www.osha.gov/pls/oshaweb/owadisp.show_document?p_table=STANDARDS&p_id=10027 (accessed 3/20/2006).

7. OSHA. *Respiratory Protection.* 29 CFR 1910.134. Available at http://www.google.com/search?hl=en&lr=&q=29+CFR+1910.134&btnG=Search (accessed 3/20/2006).

8. *NIOSH Guide to the Selection and Use of Particulate Respirators Certified Under 42 CFR 84.* HHS (NIOSH) Publication 96–101. Available at http://www.cdc.gov/niosh/userguid.html (accessed 3/20/2006).

9. U.S. Department of Labor, Bureau of Labor Statistics. *Accidents Involving Head Injuries.* Report 605. Washington, DC: U.S. GPO, 1980.

10. OSHA. *Hearing Conservation.* Publication 3074. Available at http://www.osha.gov/Publications/osha3074.pdf (accessed 3/20/2006).

11. OSHA. *Personal Protective Equipment.* 29 CFR 1932(f)(4). Available at http://www.osha.gov/pls/oshaweb/owadisp.show_document?p_table=STANDARDS&p_id=9777 (accessed 3/21/2006).

CHAPTER 10

ERGONOMICS

I now wish to turn to workers in whom certain morbid affections gradually arise from some particular posture of the limbs or unnatural movements of the body called for while they work. Such are the workers who all day long stand or sit, stoop or are bent double; who run or ride or exercise their bodies in all sorts of ways.

Bernardino Ramazzini[1]

The first thing in the morning, after breakfast, I sponge her and I give her a backrub. And I keep her clean. She's supposed to be turned every two hours. If we don't turn her every two hours, she will have sores. Even though she's asleep, she's got to be turned.

Carmelita Lester (quoted in Studs Terkel, *Working*)[2]

Ramazzini observed work with the keen eye of a clinician. His few words capture the side of work that, despite 300 years of technological advances, remains a principal cause of workplace injuries and illnesses today. Though Ramazzini's observation concerned jobs that were more demanding in many ways than they are now, the simple narration of Carmelita Lester, as she turns her patient every two hours whether she is awake or asleep, makes it clear that today's health care workers are still subject to the aches and pains of the "particular posture of the limbs or unnatural movements of the body."

Today we call this interaction between humans and the work environment "ergonomics." The Occupational Safety and Health Administration (OSHA) describes ergonomics as:[3]

> the science of fitting the job to the worker. When there is a mismatch between the physical requirements of the job and the physical capacity of the worker, work-related musculoskeletal disorders (MSDs) can

result. Ergonomics is the practice of designing equipment and work tasks to conform to the capability of the worker; it provides a means for adjusting the work environment and work practices to prevent injuries before they occur.

Injuries associated with ergonomic factors have been referred to as cumulative trauma disorders (CTDs), repetitive stress injuries (RSIs), and musculoskeletal disorders (MSDs). Of these terms, MSD is the most commonly used and will be used in this chapter.

Some careers involve greater physical strain and repetitive motion than others. The Occupational Safety and Health Administration has identified health care facility workers, especially those in nursing homes, as having a greater incidence of MSDs than workers in any other industry sector in the United States.

In health care facilities, there are several tasks that can be considered a challenge to proper workplace ergonomics. It is easy to understand how nurses such as Carmelita Lester can be affected. However, what is often not considered are the tasks of nonmedical personnel. For example, office staff typically remain seated in front of a display terminal for protracted periods, and housekeeping, dietary, and maintenance staff perform lifting, reaching, and pushing tasks throughout the day.

In 2003 about 270,000 hospital workers (SIC 806, NAICS 622) sustained injuries that were reported to OSHA. An additional 211,000 workers in nursing and residential facilities (SIC 805, NAICS 623) were also injured. Of those 481,000 recordable injuries, about 25 percent (101,640) can be considered MSDs. Table 10-1 lists the types of injuries and the numbers of health care workers who incurred them. For example, of the 12,900 health care workers who reported soreness and pain, 5,180 reported the back as the location. Table 10-2 describes how the injuries occurred and the number of workers who were injured in each category.[4] This table reveals that of the 58,440 injuries caused by overexertion, 27,750 occurred during lifting.

When employees suffer a traumatic injury on the job, the cause is usually known and the injury can be easily observed. A traumatic injury such as a broken bone may require an x-ray to determine its extent. However, MSDs are not easily observed because they are generally soft-tissue injuries. Furthermore,

Table 10–1. MSD-Related Injuries Reported to OSHA in 2003 for Health Care Workers

Type of Injury	Number of Workers (SIC 805 and 806, NAICS 622 and 623)
Sprains and strains	78,600
Carpal tunnel syndrome	7,180
Tendonitis	2,700
Soreness with pain	12,900

Table 10–2. Causes of MSD Injuries

Cause of Injury	Number of Workers (SIC 805 and 806, NAICS 622 and 623)
Fall to lower level	3,110
Fall on same level	21,760
Slips, trips	2,270
Overexertion	58,440

traumatic injuries are immediate, whereas MSDs may develop over weeks, months, or years.

Physical and environmental factors that can lead to MSDs include:

☐ Repetitive twisting movements combined with poor body position

☐ Excessive standing with no chance to lean, sit, or comfortably reposition the body

☐ Repetitive motions that place a constant strain on a joint, muscle, or tendon

☐ Working in an awkward position

☐ Lifting beyond one's ability

☐ Lifting using an awkward position or one that places undue strain on the musculoskeletal system

☐ Poor-quality air, which may cause headaches, congestion, or fatigue

☐ Improper lighting, which can cause eyestrain and headaches

The National Institute for Occupational Safety and Health (NIOSH) document *Elements of Ergonomics Programs*[5] [CD-ROM 10.1] reports that work-related MSDs are under-reported. Therefore, it is particularly important to recognize early signs and symptoms of MSDs and to be aware of MSD hazards in the workplace. Reasons for the under-reporting of work-related MSDs include:

☐ The difficulty of linking symptoms, such as pain and tingling, to workplace risk factors

☐ The belief that pain is a part of the job and that nothing can be done about it

☐ Intentional or unintentional discouragement of reporting by management

☐ Employee fear of reprisal for reporting

☐ Employee discouragement from filing a workers' compensation claim

☐ The hassle of filing a workers' compensation claim

☐ The preference (or encouragement by employers) to use the employer's or the employee's own health insurance rather than the workers' compensation insurance system

Individual physical factors, work organization issues, psychosocial factors, and sociocultural factors can all contribute to the development of an MSD.[6]

INDIVIDUAL RISK FACTORS ASSOCIATED WITH MSDs

In its review of the literature reported in *Musculoskeletal Disorders and Workplace Factors: A Critical Review of Epidemiologic Evidence for Work-Related Musculoskeletal Disorders of the Neck, Upper Extremity, and Low Back*[7] [CD-ROM 10.2], NIOSH concludes that a number of factors can influence a person's response to risk factors for MSDs in the workplace and elsewhere. Among these are age, gender, smoking, physical activity, strength, and anthropometry (measurement of the human body to determine differences between groups and individuals). Certain epidemiologic studies have used statistical methods to take into account the effects of these individual factors.

A worker's ability to respond to external work factors may be modified by the worker's own capacity, such as tissue resistance to deformation when exposed to high force demands. The level, duration, and frequency of the loads imposed on tissues, as well as the adequacy of recovery time, are critical components in determining whether increased tolerance (training or conditioning effect) occurs or whether reduced capacity that can lead to MSDs occurs.

OSHA's ERGONOMICS GUIDELINES

There continues to be considerable debate regarding the need for an OSHA standard for ergonomic risks in the workplace. Until the issues under discussion are settled, OSHA plans to develop industry- and task-specific guidelines to assist employers and employees in recognizing and controlling potential ergonomic hazards.

The scope, form, and content of the guidelines will vary because the types of ergonomic hazards, injuries, and controls vary from industry to industry and task to task. Additional information can be found in OSHA's ergonomics guidelines protocol.[8] [CD-ROM 10.3]

The same principles that apply to OSHA's *Safety and Health Program Management Guidelines*[9] [CD-ROM 10.4] apply to a viable ergonomics program, including recognition, evaluation, and control of signs that may indicate problems.

Whether or not ergonomics becomes a separate OSHA standard, OSHA holds workplaces accountable for ergonomics-related injuries and illnesses under the Occupational Safety and Health Act (OSH Act) general duty clause.[10] [CD-ROM 10.5]

Sec. 5. Duties

a) Each employer—

1. shall furnish to each of his employees employment and a place of employment which are free from recognized hazards that are causing or are likely to cause death or serious physical harm to his employees.

NIOSH ELEMENTS OF ERGONOMICS PROGRAMS

The National Institute for Occupational Safety and Health operates an 800 number to provide workers, employers, and organizations with information about various workplace safety and health concerns. Over the past several years, the volume of NIOSH 800-number calls concerning work-related MSDs has grown; they are now second only to questions about chemical hazards. In 1997 NIOSH prepared a primer, *Elements of Ergonomics Programs*[11] [CD-ROM 10.6], describing the basic elements of a workplace ergonomics program. The text is largely built around NIOSH experiences in evaluating the risks of MSDs in a variety of workplaces.

In the primer, NIOSH presents seven elements of an effective ergonomics program that comprise a "pathway" for evaluating and addressing musculoskeletal concerns in an individual workplace. Each step is explained in detail. The seven steps are as follows:

1. Looking for signs of a potential musculoskeletal problem in the workplace, such as frequent worker reports of aches and pains, or job tasks that require repetitive, forceful exertions
2. Showing management commitment to addressing possible problems and encouraging worker involvement in problem-solving activities
3. Offering training to expand management and worker ability to evaluate potential musculoskeletal problems
4. Gathering data to identify jobs or work conditions that are most problematic, using sources such as injury and illness logs, medical records, and job analyses
5. Identifying effective controls for tasks that pose a risk of musculoskeletal injury, and evaluating these approaches once they have been instituted to see if they have reduced or eliminated the problem
6. Establishing health care management to emphasize the importance of early detection and treatment of musculoskeletal disorders in preventing impairment and disability
7. Minimizing risk factors for musculoskeletal disorders when planning new work processes and operations; it is less costly to build good design into the workplace than to redesign or retrofit later

Step 1: Looking for Signs of Work-Related Musculoskeletal Problems. What clues or tip-offs exist that point to MSDs as a real or possible workplace problem? Some signs are obvious while others are subtler. The first step is to look for signs or clues.

Step 2: Setting the Stage for Action. As with other workplace safety and health issues, managers and employees play key roles in developing and carrying out an ergonomics program. Ergonomics problems typically require a response that cuts across a number of organizational units. Hazard identification through job risk analyses and review of injury records or symptoms surveys, as well as the development and implementation of control measures, can require input from safety and industrial hygiene personnel, health care providers, human resources personnel, engineering personnel, and ergonomics specialists.

Step 3: Training—Building In-House Expertise. Identifying and solving workplace MSD problems require some level of ergonomic knowledge and skills. Recognizing and filling different training needs is an important step in building an effective program.

Step 4: Gathering and Examining Evidence of MSDs. Once a decision has been made to initiate an ergonomics program, a necessary step is to gather information to determine the scope and characteristics of the problem or potential problem. A variety of techniques and tools have been used. Many provide the basis for developing solutions to identified problems, such as health and medical indicators, and risk factors.

Step 5: Developing Controls. Analyzing jobs to identify factors associated with risks for MSDs lays the groundwork for developing ways to reduce or eliminate ergonomic risk factors for MSDs.

Step 6: Health Care Management. Facility health care management strategies and policies and health care providers can be important parts of the overall ergonomics program. In general, health care management emphasizes the prevention of impairment and disability through early detection, prompt treatment, and timely recovery. Medical management responsibilities fall on employers, employees, and health care providers.

Step 7: Proactive Ergonomics. Proactive approaches to workplace ergonomics programs emphasize the prevention of MSDs through recognizing, anticipating, and reducing risk factors in the planning stages of new work processes.

MAJOR CATEGORIES OF ERGONOMIC INJURIES

A significant number of work-related MSDs occur in health care facilities. The hospital web-based training tool available from OSHA[12] [CD-ROM 10.7] provides examples of some of the activities that can contribute to work-related MSDs.

Overexertion

Overexertion is one of the principal factors in back injuries among health care workers. Many patients are totally dependent on staff members like Carmelita Lester for activities of daily living, such as dressing, bathing, feeding, and toileting. Each of these activities may require frequent interaction between staff and patients, which increases the risk of injury. Other health care workers have jobs that also require lifting. Lifting even a light object can lead to an injury if insufficient attention is given to posture and body mechanics. Some of the more common sources of back injuries are listed in figure 10-1.

Slips, Trips, and Falls

Slips, trips, and falls also account for a significant proportion of recordable injuries in health care facilities. Slips, trips, and falls often involve slippery or wet floors, uneven floor surfaces, and cluttered or obstructed work areas

Figure 10–1. Common Sources of Back Injuries

- ☐ Trying to stop a patient from falling or picking a patient up from the floor or bed
- ☐ Multiple instances of lifting per shift
- ☐ Lifting alone when no other staff are available to help
- ☐ Lifting uncooperative, confused patients
- ☐ Lifting patients who cannot support their own weight
- ☐ Lifting bariatric patients
- ☐ Expecting employees to perform work beyond their physical capabilities
- ☐ Reaching to lift, which, even for lightweight objects, is more stressful than simple lifting, if the body is not properly positioned
- ☐ Awkward posture required by the activity
- ☐ Inadequate training of employees in proper body mechanics and lifting techniques
- ☐ Failure to train employees in significant factors such as stress, tension, physical strength and flexibility, correct body movement, fitness, proper breathing, and mental focus during physical exertion

or passageways. Poorly maintained walkways and broken or uneven pavement also contribute to slips, trips, and falls.

Statistics show that the majority (60 percent) of falls are to the same level and result from slips or trips. The remaining 40 percent are falls from a height, such as from ladders or roofs, down stairs, or from jumping to a lower level. [CD-ROM 10.8]

Awkward Postures

When workers use awkward postures to move or lift patients, boxes, furniture, or any other object, abnormal stress is placed on muscles and joints, which can lead to sprains and strains. Forces on the spine increase during the act of lifting, lowering, or handling objects when the back is bent or twisted. Bending and twisting prevents the muscles from working as designed, causing more force to be exerted in the performance of the task. Awkward postures include twisting while lifting, bending over to lift, and lateral or side bending. Awkward postures also include back hyperextension or flexion, reaching forward or twisting to support patients from behind to assist them in walking, and reaching forward or twisting when carrying heavy objects.

Video Display Terminal Use

The applications of computer technology and the accompanying use of video display terminals (VDTs) have revolutionized workplaces, and VDT use will continue to grow in the future. Along with the use of VDTs have come reports of adverse health effects for VDT operators. To help inform employers and employees, OSHA produced *Working Safely with Video Display Terminals*.[13] This booklet briefly examines potential hazards relating to the harmful effects of working with VDTs. A summary follows: [CD-ROM 10.9]

> VDTs are comprised of a display screen, a keyboard, and a central processing unit. The VDT operates at high voltages, but the power supplies generating these voltages produce very little current. To date, however, there is no conclusive evidence that the low levels of radiation emitted from VDTs pose a health risk to VDT operators.

With the expanding use of VDTs, concerns have been expressed about their potential health effects. Complaints include excessive fatigue; eyestrain and eye irritation; blurred vision; headaches; stress; and neck, back, arm, and muscle pain. Research has shown that these symptoms can result from problems with the equipment, workstation, office environment, job design, or a combination of these. Concerns about the potential exposure to electromagnetic fields also have been raised.

Visual Problems

Visual problems, such as eyestrain and eye irritation, are among the most frequently reported complaints by VDT operators. These visual symptoms can result from improper lighting, glare from the screen, poor user positioning in relation to the screen, or display material that is difficult to read.

Fatigue and Musculoskeletal Problems

Work performed at VDTs may require sitting still for a considerable period of time and usually involves frequent, limited movements of the eyes, head, arms, and fingers. Maintaining a fixed posture over long periods of time causes muscle fatigue and, if this practice is consistent, can eventually lead to muscle pain or injury.

Visual display terminal operators also are subject to the risk of developing various musculoskeletal disorders such as carpal tunnel syndrome and tendonitis. Musculoskeletal disorders are injuries to the muscles, joints, tendons, or nerves that are caused or aggravated by work-related risk factors. Early symptoms of musculoskeletal disorders include pain and swelling, numbness and tingling (hands falling asleep), loss of strength, and reduced range of motion.

Demands on the Neck

The use of the telephone handset is responsible for the most significant work-related disorders of the neck. When the seemingly innocuous act of squeezing the handset between the shoulder and neck to keep the hands free is performed routinely, or continued for long periods of time, complications ranging from discomfort to structural tissue damage can occur.

Other Ergonomic Hazards

Employee exposure to ergonomic stressors in health care facilities occurs not only during patient handling but also with performance of tasks in the kitchen, laundry, engineering, and housekeeping areas of facilities. Figure 10-2 lists examples of health care tasks that are associated with ergonomic stressors.

APPROACHES TO SOLVING ERGONOMIC PROBLEMS

The performance of physically demanding tasks may not present problems in all circumstances. However, the duration, frequency, and magnitude of employee exposure to forceful exertions, repetitive activities, and awkward postures should be considered. In the majority of cases, the risks associated

Figure 10–2. Examples of Health Care Tasks That Are Associated with Ergonomic Stressors

- Transporting equipment such as IV poles, wheelchairs, oxygen canisters, respiratory equipment, dialysis equipment, and x-ray machines, or multiple items at the same time
- Reaching into deep sinks or containers
- Lifting trash, laundry, or other bagged materials
- Moving heavy dietary, laundry, housekeeping, or other carts
- Using hand tools in maintenance areas
- Housekeeping tasks

with a particular job can be assessed by observing employees performing the task, by discussing the activities and conditions associated with difficulties, and by checking injury records. Observation provides general information about workstation layout, tools, equipment, and general environmental conditions in the workplace. Discussing tasks with employees helps to ensure a complete understanding of the job. Employees who perform a given task are also often the best resources for identifying the cause of a problem and developing the most practical and effective solutions. The Occupational Safety and Health Administration's hospital web-based training tool[14] provides examples of activities that can help to prevent work-related MSDs.

Lifting

Health care facilities should establish a prevention program that addresses hazards and specifies criteria in relation to patient lifting. In its guidelines for nursing homes, OSHA recommends minimizing manual lifting of patients in all cases and eliminating lifting whenever possible.[15] [CD-ROM 10.10] These guidelines also apply to health care facilities. In addition, the OSHA guidelines provide information that can be used to determine the safest methods for lifting and repositioning patients without injuring workers. A list of sample solutions involving the use of equipment for patient lifting and repositioning tasks is also included in the guidelines.

Employees should be provided with proper assist devices and equipment to reduce hazards associated with excessive lifting. Proper equipment selection depends on the specific needs of the facility, patients, staff, and management. Table 10-3 illustrates how equipment is properly used to reduce injuries. In the absence of lifting devices, employees should be trained in the use of safe lifting techniques, including team lifting.

Some workplaces continue to use back belts to provide support during lifting; however, their effectiveness in reducing back injury remains unproven. If employees falsely believe that they are protected when wearing back belts,

Table 10–3. Examples of Equipment That Can Be Used to Lift or Move Patients

Device	Use	Benefit
Shower chair	Fits over the toilet.	Use of this device can eliminate multiple transfers, sparing employees multiple lifts. The patient can be moved to the shower chair, toileted, showered, and transferred back to the wheelchair.
Shower stall	Allows for chairs to be pushed in and out on level floor surfaces.	This is a standard shower without the front lip to allow easy access.
Toilet seat riser	Used on toilets.	Equalizes the height of the wheelchair and toilet seat, making it a lateral transfer rather than a lift up from and back into the wheelchair.
Mechanical lift equipment	Helps lift patients who cannot support their own weight.	Choosing a lift that does not require manual pumping avoids possible repetitive-motion disorders to workers' arms or shoulders.
Overhead track-mounted patient lifter	Track system built into the ceiling to which sling lifts attach.	Provides the patient with mobility from room to room without manual lifting.
Lateral transfer device	Transfers patient, for example, from bed to gurney. Usually requires multiple staff members to help with the lifting.	Helps prevent back injuries among staff.
Sliding board	Slick board used under patients t help reduce need for lifting during transfer of patients from bed to chair, or chair to chair.	Patients are slid rather than lifted.
Slip sheet/roller sheet	Helps to reduce friction while patients are laterally transferred or repositioned in bed.	Reduces the force employees need to exert to move the patient.
Repositioning device	Mechanically pulls the patient up in bed.	Eliminates manual maneuvering by staff.
Height-adjustable electric bed	Height controls allow for easy transfers from bed height to wheelchair height.	Beds can be kept low to the ground for patient safety and then raised for interaction with staff. Avoid hand-cranked beds, which can lead to wrist/shoulder musculoskeletal disorders such as strain or repetitive-motion injuries.

(Continued on next page)

Table 10–3. *(Continued)*

Device	Use	Benefit
Trapeze lift	Bar device suspended above the bed, which allows patients with upper muscle strength to help reposition themselves.	Useful with adjustable beds and armless wheelchairs.
Walking belt or gait belt (with handles)	Provides stabilization for ambulatory patients.	Allows employees to hold onto the belt and support patients when walking. Not designed for lifting patients.
Wheelchairs with removable arms	Especially useful with height-adjustable bed.	Allows for easier lateral transfers.
Descent control system (DCS)	Emergency evacuation or retrieval from older or disabled structures may require the use of stairs or negotiation of rough terrain when moving patients.	Allows ambulance technicians or emergency evacuation personnel to safely move a loaded cot or gurney down stairs or any steep decline.
Roll-on weight scale	Patients who cannot stand can be weighed in their wheelchairs.	Avoids multiple lifting or transferral of patients.
Pivot transfer disk device	Used for standing pivot transfers and seated pivot transfers for patients who have weight-bearing capacity and are cooperative.	Some are designed for heavy patients. Lightweight. Reduces back strain on patient and caregiver. Turning discs reduce the forces required to rotate or pivot patients.

they may attempt to lift more weight than they would without a belt and thereby increase their risk of incurring an injury.[16] [CD-ROM 10.11]

Slips, Trips, and Falls

Both slips and trips result from some unintended or unexpected change in the contact between the feet and the ground or walking surface. Good housekeeping, quality of walking surfaces (flooring), selection of proper footwear, and appropriate pace are critical in preventing fall accidents.[17] [CD-ROM 10.12]

Housekeeping

Good housekeeping is the first and the most important (fundamental) step in preventing falls due to slips and trips. It includes:

□ Cleaning spills immediately
□ Marking spills and wet areas

> ☐ Mopping or sweeping debris from floors
> ☐ Keeping walkways free of obstacles and clutter
> ☐ Securing (tacking, taping, etc.) mats, rugs, and carpets that do not lay flat
> ☐ Keeping file cabinet or storage drawers closed
> ☐ Covering cables that cross walkways
> ☐ Keeping working areas and walkways well lit
> ☐ Replacing used light bulbs and faulty switches

Without good housekeeping practices, other preventive measures such as installation of sophisticated flooring, specialty footwear, or training on techniques of walking and safe falling will never be fully effective.

Flooring

Changing or modifying walking surfaces is the next step in preventing slips and trips. Recoating or replacing floors, and installing mats or pressure-sensitive abrasive strips can further improve safety and reduce the risk of falling. However, high-tech flooring requires good housekeeping as much as does any other flooring. In addition, resilient, non-slippery flooring prevents or reduces foot fatigue and contributes to slip prevention measures.

Footwear

In workplaces where floors may be oily or wet or where workers spend considerable time outdoors, accident prevention should focus on the selection of proper footwear. Since there is no footwear with anti-slip properties that cover every condition, employees should consult manufacturers. Properly fitting footwear increases comfort and prevents fatigue, which in turn improves safety for employees.

Video Display Terminal Use

There are a variety of interventions that health care facilities can implement to reduce or prevent harmful effects associated with VDT use. Video display terminal operators can reduce eyestrain by taking breaks after each hour or so of VDT operation. Changing focus is another way to give eye muscles a chance to relax. The employee need only glance across the room or out the window from time to time and look at an object at least 20 feet away. The Occupational Safety and Health Administration's *Working Safely with Video Display Terminals* provides additional approaches to protecting employees from the harmful effects of working with VDTs, and some of these are outlined in the following sections. [CD-ROM 10.13]

Lighting

Light should be directed so that it does not shine into the operator's eyes when the operator is looking at the display screen. Further, lighting should be adequate for the operator to see the text and the screen, but not so bright as to cause glare or discomfort.

Four basic lighting factors must be controlled to ensure suitable office illumination and prevent eyestrain: quantity, contrast, direct glare, and reflected glare.

Workstation Design

Proper workstation design will minimize visual and musculoskeletal discomfort associated with VDT use when the following work practices are observed:

- ☐ The operator employs a comfortable sitting position sufficiently flexible to reach, use, and observe the display screen, keyboard, and document.
- ☐ Posture support is provided for the back, arms, legs, and feet, and display screens and keyboards are adjustable.
- ☐ VDT tables or desks are vertically adjustable.
- ☐ The setup allows for proper chair height and support to the lower region of the back.
- ☐ Document holders allow the operator to position and view material without straining the eyes or neck, shoulder, or back muscles.

The type of task performed at the VDT may also influence the development of fatigue. In designing a workstation, the type of task involved should be a factor determining the placement of the display screen and keyboard. For example, if the job requires that the operator look mainly at the source document and not at the display screen, the source document should be positioned in front of the operator and the screen to the side.

The employee must have adequate workspace to perform each of the tasks required by the job. Individual body size will influence the design of the workstation and the operator's access to various resources.

In general, VDT workstations should provide as many adjustable features as possible. Also, adequate legroom should be available for the employee to stretch out and relieve some of the static load that results from sitting with the legs in a fixed position for long periods.

VDT Design

Display screens should have user controls for character brightness. Screens that swivel horizontally and tilt or elevate vertically enable the operator to select the optimal viewing angle. The topmost line of the screen should be no higher than the user's eyes. The screen and document holder should be the same distance from the eye (to avoid constant changes in focus) and close enough together that the operator can look from one to the other without excessive movement of the neck or back. People who wear bifocals often must tilt the head back to read through the bottom portion of their lenses. They should avoid head tilting by lowering the display or by using single-lens glasses while using the VDT.

Keyboards should be detachable and adjustable to ensure proper position, angle, and comfort for the operator. A lower-than-normal work surface may be necessary to keep the operator's arms in a comfortable position. This can be achieved by installing a keyboard extender or tray. The thickness and slope of the keyboard are critical in determining the proper height.

The preferred working position for most keyboard operators is having the forearms parallel to the floor and elbows at the sides, which allows the hands to move easily over the keyboard. The wrist should be in line with the forearm. A padded and detachable wrist rest can help keep the keyboard operator's wrists and hands in a straight position.

The operator should work with the mouse positioned at the side and with the arm close to the body for support, while maintaining a straight line between the hand and forearm. The upper arm should not be elevated or extended while using the mouse. The top surface of the wrist should be flat, not angled. A mouse pad or rest can be used to help keep the wrists straight.

Work Practices and Job Organization

Operating a VDT, like any other form of sustained physical or mental work, may lead to visual, muscular, or mental fatigue. Rests to alleviate or delay the onset of fatigue are necessary. The National Institute for Occupational Safety and Health recommends a 10-minute rest break after two hours of continuous VDT work for operators under moderate visual demands, and a 15-minute rest break after one hour of continuous VDT work where there is a high visual demand or a repetitive work task. Jobs should be designed so that employees can alternate VDT tasks with non-VDT tasks. In addition, open and positive working relationships between worker and manager, and involvement of employees in workplace decisions and practices, can be factors in reducing muscle tension and musculoskeletal disorders.

Demands on the Neck

Stretching exercises and frequent changes in position can help employees to relieve pain and prevent repetitive task injuries. However, sometimes these activities are not enough.

The use of telephone headsets is beneficial for improving head and neck postures. With the freedom a headset affords, users can avoid awkward and prolonged static postures of the head, neck, and shoulders. In addition, the freedom of hand movement allows workers extra mobility, reduces static loads on the entire body, and contributes to worker comfort and productivity. Headsets are known to alleviate stress on the neck for all-day users, as well as for those who use the telephone only sporadically throughout the day.

Worn only by telephone operators back in the 1950s, headsets today are finding their way into offices across the world, and with good reason. Headsets reduce neck, upper back, and shoulder tension by as much as 41 percent. Adding hands-free headsets to office telephones improves productivity. Headsets are known to reduce the chances of work-related physical disorders, specifically injuries of the neck and upper body, thus reducing workers' compensation costs. The provision of telephone headsets is a proactive measure in preventing one of the most common sources of neck and back pain—cradling the telephone handset between the ear and shoulder. The process of choosing the right headset is just as important as buying the right pair of shoes.

Research has shown that the use of telephone headsets can reduce neck pain, back pain, and headaches in employees who use the phone and computer simultaneously for a minimum of two hours a day.

Other Ergonomic Solutions

Transferring Equipment

To reduce the hazards associated with transferring equipment:

- ☐ Place equipment on a rolling device, if possible, to allow for easier transport, or attach wheels to the equipment.
- ☐ Push rather than pull equipment, when possible. Keep arms close to the body and push with the whole body, not just the arms.
- ☐ Ensure that passageways are unobstructed.
- ☐ Attach handles to equipment to help with the transfer process.
- ☐ Get help with moving heavy, bulky, or tall equipment.
- ☐ Do not transport multiple items alone. Get help when moving a patient in a wheelchair with an IV pole and/or other equipment.

Reaching into Deep Sinks or Containers

Limit excessive reaching and back flexion when washing dishes or laundry, or when working in maintenance areas and using a deep sink, by:

- ☐ Placing an object such as a plastic basin in the bottom of the sink to raise the surface used for washing items in the sink
- ☐ Moving objects to be washed into a smaller container on the counter for scrubbing or soaking, and placing them back in the sink for the final rinse

Lifting Trash, Laundry, or Other Bagged Material

Limit lifting hazards by:

- ☐ Using handling bags for laundry, garbage, and housekeeping that have side openings to allow for easy disposal
- ☐ Sliding bags off carts rather than lifting them
- ☐ Limiting the size and weight of bags
- ☐ Using garbage cans that have a frame, rather than a solid can, to prevent plastic bags from sticking to the inside of the can, or using products that are stuck to the inside of the garbage can to prevent the bag from sticking
- ☐ Restricting container size to limit the weight of the load that must be lifted
- ☐ Using mechanized platforms for lifting heavy items

Reaching and Pushing

Limit reaching and pushing hazards by:

- ☐ Keeping carts, hampers, gurneys, or other carts well maintained to minimize the amount of force exerted in using these items
- ☐ Using carts with large, low–rolling-resistance wheels; these usually roll easily over mixed flooring as well as over gaps between elevators and hallways
- ☐ Keeping the handles of devices to be pushed at waist to chest height
- ☐ Using handles to move carts, rather than the side of the cart, to prevent the smashing of hands and fingers
- ☐ Keeping floors clean and well maintained
- ☐ Pushing rather than pulling whenever possible
- ☐ Removing malfunctioning carts from use
- ☐ Getting help with heavy or bulky loads

Using Hand Tools in Maintenance Areas

Limit strains and sprains of maintenance workers' wrists, arms, and shoulders by choosing hand tools carefully. Hand tools should:

- ☐ Be properly designed and fit to the user
- ☐ Have padded non-slip handles
- ☐ Allow the wrist to remain straight in the performance of finger-intensive tasks (e.g., ergonomic knives or bent-handled pliers)

□ Have minimal weight

□ Involve minimal vibration (or be used with vibration-dampening devices and gloves)

□ Use trigger bars rather than single-finger triggers

□ Not be used for performing highly repetitive manual motions (e.g., use power screwdrivers instead of manual screwdrivers)

Performing Housekeeping Tasks

To decrease ergonomic stressors when performing cleaning tasks, employees should:

□ Alternate the leading hand to distribute the force

□ Avoid tight and static grip, and use padded non-slip handles

□ Clean objects at waist level, if possible, rather than bending over them (e.g., push wheelchairs up a ramped platform to perform cleaning work, or raise beds to waist level before cleaning)

□ Use kneepads when kneeling

□ Use tools with extended handles, or use step stools or ladders to avoid or limit overhead reaching

□ When sweeping or dusting, use flat-head dusters and push with the leading edge; sweep everything into one pile and pick it up with a vacuum

□ Soak soiled items in chemical or water-based cleaners to minimize the force needed for scrubbing

□ Frequently change mopping styles (e.g., push/pull, figure 8, and rocking side to side) to alternate stress between muscles

□ Be sure that buckets, vacuum cleaners, and other cleaning tools have wheels, or are set in wheeled containers with functional brakes

□ Alternate tasks or rotate employees through stressful tasks

□ Avoid awkward postures (e.g., twisting and bending)

□ Use carts to transport supplies rather than carrying them

□ Use floor buffers and vacuum cleaners that employ lightweight construction and adjustable handle height

□ Use spray bottles and equipment that use trigger bars rather than single-finger triggers

ERGONOMIC SUCCESS STORIES

Though debate continues about the nature and causes of ergonomic injuries, there are documented examples of well-managed ergonomics programs that have reduced injuries, illnesses, and costs.

Example 1

One ergonomics program driven by employee participation resulted in significant decreases in injuries in one 1,500-employee health care facility.[18] The facility sought to reduce the risk of ergonomics-related injuries below the level typically found in the health care industry, and came up with the following solution:

> Each job within the company was evaluated for ergonomic risk factors, and employees received training in the use of proper body mechanics and injury avoidance. Assistive devices were made available for lifting and transferring patients, and stationary workstations were individualized. The facility emphasized employee involvement as the most important element of the program. Employees participated in every aspect of safety management from risk assessment to program evaluation.

The company's injury incident rate decreased 66 percent in 2002 compared with the rate at the beginning of the program.

Example 2

Injuries to caregivers and other workers in a 2,400-employee facility from resident handling included back, shoulder, and knee injuries.[19] To reduce the number and severity of work-related injuries, the facility decided to modify working conditions to improve ergonomics.

The organization's workers' compensation carrier provided a risk management consultant, who developed a "no lift" program for the organization's nursing homes. Although the equipment was costly, the facility decided that the projected results made the start-up costs well worth the expense. The facility initially hoped that the program would improve employee morale and lead to fewer injuries and decreased workers' compensation costs.

Under the "no lift" policy, employees no longer had to lift residents, and manual transfers were performed only if the resident was ambulatory and the transfer required no lifting. Instead, a machine lifted the residents. Each resident was evaluated by the facility, and the type of care required by the resident (e.g., sit-to-stand lift or full lift) was recorded on a picture board in the resident's room.

When new equipment arrived, the staff were trained in its proper use. Compliance with the "no lift" policy became mandatory. Each facility also had at least two "product champions," who served as the model employees for demonstrating the policy. They were put in charge of orienting new employees to the machines and reeducating existing employees, as necessary, to ensure proper compliance with the policy and training for all other employees. Maintenance employees were responsible for ensuring that the batteries for the lifts were kept charged and available. Designated laundry employees were responsible for inspecting the slings for fraying, seam problems, or tears.

As a result of the "no lift" program, the certified nurse's aides (CNAs) reported feeling better and less fatigued at the end of the day. Their morale improved, and they were more active after work since they were not as tired as they had been before the "no lift" program was instituted. In addition, they reported feeling less stressed at the end of the day. Another positive outcome was that the CNAs were able to spend more time interacting with the residents because they spent less time lifting them. Work-related injuries and associated expenses also decreased as a result of the new "no lift" policy.

Resources Available for Ongoing Awareness

As more evidence is gathered and newer solutions are provided, what once might have seemed a hopeless problem may now have simple and economically feasible solutions. A variety of resources that provide literature and technical expertise are now available. Many publications, informational materials, and training courses are available from OSHA regional and state offices, or online at OSHA's website,[20] and OSHA also provides free on-site consultation services to employers who request help in implementing their ergonomics programs. A significant amount of information is also available from NIOSH.[21]

Some major insurance carriers now offer consultation and seminars, universities offer courses on ergonomics, and companies provide consultation. The Internet and safety-related websites are additional ways of staying abreast of safety and health breakthroughs. There are also Internet resources that can help to focus a search for ergonomics information specific to health care facilities.

Each year more companies produce ergonomically designed tools and equipment to prevent MSDs, including air-powered hand tools; height- and back-adjustable chairs, stools, and worktables; and floor mats. A new health care facility should consider installing ergonomically designed office furniture, tools and equipment, and examination room equipment. The initial purchase of ergonomically correct furniture, fixtures, and equipment can be considerably less expensive than replacing or retrofitting these items at a later date. Many computer-related ergonomic problems can also be prevented with adjustable chairs and desk surfaces, accessories such as no-glare screens for the display, and ergonomically redesigned keyboards.

One of the essential tools in preventing MSDs is physical fitness.[22] Ergonomic injuries are less likely to occur if employees maintain good physical health. There are several ways the employer can participate in this effort. Employers can provide information and training on the importance of physical fitness and proper body mechanics.

HOW THE JOINT COMMISSION PROMOTES SOUND ERGONOMIC PRACTICES

Because of the excessive rate of injuries due to overexertion (4.5 times greater than in any other industry), the Joint Commission has included injuries due to transferring patients as one of its National Patient Safety Goals for 2006 for long-term care, critical access hospitals, disease-specific care organizations, and other health care organizations. The 2006 National Patient Safety Goals require health care facilities to implement a fall reduction program, and implementation expectations included in 9B require a protocol for transferring patients.

The Joint Commission monitors a facility's awareness of the ergonomic hazards confronting health care workers under safety management (EC.1.10). Standard EC.1.10, specifically Elements of Performance (EP) 4 and 5, address ergonomic issues. Under EP4, health care facilities are required to conduct comprehensive, proactive risk assessments that evaluate the potential adverse impact of buildings, grounds, equipment, occupants, and internal physical systems on the safety and health of patients, staff, and other people coming to the facility. Under EP5, health care facilities are required to use the risks identified in EP4 to select and implement procedures and controls to achieve the lowest potential for adverse impact on the safety and health of patients, staff, and others coming to the facility.

THE ROLE OF THE ENVIRONMENTAL HEALTH AND SAFETY DEPARTMENT IN ERGONOMICS

The Environmental Health and Safety Department has a critical role in reducing injuries and illnesses associated with ergonomic hazards. Like other workplace hazards, ergonomic hazards require a process of management leadership and employee participation. This process includes collecting data, reviewing records, analyzing job-related tasks, preventing hazards through administrative and engineering controls, and administering a medical management program to oversee the care of those injured.

The Environmental Health and Safety Department should identify and address ergonomic stressors in the facility's safety and health plan. As they become aware of early warning signs of ergonomic hazards (employee fatigue or discomfort, reports of problems, or high levels of absenteeism), employees should be taught how to minimize factors that may contribute to musculoskeletal disorders at the design stage of the work process, if possible. Early action is particularly important in addressing MSDs, because they tend to be treatable and less expensive in the early stages, but irreversible and very expensive later.

The Environmental Health and Safety Department should conduct a thorough review of existing records and ensure that each injury related to an ergonomic problem is recorded. Accurate and consistent incident reporting will help identify ergonomic problems and the departments in which they are occurring.

Records of injuries and illnesses should be analyzed to identify patterns that appear over time, enabling the hazards to be addressed and prevented. This process includes reviewing OSHA Form 300 logs and workers' compensation reports. If a series of injuries can be traced to a single source, such as lifting patients, a job hazard analysis (JHA) should be performed for that job and a course of action to prevent future incidents should be determined and implemented. Routine analysis of workers' compensation reports will also help identify problem areas.

Even if there have been no incident reports or workers' compensation claims over the past year in a specific department, the occurrence of lost workdays should be reviewed periodically. Although the injury resulting in a lost workday may or may not be job related, it should be investigated to eliminate the worksite or job factors as the source of the problem.

Another way to gather information is to observe body language, which often reveals problems with muscles, eyestrain, headaches, and other symptoms associated with an MSD.

Table 10-4 presents some factors to consider in conducting a JHA for ergonomics. For example, a single employee who is absent several times a year because of a strained back muscle should receive a medical evaluation and perhaps be reassigned. Likewise, if numerous employees complain about shooting pains in one or both wrists, a JHA should be performed to determine if repetitive motion is the cause.

A training program designed and implemented by qualified personnel should be established to provide continuing education. Training about ergonomic hazards and controls should be provided for all employees, including managers and supervisors. Training should be updated as changes occur and presented at a level of understanding appropriate for those individuals being trained.

A receptive atmosphere that promotes employees' participation and encourages them to report MSDs is important to the success of the program. Involving the entire staff in finding job hazard solutions strengthens the program and helps employees understand that the effort is critical to their well-being. Even if an employee changes career direction several years later, the cumulative effects of a decade of repetitive tasks will remain.

Employees must take individual responsibility for their well-being. Employees who slouch, for example, are likely candidates for back problems later in life. Seated employees are inviting circulatory problems when they wrap their ankles around the base of the chair, cross their legs, or put added pressure on their thighs against the seat of the chair. For employees who stand all day, wearing ill-fitting or inappropriate shoes can also lead to cumulative disorders.

Work habits can sometimes be corrected by briefly chatting with employees. Otherwise, training on the physiological effects of poor posture or unnatural body positioning in the performance of certain tasks may be necessary.

Table 10–4. Sample Factors to Consider in a Job Hazard Analysis

Physical Work Activities and Conditions	Ergonomic Risk Factors That May Be Present
Exerting considerable physical effort to complete a motion	Force Awkward postures Contact stress
Using the same motion over and over again	Repetition Force Awkward postures Cold temperatures
Performing motion(s) constantly, without short pauses or breaks in between	Repetition Force Awkward postures Static postures Contact stress
Maintaining the same position or posture while performing tasks	Awkward postures Static postures Force Cold temperatures
Sitting for a long time	Awkward postures Static postures Contact stress
Objects or people moved are heavy	Force Repetition Awkward postures Static postures Contact stress
Bending or twisting during manual handling	Force Repetition Awkward postures Static postures
Poor workstation design, including using telephone handsets for extended periods	Eyestrain Neck, muscle, back problems Fatigue Insomnia
Poorly illuminated computer monitors	Eyestrain Blurred vision Teary or itchy eyes
Excessive computer use	Eye pain Primary color reversal (seeing green as red and red as green) Wrist tendonitis

Source: Adapted from www.osha.gov, proposed ergonomics standard.

As with other safety and health issues, MSD reports may increase temporarily, giving the appearance that the program is creating more problems than solutions. But as the program gains recognition, the number and frequency of MSDs will decrease, as will workers' compensation claims.

References

1. Ramazzini, Bernardino. *De Morbis Artificum Diatriba* (*Diseases of Workers*) (from the Latin text of 1713, revised, with translation and notes by Wilmer Cave Wright). Chicago: University of Chicago Press, 1940.

2. Terkel, Studs. *Working*. New York: New Press, 1974.

3. Occupational Safety and Health Administration. *Hospital eTool*, p. 1. Available at http://www.osha.gov/SLTC/etools/hospital/hazards/ergo/ergo.html (accessed 3/25/2005).

4. Table R4. Available at http://www.stats.bls.gov/iif/oshwc/osh/case/ostb1159.pdf (accessed 3/20/2006).

5. National Institute for Occupational Safety and Health. *Elements of Ergonomics Programs*. HHS (NIOSH) Publication No. 97–117. Cincinnati: NIOSH, 1997.

6. National Institute for Occupational Safety and Health. *Musculoskeletal Disorders and Workplace Factors: A Critical Review of Epidemiologic Evidence for Work-Related Musculoskeletal Disorders of the Neck, Upper Extremity, and Low Back* (second printing). HHS (NIOSH) Publication No. 97–141. Cincinnati: NIOSH, 1997. Available at http://www.cdc.gov/niosh/ergosci1.html (accessed 3/20/2006).

7. National Institute for Occupational Safety and Health. *Musculoskeletal Disorders and Workplace Factors: A Critical Review of Epidemiologic Evidence for Work-Related Musculoskeletal Disorders of the Neck, Upper Extremity, and Low Back* (second printing). HHS (NIOSH) Publication No. 97–141. Cincinnati: NIOSH, 1997. Available at http://www.cdc.gov/niosh/ergosci1.html (accessed 3/20/2006).

8. Occupational Safety and Health Administration. *Ergonomics: Guidelines. OSHA Protocol for Developing Industry-Specific and Task-Specific Ergonomics Guidelines* (revised December 16, 2002). Available at http://www.osha.gov/SLTC/ergonomics/protocol.html (accessed 3/20/2006).

9. Occupational Safety and Health Administration. "Safety and Health Program Management Guidelines: Issuance of Voluntary Guidelines," *OSHA Federal Register Notice* (January 26, 1989), 54 (18), pp. 3908–3916.

10. Occupational Safety and Health Administration. *OSH Act* (1970). Available at http://www.osha.gov/pls/oshaweb/owasrch.search_form?p_doc_type=OSHACT (accessed 3/20/2006).

11. NIOSH. *Elements of Ergonomics Programs. A Primer Based on Workplace Evaluations of Musculoskeletal Disorders*. HHS (NIOSH) Publication 97-117. Cincinnati: NIOSH, 1997.

12. Occupational Safety and Health Administration. *Hospitals, Healthcare-Wide Hazards, Ergonomics*. OSHA eTool. Available at http://www.osha.gov/SLTC/etools/hospital/index.html (accessed 3/20/2006).

13. Occupational Safety and Health Administration. *Working Safely with Video Display Terminals*. OSHA 3092 1997 (revised). Available at http://www.osha.gov/Publications/osha3092.pdf (accessed 3/20/2006).

14. Occupational Safety and Health Administration. *Hospitals, Healthcare-Wide Hazards, Ergonomics*. OSHA eTool. Available at http://www.osha.gov/SLTC/etools/hospital/index.html (accessed 3/20/2006).

15. Occupational Safety and Health Administration. *Guidelines for Nursing Homes: Ergonomics for the Prevention of Musculoskeletal Disorders*. OSHA 3182 2003. Available at http://www.osha.gov/ergonomics/guidelines/nursinghome/final_nh_guidelines.pdf (accessed 3/20/2006).

16. NIOSH. *Backbelts: Do They Prevent Injury?* HHS (NIOSH) Publication No. 94–127. Cincinnati: NIOSH, 1994.

17. Canadian Centre for Occupational Health and Safety. *Prevention of Slips, Trips and Falls*. Available at http://www.ccohs.ca/oshanswers/safety_haz/falls.html (accessed 3/20/2006).

18. Citizens Memorial Healthcare, Bolivar, Missouri (February 2003).

19. Heritage Enterprises, Inc., Bloomington, Illinois (July 2002).

20. www.osha.gov.

21. www.cdc.gov/niosh.

22. Mulry, Ray. *In the Zone*. Arlington, VA: Great Ocean, 1995.

CHAPTER 11

WORKPLACE VIOLENCE

There was an old sow with three little pigs, and as she had not enough to keep them, she sent them out to seek their fortune. The first that went off met a man with a bundle of straw, and said to him, "Please, man, give me that straw to build me a house." Which the man did, and the little pig built a house with it.

Presently came along a wolf, and knocked at the door, and said, "Little pig, little pig, let me come in."

To which the pig answered, "No, no, not by the hair of my chinny chin chin."

The wolf then answered to that, "Then I'll huff, and I'll puff, and I'll blow your house in." So he huffed, and he puffed, and he blew his house in, and ate up the little pig.

Three Little Pigs, nineteenth-century English fairy tale

In turn, each of the three little pigs was harassed, stalked, bullied, threatened, and assaulted by the wolf. Two of them had their homes destroyed, and the lives of all three and their mother were changed forever. Being eaten by a wolf is, after all, a significant life-altering event. The last little pig, whom we believe to be the wisest, built his house of brick to deter the wolf, and then found clever solutions to deceive him so that he could go about his business. When, as a last resort, the wolf launched a full-scale attack by trying to break into the house through its chimney, the last little pig found a clever way to turn the tables on the wolf.

The last little pig had observed what happened to his brothers and prepared himself. He understood the wolf's methods and knew that the wolf would do him harm if given the chance. He knew that he must take an active role in his personal safety in order stop the bullying, harassment, threats, and assault that his brothers had experienced.

WORKPLACE VIOLENCE

The story of the *Three Little Pigs* is a fairy tale, but it has a real-world message. The little pigs had a plan for their personal safety because they knew that the wolf was lurking and intended to do them harm. For the health care worker, however, it may be difficult to predict when a patient, a visitor, an employee, or an ex-employee may become violent or what form the violence may take. A visitor may become verbally abusive, one employee may bully another, an incoherent patient might suddenly become physically violent, or an employee may be sexually assaulted in an isolated area of the facility.

Violence between staff members consisting of threats and harassment occurs more often in organizations that have poor human resources practices and policies and that lack workplace violence prevention policies and programs.[1] Workplace violence can be reduced when employees are treated fairly and equitably, are valued, are kept informed of issues that affect their work conditions, and are shown appreciation for their efforts.

Organizational Structure

Although workplace violence has become a concern of the occupational safety and health community throughout the world, the traditional tools used to solve occupational health and safety problems are generally ill suited to workplace violence. The Human Resources and Security departments are far better qualified in terms of expertise to address workplace violence and apply surveillance, training, and engineering approaches to workplace violence issues. Those departments have the infrastructure needed to handle potentially violent situations, to prevent difficult situations from getting out of control, and to screen new employees who may have a history of violence.

Unless the Security Department reports administratively to the Environmental Health and Safety Department, the role of the Environmental Health and Safety director should be to provide support within the function and structure of the facility's employee health and safety program.

Some health care facilities combine the safety and security functions in one department. In health care facilities with over 100 beds, this practice should be closely evaluated by senior administration. In today's environment, the Environmental Health and Safety director's responsibilities are immense. Correspondingly, a trained professional should direct the Security Department. However, because a single individual sometimes has the dual role of safety and health director and security director, this chapter provides guidelines that Environmental Health and Safety staff can use for preventing and responding to incidents of workplace violence.

Workplace Violence Statistics

In 1999 the Bureau of Labor Statistics (BLS) reports that there were 2,637 assaults and other violent acts in hospitals that resulted in days away from work. In 2002 BLS reported that the number of assaults and violent acts in hospitals exceeded 4,100. In 2003 more than 3,500 health care workers were the victims of assaults or other violent acts that resulted in days away from work.

The rate at which health care workers were injured in 2003 as a consequence of an assault or other violent act was more than three times the rate for all of private industry (8.5 per 10,000 for full-time health care employees vs. 2.6 per 10,000 for all other full-time employees). These statistics include only incidents that were reported to the Occupational Safety and Health Administration (OSHA) on Form 300, Log of Work-Related Injuries and Illnesses, and resulted in days away from work. Therefore, it is reasonable to assume that the true number of cases is much greater. Moreover, there is no way of knowing how many other acts of violence, such as harassment, bullying, or stalking, occur each year because there is no requirement to record them.

TYPES OF WORKPLACE VIOLENCE

In developing its guidelines, OSHA relied on a definition of workplace violence that has been proposed by the National Institute for Occupational Safety and Health (NIOSH):

> Violent acts (including physical assaults and threats of assaults) directed toward persons at work or on duty.[2]

There are several problems with this definition. First, it is too narrow to address the full scope of workplace violence problems. Second, the definition includes acts of terrorism, which is not typically considered to be an issue of workplace violence. Therefore, the description of workplace violence offered by the Canadian Initiative on Workplace Violence is the basis for this chapter. The chapter focuses on those acts of violence that occur in health care facilities but excludes acts of terrorism perpetrated by political entities. According to the Canadian Initiative, workplace violence and aggression are more than physical acts and include:[3]

Harassment
Bullying and intimidation
Physical assaults
Stalking

All four of these elements can be present in domestic violence.

Harassment

Harassment is discrimination and is therefore against the law. Human rights commissions throughout the United States and around the world define harassment as unwelcome physical, visual, or verbal conduct that may involve the items listed in figure 11-1.

Figure 11–1. Conduct That Contributes to Harassment

    □ Unwelcome physical contact such as touching, stroking, pushing, and pinching

    □ Practical jokes

    □ Insults

    □ Threats

    □ Personal comments or innuendo

    □ Physical assault

    □ Unwelcome sexual acts, comments, or propositions

Any behavior that insults or intimidates can be considered harassment, if a reasonable person should have known that the behavior is unwelcome.

Bullying and Intimidation

Bullying is an offensive behavior characterized by vindictive, cruel, malicious, or humiliating attempts to undermine an individual or group of employees, and can include threats of reprisal in the form of demotions and poor performance appraisals. These persistently negative attacks are typically unpredictable, irrational, and unfair. Bullying and intimidation can happen at every level of an organization and are sometimes tolerated by managers who are under pressure to obtain results in a highly competitive market. On rare occasions, an employee's retaliation can be deadly.

Examples of bullying include:

□ Punishing others by constantly criticizing them, removing their responsibilities, or assigning them trivial tasks

□ Shouting at staff

□ Persistently picking on or berating co-workers, either in front of others or in private

□ "Keeping people in their place" by blocking their promotion

□ Overloading an individual with work and reducing time frames for completion

Physical Assaults

A physical assault, or the threat of one, is a criminal matter and should never be tolerated either inside or outside the workplace. Health care workers run the risk of physical assault on a daily basis. Every effort should be made to ensure that safety precautions are in place to protect employees and that swift action is taken against those who commit or threaten violent acts.

Physical assaults may occur either inside or outside the health care facility. Health care workers are at risk of assault by unruly patients, frustrated family and friends, or other employees. Conflicts can arise between employees because of personality differences or perceived or actual harassment, bullying, or intimidation. Family or friends of patients, disgruntled current or former employees, or sexual predators can perpetrate physical assaults.

Stalking

A recent study by the National Institute of Justice found that 8 percent of American women and 2 percent of American men reported being stalked at least once in their lifetime.[4] This translates into approximately 1.4 million American stalking victims every year. Although the majority of these stalkers had been in relationships with their victims, a significant percentage were either strangers or acquaintances, such as neighbors, friends, or co-workers.

Stalking victims often do not think of themselves as victims and consequently fail to report incidents of stalking. Stalking can cause anxiety, erode confidence, and have a negative impact on job performance.

RISK FACTORS

The Occupational Safety and Health Administration has identified a number of risk factors confronting health care workers:

- □ The prevalence of handguns and other weapons among patients and their families or friends
- □ The increasing use of hospitals by police and the justice system for criminal detentions and for the care of acutely disturbed, violent individuals
- □ The increasing number of acute and chronic mentally ill patients being released from hospitals without follow-up care (these patients have the right to refuse medicine and can no longer be hospitalized involuntarily unless they pose an immediate threat to themselves or others)
- □ The availability of drugs or money at hospitals, clinics, and pharmacies, making them likely robbery targets
- □ Unrestricted public movement in clinics and hospitals, and long waits in emergency or clinic areas, which can lead to client frustration
- □ The increasing presence of gang members, drug or alcohol abusers, trauma patients, and distraught family members in health care facilities
- □ Low staffing levels during times of increased activity, such as mealtimes, visiting times, and when employees are transporting patients

□ Isolation with clients during examinations or treatment

□ Solo work, often in remote locations with no backup or means to summon assistance, such as communication devices or alarm systems

□ Lack of staff training in the recognition and management of hostile behavior

□ Poorly lit parking areas

□ Working late at night or during early morning hours

THE COST OF VIOLENCE AT WORK

A 2001 report on violence and stress in the workplace, commissioned by the International Labour Organization (ILO), determined that there are both tangible and intangible costs associated with workplace violence.[5] [CD-ROM 11.1] The tangible costs include lost workdays, loss of income, and the cost of medical care. The intangible costs, however, extend well beyond those paid by the victims. The ILO report suggests that the impact of a violent act ripples through the organization and the community, causing both physical and mental stress. The outcomes may include absenteeism, sickness, loss of productivity, and increased turnover rates. Other effects may include poor concentration, diminished self-confidence, personal withdrawal, and social isolation. In such situations victims of violence are often skeptical about receiving any assistance, which makes treatment more difficult and prolongs recovery.

The factors listed in figure 11-2 also need to be considered in assessing the cost of stress and violence to the organization.

PREVENTING WORKPLACE VIOLENCE

The Occupational Safety and Health Administration (OSHA) has no specific standard that is designed to prevent workplace violence. However, in *Guidelines for Preventing Workplace Violence for Health Care & Social Service Workers*,[6]

Figure 11–2. Factors to Consider in Assessing the Cost of Violence

---

□ Absence due to illness

□ Premature retirement

□ Increased turnover and replacement costs

□ Grievance and litigation costs

□ Compensation costs

□ Cost of repairing damaged equipment or infrastructure

□ Reduced productivity

□ Loss of public goodwill and reputation

OSHA states, "Workplace violence policies indicate a zero-tolerance for all forms of violence from all sources" [CD-ROM 11.2], and OSHA also states that in lieu of a specific standard for workplace violence, Section 5(a)(1) of the Occupational Safety and Health Act (OSH Act) will apply: [CD-ROM 11.3]

Sec. 5. Duties

a) Each employer—
   1. shall furnish to each of his employees employment and a place of employment which are free from recognized hazards that are causing or are likely to cause death or serious physical harm to his employees.

In the guidelines, OSHA noted that in 2000:

48 percent of all non-fatal injuries from occupational assaults and violent acts occurred in health care and social services. Most of these occurred in hospitals, nursing and personal care facilities, and residential care services. Nurses, aides, orderlies and attendants suffered the most non-fatal assaults resulting in injury.

The guidelines also state:

Incidents of violence are likely to be underreported, perhaps due in part to the persistent perception within the healthcare industry that assaults are part of the job. Underreporting may reflect a lack of institutional reporting policies, employee beliefs that reporting will not benefit them or employee fears that employers may deem assaults the result of employee negligence or poor job performance.

Because of these conditions, OSHA recommends:

- Adopting a zero-tolerance policy for workplace violence, including verbal and nonverbal threats and related actions
- Ensuring that managers, employees, patients, visitors, and vendors are aware of the zero-tolerance policy
- Ensuring that there are no reprisals for reporting policy violations
- Encouraging prompt reporting of violent acts
- Encouraging and ensuring that records of violent acts are maintained
- Developing a comprehensive security plan that includes liaison with local law enforcement authorities and others who can help identify ways to prevent and mitigate workplace violence
- Assigning program authority to individuals with the appropriate training and skills, and ensuring that adequate resources for operating the program are provided
- Ensuring that management commitment to the program is visible and proactive, and affirming management commitment to a

worker-supportive environment that places as much importance on employee safety and health as on serving the patient

☐ Setting up a facility briefing as part of the initial effort to address issues such as preserving safety, supporting affected employees, and facilitating recovery

Employees must understand that the OSH Act applies to protected activity involving the hazard of workplace violence as much as it does to other health and safety matters, and that they are protected by the anti-discrimination (whistle-blower) provisions of the OSH Act:

Sec. 11.(c)

1. No person shall discharge or in any manner discriminate against any employee because such employee has filed any complaint or instituted or caused to be instituted any proceeding under or related to this Act or has testified or is about to testify in any such proceeding or because of the exercise by such employee on behalf of himself or others of any right afforded by this Act.

OSHA's RECOMMENDED SAFETY AND HEALTH PROGRAM MANAGEMENT GUIDELINES

Voluntary, generic safety and health program management guidelines were issued by OSHA for all employers to use as a foundation for their safety and health programs, which can include workplace violence prevention programs. The violence prevention guidelines extend these generic guidelines by identifying common risk factors and describing some feasible solutions. Although not exhaustive, the workplace violence guidelines include policy recommendations and practical corrective methods to help prevent and mitigate the effects of workplace violence.

Guidelines for Preventing Workplace Violence for Health Care & Social Service Workers suggests that the successful violence prevention program will have five components. These same components are presented in OSHA's *Safety and Health Program Management Guidelines:*[7] [CD-ROM 11.4]

Management commitment and employee involvement
Worksite analysis
Hazard prevention and control
Safety and health training
Recordkeeping and program evaluation

As is the case for OSHA's safety and health program management guidelines, a key element in the violence prevention program is the firm and proactive commitment of management and employees.

Management Commitment

Management must take the lead and demonstrate its willingness to do the difficult work of effectively communicating the facility's policy to employees, patients, and visitors. Management can show its commitment by:

- Demonstrating organizational concern for employees' emotional and physical safety and health
- Demonstrating that its commitment extends to workers, patients, and visitors alike
- Assigning responsibility for the various aspects of the workplace violence prevention program
- Ensuring that all managers, supervisors, and employees understand their obligations
- Allocating appropriate authority and resources to all responsible parties
- Maintaining a system of accountability for managers, supervisors, and employees
- Establishing a comprehensive program of medical and psychological counseling and debriefing for employees experiencing or witnessing assaults and other violent incidents
- Supporting and implementing appropriate recommendations from safety and health committees
- Encouraging employee involvement and feedback, and providing a non-threatening atmosphere for employees to openly express their concerns and ideas

Employee Involvement

Employees have an obligation to be actively involved in the violence prevention program to facilitate its success. Employees must:

- Understand and comply with the workplace violence prevention program and other safety and security measures
- Participate in employee complaint or suggestion procedures that address personal safety and security concerns
- Report violent incidents promptly and accurately
- Participate on the Environmental Health and Safety Committee or on teams that receive reports of violent incidents or security problems
- Participate in facility inspections and help develop recommendations for corrective strategies
- Take part in continuing education programs that cover techniques for recognizing escalating agitation, violent behavior, or criminal intent, and that discuss appropriate responses

Worksite Analysis

Just as there must be a worksite analysis for the employee health and safety program, those with responsibility for the workplace violence program should conduct a thorough examination of the workplace to identify conditions that may foster or contribute to workplace violence. This analysis can be conducted by a trained threat assessment team or similar interdisciplinary team experienced in assessing the facility's vulnerabilities and in determining appropriate preventive actions. This group may also be responsible for implementing the workplace violence prevention program. The team should include representatives from senior management, employee assistance, security, occupational safety and health, legal and human resources staff, as well as representatives from departments in the facility.

The worksite analysis should focus on:

☐ Analyzing and tracking records
☐ Screening surveys
☐ Analyzing workplace security

Records Analysis and Tracking

For certain incidents, information will be collected on OSHA Form 300. But the system that is developed for information collection must also be able to accommodate information on other acts of violence, such as bullying, harassment, stalking, and those physical assaults not reported on OSHA Form 300. The data collected in such a system will be crucial to developing intervention strategies and assessing their success and appropriateness.

This analysis should include a review of safety, workers' compensation, police reports, and the OSHA Form 300 to identify and analyze trends in assaults specific to:

☐ Departments
☐ Units
☐ Job titles
☐ Unit activities
☐ Workstations
☐ Times of day

Review of these data will help identify the frequency, severity, and locations of incidents to determine if there are particular areas that require immediate attention and to establish a baseline for measuring improvement. Several years of data should be used, if possible, to trace trends of injuries and incidents of actual or potential workplace violence.

Screening Surveys

Properly constructed surveys or employee questionnaires that ensure the anonymity of participants can be used to elicit information about existing security problems or potential problems within particular departments, units, or areas of the facility. Detailed baseline screening surveys can help pinpoint tasks that put employees at risk. Periodic surveys—conducted at least annually, or whenever operations change or incidents of workplace violence occur—help identify new or previously unnoticed risk factors and deficiencies or failures in work practices, procedures, or controls. Also, the surveys help in assessing the effects of changes in the work processes. The periodic review process should also include feedback and follow-up.

The Environmental Health and Safety Department and other independent reviewers, such as law enforcement or security specialists and insurance safety auditors, may offer advice or provide fresh perspectives to strengthen the program.

Analyzing Workplace Security

The threat assessment team should periodically inspect the workplace and evaluate employee tasks to identify hazards, conditions, operations, and situations that could lead to violence.

To find areas requiring further evaluation, the team or coordinator should:

☐ Analyze incidents to understand the characteristics of assailants and victims, what happened before and during the incident, and the relevant details of the situation and its outcome.

☐ Identify jobs or locations with the greatest risk of violence as well as processes and procedures that put employees at risk of assault, including identifying how often and when.

☐ Note high-risk factors such as types of patients (e.g., those with psychiatric conditions or who are disoriented by drugs, alcohol, or stress); physical risk factors related to building layout or design; isolated locations and job activities; lighting problems; lack of phones and other communication devices; and areas characterized by easy, unsecured access or previous security problems.

☐ Evaluate the effectiveness of existing security measures, including engineering controls; determine if risk factors have been reduced or eliminated, and take appropriate action.

Hazard Prevention and Control

After hazards have been identified through the systematic worksite analysis, engineering and administrative solutions can be coupled with new work practices to prevent or control the risk of violent acts. If violence does occur, the response can be an important tool in preventing future incidents.

Engineering Controls

Engineering controls remove the hazard from the workplace or create a barrier between the worker and the hazard. The third little pig found an engineering solution to his problem when he built his house using bricks; in the workplace, engineering solutions can also be used to prevent violent acts. The selection of measures should be based on the hazards identified in the security analysis of the facility.

Among other options, engineering controls include:

- Plans for new construction or physical changes to the facility that eliminate or reduce security hazards
- Use of alarm systems, panic buttons, handheld alarms, cellular phones, or private-channel radios where risk is apparent or may be anticipated
- A reliable response in the event that an alarm is triggered
- Metal detectors, where appropriate, to detect weapons
- Closed-circuit video recording in high-risk areas on a 24-hour basis (public safety is of greater concern than privacy in these situations)
- Curved mirrors at hallway intersections or next to concealed areas
- Enclosed nurses' stations and deep service counters or bullet-resistant, shatterproof glass in reception, triage, and admitting areas or client service rooms
- Employee "safe rooms" for use during emergencies
- "Time-out" or seclusion areas that have high ceilings without supporting grids (which could be used as weapons) for patients who "act out"
- Separate rooms for criminal patients
- Comfortable client or patient waiting rooms designed to minimize stress
- Locked staff counseling rooms and treatment rooms to limit access
- Furniture arranged to prevent entrapment of staff
- If possible, furniture without sharp corners (perhaps attached to the floor) in interview rooms or crisis treatment areas; limited numbers of pictures, vases, ashtrays, or other loose items that could be used as weapons
- Lockable, secure bathrooms for staff members separate from patient/client and visitor facilities
- Locked unused doors to limit access—in compliance with local fire codes

❑ Bright and effective lighting, both indoors and outdoors

❑ Replacing burned-out lights and broken windows and locks as soon as they are discovered

❑ Proper maintenance of automobiles used in the field

❑ Promotion of the importance of locking automobiles

Administrative Controls

Administrative and work practice controls affect the way people perform their jobs. Examining how jobs are performed can lead to the development and implementation of changes to prevent violent acts. Examples of administrative and work practice controls include:

❑ Stating clearly to patients, clients, employees, and the public that violence is not permitted or tolerated

❑ Establishing liaison with local police and state prosecutors, reporting all incidents of violence, and equipping police with physical layouts of facilities to expedite investigations

❑ Requiring employees to report all assaults or threats to a supervisor, to security, or to a member of the threat assessment team; and keeping log books and reports of such incidents to determine necessary preventive measures

❑ Advising employees of procedures for requesting police assistance in case of assault, and providing management support during emergencies

❑ Responding promptly to all complaints

❑ Using properly trained security officers to deal with aggressive behavior

❑ Following written security procedures

❑ Ensuring that adequate and properly trained staff are available to restrain patients or clients, if necessary

❑ Enforcing visitor hours and procedures

❑ Using case management conferences with co-workers and supervisors to discuss ways to effectively treat potentially violent patients

❑ Ensuring that nurses and physicians are not alone when performing intimate physical examinations of patients

❑ Discouraging employees from wearing necklaces or chains to help prevent possible strangulation in confrontational situations

❑ Surveying the facility to remove tools or possessions left by visitors or maintenance staff that could be used inappropriately by patients

❑ Providing staff members with security escorts to parking areas in evening or late hours, and ensuring that parking areas are highly visible, well lit, and safely accessible from the building

Figure 11–3. Consequences of Workplace Violence Victims Suffer in Addition to Physical Injuries

□ Short- and long-term psychological trauma
□ Fear of returning to work
□ Changes in relationships with co-workers and family
□ Feelings of incompetence, guilt, and powerlessness
□ Fear of criticism by supervisors or managers

Employer Responses to Incidents of Violence

Post-incident response and evaluation are essential to an effective violence prevention program. All workplace violence programs should provide comprehensive treatment for employees who are victimized personally or may be traumatized by witnessing a workplace violence incident. Injured staff should receive prompt treatment and psychological evaluation whenever an assault takes place, regardless of its severity.

Victims of workplace violence suffer a variety of consequences in addition to their actual physical injuries. These may include the fears and feelings listed in figure 11-3. A strong follow-up program for these employees will not only help them to deal with these problems but also help prepare them to confront or prevent future incidents of violence.

Several types of assistance can be incorporated into the post-incident response. For example, trauma crisis counseling, critical-incident stress debriefing, or employee assistance programs may be provided to victims.

Counselors should be well trained and have a good understanding of the issues and consequences of assaults and other aggressive, violent behavior. Appropriate and promptly conducted post-incident debriefings and counseling reduce acute psychological trauma and general stress levels among victims and witnesses. In addition, this type of counseling educates staff about workplace violence and positively influences workplace and organizational cultural norms to reduce trauma associated with future incidents.

Safety and Health Training

Regular and updated training is essential to the prevention of violence and can help foster interpersonal and communication skills that employees can use to defuse potentially threatening situations.

Training for All Employees

Employees should learn to identify potentially violent situations and people, and should understand the nature of aggression and how to respond to emotional individuals.

Every employee should understand the concept of "universal precautions for violence"—that violence should be expected but can be avoided or mitigated through preparation. Frequent training also can reduce the likelihood of being assaulted.[8]

Employees who may face safety and security hazards should receive formal instruction on the specific hazards associated with the unit or job and the facility. This includes information on the types of injuries or problems that have been identified in the facility and the methods to control specific hazards. It also includes instructions to limit physical interventions in workplace altercations whenever possible, unless enough staff or emergency response teams and security personnel are available. In addition, all employees should be trained to behave compassionately toward co-workers when an incident occurs.

All employees, including supervisors and managers, should receive training that includes at least the following elements:

- The workplace violence prevention policy
- Risk factors associated with assaults
- How to recognize the warning signs or situations that may precede assaults
- Prevention and control of volatile situations or aggressive behavior
- Anger management
- The facility's action plan for response, including how to call for assistance, how to react to alarm systems, and how to follow communication procedures
- How to deal with hostile relatives and visitors
- Progressive behavior control methods
- The "buddy system" as a tool for protection
- Policies and procedures for reporting incidents
- Information on multicultural diversity to increase staff sensitivity to racial and ethnic issues and differences
- Policies and procedures for obtaining medical care, counseling, workers' compensation, or legal assistance after a violent episode or injury

Training for Supervisors and Managers

Supervisors and managers need to learn to recognize high-risk situations that place employees in situations that compromise their safety. They also need training to encourage employees to report incidents.

Supervisors and managers should learn how to reduce security hazards and ensure that employees receive appropriate training. Following training, supervisors and managers should be able to recognize a potentially hazardous situation and to make any necessary changes to the physical plant, patient care treatment program, and staffing policy and procedures to reduce or eliminate the hazards.

Training for Security Personnel

Security personnel need specific training, including verbal intervention skills for handling aggressive and abusive patients. Their training should also include alternative means of handling aggression and defusing hostile situations.

The training program should be evaluated at least annually. The content, methods, and frequency of training should be reviewed. Individuals should demonstrate competency. Program evaluation may involve supervisor and employee interviews, testing and observing, reviewing reports of behavior of individuals in threatening situations, and the responses of those individuals.

Recordkeeping and Program Evaluation

Recordkeeping and evaluation of the violence prevention program are necessary to determine its overall effectiveness and to identify any deficiencies or changes that should be made. All reports must protect employee confidentiality. Data should be presented only in aggregate or summary form, and all personal identifiers must be removed.

Recordkeeping

Recordkeeping for workplace injuries and illnesses assists in the determination of the success of the employee health and safety program. Accurate recordkeeping of violent acts will provide a tool for the evaluation of the successes and failures of the violence prevention program. The following logs and reports are essential components of the recordkeeping process:

- □ OSHA Form 300, Log of Work-Related Injuries and Illnesses. Employers who are required to keep this log must record any new work-related injury that results in death, days away from work, days of restriction or job transfer, medical treatment beyond first aid, loss of consciousness, or a significant injury diagnosed by a licensed health care professional. Injuries caused by assaults must be entered in the log if they meet the recording criteria. All employers must report, within 24 hours, a fatality or an incident that results in the hospitalization of three or more employees.[9]
- □ Medical reports of work injury and supervisors' reports for each recorded assault. These records should describe the type of assault, such as an unprovoked sudden attack or patient-to-patient altercation; who was assaulted; and all other circumstances of the incident. The records should include a description of the environment or location, potential or actual cost, lost work time that resulted, and the nature of injuries sustained. These medical records are confidential documents and must be kept in a locked location under the direct responsibility of a health care professional.
- □ Records of incidents of abuse, verbal attacks, or aggressive behavior that may be threatening, such as pushing or shouting, and acts of

aggression toward other patients or employees. This may be kept as part of an assaultive incident report, and the records must be evaluated routinely. These types of incidents are not reported on the OSHA Form 300.

☐ Information relating to a history of violence, drug abuse, or criminal activity recorded on the patient's chart. All staff who care for a potentially aggressive, abusive, or violent patient should be aware of the person's background and history.

☐ Documentation including minutes of Environmental Health and Safety Committee meetings, records of hazard analyses, and the corrective actions recommended and taken.

☐ Records of all training programs, the attendees, and the qualifications of trainers.

Program Evaluation

The violence prevention program should undergo routine and periodic evaluation to determine whether the measures that have been instituted have been effective in reducing acts of violence. Program evaluation begins with an examination of the appropriate records to determine if the number of violent acts has increased, decreased, or remained constant. Based on the review, corrective actions can be taken to remedy any deficiencies that have appeared. Though it is the Security and Human Resources departments that will be primarily responsible for the violence prevention program, its evaluation should take place during the facility's Environmental Health and Safety Committee meetings or with union representatives or other employee groups. Program evaluation reports should be made available to all employees.

Processes involved in an evaluation include:

☐ Regularly reviewing reports

☐ Reviewing reports and minutes on safety and security issues and incidents

☐ Analyzing trends and rates in illnesses, injuries, or fatalities caused by violence relative to initial or "baseline" rates

☐ Measuring improvement based on lowered frequency and severity of workplace violence

☐ Keeping up-to-date records of changes in administrative and work practice to prevent workplace violence to evaluate how well they work

☐ Surveying employees before and after job or worksite changes, or following the installation of security measures or new systems, to determine their effectiveness

☐ Complying with OSHA and state requirements for recording and reporting deaths, injuries, and illnesses

☐ Requesting periodic law enforcement or outside consultant review of the worksite for recommendations on improving employee safety

An important goal of program evaluation is to determine if facility personnel are aware of any new strategies or best practices to deal with violence in the health care arena. Periodic surveys of employees can also help the program coordinator gauge the strengths and weaknesses of the existing program and identify areas in which improvement is needed.

OSHA Violence Prevention Checklists and Violence Incident Report Forms

Appendixes A and B of OSHA's *Guidelines* provide samples of checklists and forms that can be used or modified by health care facilities as part of their effort to prevent workplace violence.[10]

THE JOINT COMMISSION SECURITY STANDARD AS A DETERRENT TO WORKPLACE VIOLENCE

The Environment of Care (EC) standards of the Joint Commission on Accreditation of Healthcare Organizations require health care facilities to have a written security plan that addresses security issues for the facility and that provides for orientation and education of staff.[11] Each facility must have a security program along with performance standards and a plan for periodic evaluation of the security program. Each facility must also maintain records of the program's performance and make improvements as needed. The elements of this requirement are very similar to the elements described in OSHA's *Guidelines* and provide a sound process for planning, employee training, and performance monitoring.

According to the Joint Commission, the most common pattern of violence in a health care setting is care recipient against staff, followed closely by visitor against staff, and third, staff against care recipient. To address the problem of violence in health care facilities, the Joint Commission suggests developing a workplace violence prevention program that has the following elements:

- ☐ Effective leadership and employee involvement
- ☐ Worksite analysis
- ☐ Hazard prevention and control
- ☐ Training and education
- ☐ Recordkeeping and evaluation of the program

The Joint Commission has a number of standards that address violence in health care facilities. As is the case with most health care facility safety issues, the overarching Joint Commission standard is safety management (EC.1.10). The standard that most specifically addresses violence in the health care facility is security management (EC.2.10). Standard EC.2.10 specifically requires the organization to manage the potential for violence to patients and staff in the workplace and in the community. The Joint Commission also addresses aspects of violence prevention in:

- ☐ Emergency management (EC.4.10)
- ☐ Monitoring environmental conditions (EC.9.10)
- ☐ Analyzing environmental issues (EC.9.20)
- ☐ Improving the environment (EC.9.30)
- ☐ Staff qualifications (HR.1.20)
- ☐ Staff initial job training (HR.2.10)
- ☐ Staff roles and responsibilities (HR.2.20)

THE ROLES OF COMMUNICATION AND WORK ORGANIZATION IN PREVENTING VIOLENT ACTS

Effective communication and work organization considerations are integral in preventing violent acts.

Information and Communication

Open communication and information sharing can reduce the risk of workplace violence by defusing tension and frustration among workers. Information sessions, personnel meetings, and group discussions can be effective ways for employees to obtain accurate information, share concerns, and develop solutions for preventing violent acts or mitigating potential hazards. Effective communication with patients, their families, and visitors can also help prevent violence. This is particularly true in cases in which patients or their families or friends are distressed or have waited for long periods without receiving information.

Part of an effective communication strategy is the conflict resolution process. Human Resources and Security professionals who are trained in conflict resolution can train employees in techniques that defuse antagonistic situations that have the potential to escalate. Training in conflict resolution, coupled with a dispute resolution process, will increase the likelihood that a minor disagreement will not become serious. In some cases, a neutral party from outside the organization may be more effective than an individual perceived to have a "corporate bias."

Work Organization

Work organization is simply the act of giving consideration to how work is performed and the impediments to its conduct. Work organization considerations can help prevent workplace violence by ensuring that:

□ Staffing levels are appropriate

□ Tasks are assigned according to workers' experience and competence

□ Tasks are clearly defined

□ Working hours are not excessive

□ Shifts are adequate for the particular requirements

In the context of violence prevention, one approach may be to limit face-to-face contact between employees and the public in those situations in which violent behavior is possible. When such contact cannot be avoided, every effort should be made to ensure that employees are trained in skills to control potentially volatile situations.[12]

THE ROLE OF THE ENVIRONMENTAL HEALTH AND SAFETY DEPARTMENT

As mentioned previously, unless the responsibility for security resides administratively in the Environmental Health and Safety Department, or the facility combines the functions of the Security and Environmental Health and Safety departments, the skills of the Environmental Health and Safety director are generally not appropriate to managing the violence prevention program. Therefore, Human Resources and Security professionals who have the necessary skills, training, and experience should direct the program. Nevertheless, the standard principle of "Recognition, Evaluation, and Control" observed by health and safety professionals is equally suited to the prevention of violent acts.

The Environmental Health and Safety Department does, however, need to work closely with the Human Resources and Security departments in data collection and maintenance. This interaction is particularly important for the accurate completion and analysis of the OSHA Form 300 log.

The prevention of violent acts includes a strategic process of planning and communication. Combining well-known prevention strategies with the program elements discussed in this chapter can greatly reduce the incidence of workplace violence. By effectively addressing workplace violence, health care facilities will reduce their costs as a result of:

□ A reduction in grievances

□ Fewer recordable injuries

□ A drop in absenteeism

□ Lowered legal costs associated with litigation

In one version of the *Three Little Pigs*, as each house is destroyed, its builder takes his knowledge and experience to the next brother, and together they build a stronger house until, finally, their combined experience and knowledge enable them to defeat the big bad wolf. The successful violence prevention program requires the same dedication to information sharing and cooperation between the various departments as was demonstrated by the three pigs.

References

1. Bowman, D. *Workplace Violence—A Real Killer*. Lincolnshire International. Available at http://www.lincolnshireintl.com/resourcedisp.php3?rescID=2002040201300435 (accessed 3/21/2006).

2. CDC/NIOSH. *Violence: Occupational Hazards in Hospitals*. 2000. DHHS 2002-101. Available at http://www.cdc.gov/niosh/2002-101.html (accessed 3/21/2006).

3. *Profit through Prevention*. Canadian Initiative on Workplace Violence. Available at http://www.workplaceviolence.ca/home.html (accessed 3/21/2006).

4. Tjaden, P., and N. Thoennes. *Stalking in America: Findings From the National Violence Against Women Survey*. National Institute of Justice and the National Center for Injury Prevention and Control, Centers for Disease Control and Prevention. Available at http://www.ncjrs.gov/txtfiles/169592.txt (accessed 3/21/2006).

5. Hoel, Helge, Kate Sparks, and Cary L. Cooper, *The Cost of Violence/Stress at Work and the Benefits of a Violence/Stress-Free Working Environment*. Report Commissioned by the International Labour Organization (ILO), Geneva. University of Manchester Institute of Science and Technology.

6. Occupational Safety and Health Administration. US Department of Labor. *Guidelines for Preventing Workplace Violence for Health Care and Social Service Workers*. OSHA 3148, 01R 2004.

7. "Safety and Health Program Management Guidelines: Issuance of Voluntary Guidelines," *OSHA Federal Register Notice* (January 26, 1989) 54 (18), pp. 3908–3916.

8. OSHA. *Guidelines for Preventing Workplace Violence for Health Care and Social Service Workers*. OSHA 3148, 01R 2004.

9. OSHA. *Recording and Reporting Occupational Injuries and Illness*. 29 CFR 1904.7 (revised 2001). Available at http://www.osha.gov/pls/oshaweb/owadisp.show_document?p_table=STANDARDS&p_id=9638 (accessed 3/21/2006).

10. OSHA. *Guidelines for Preventing Workplace Violence for Health Care and Social Service Workers*. OSHA 3148, 01R 2004. Appendixes A and B.

11. Joint Commission. 2006 Comprehensive Accreditation Manual for Hospitals. Standard EC.2.10.

12. *Profit through Prevention*. Canadian Initiative on Workplace Violence. Available at http://www.workplaceviolence.ca/home.html (accessed 3/21/2006).

CHAPTER 12

EMERGENCY MANAGEMENT

Emergency (n) A situation or occurrence of a serious nature, developing suddenly and unexpectedly, and demanding immediate attention.

The American Heritage Dictionary

One day Chicken Little was walking in the woods when—kerplunk—an acorn fell on his head, "Oh my goodness!" said Chicken Little. "The sky is falling! I must go and tell the king."

On his way to the king's palace, Chicken Little met Henny Penny. Henny Penny said that he was going into the woods to hunt for worms. "Oh no, don't go!" said Chicken Little. "I was there and the sky fell on my head! Come with me to tell the king."

On their way to warn the king, Chicken Little and Henny Penny met a few others and explained to them that the sky was falling. Eventually all the birds in the woods joined them in this most urgent journey. But then the plot thickened:

"Where are you going, my fine feathered friends?" asked Foxy Woxy. He spoke in a polite manner, so as not to frighten them.

"The sky is falling!" cried Chicken Little. "We must tell the king."

"I know a shortcut to the palace," said Foxy Woxy sweetly. "Come and follow me."

Anonymous

We all know that a bird following a fox on a shortcut through the forest is really not a very good idea. Imagine the consequences for Chicken Little and his friends if the king's hunter and his dogs had not arrived to scare Foxy Woxy away. Like most fairy tales, this one has a happy ending.

After that day, Chicken Little always carried an umbrella with him when he walked in the woods. The umbrella was a present from the king. And if—*kerplunk*—an acorn fell, Chicken Little didn't mind a bit. In fact, he didn't even notice it.

Chicken Little knew an emergency when he saw one, and the sky falling on one's head certainly qualifies. The problem was that he was not prepared. It had never occurred to him, or anyone else for that matter, that one day the sky would fall on his head. Had he prepared himself, he might first have made a list of all the possible emergencies that might arise. Once he had that list, he could have developed a plan for responding to each of the potential emergencies in order to protect himself as well as Henny Penny, Loosey Goosey, Turkey Lurkey, and anyone else who might be affected. Having the sky fall on your head is obviously a sudden and unexpected event, and Chicken Little did give it his immediate attention, but was it the right attention?

Between 1970 and 2002, there were four events that helped shape the way emergency response and management are viewed in the United States. In the 1970s there were a series of wildfires in California. In 1995 the neurotoxin sarin was released on a Tokyo subway train. In 2001 terrorists in hijacked passenger aircraft flew into the World Trade Center buildings in New York City, New York. Later that same year the East Coast of the United States was subjected to a biological attack when *Bacillus anthracis* spores were sent via the U.S. mail to members of Congress and the media.

The fires in California crossed the jurisdictional boundaries of several fire departments. Unfortunately, there was no uniform method of communicating between departments and there were often disputes concerning which department had command responsibility. In the sarin attack, local hospitals were overwhelmed by the thousands of people who self-reported. In the third event, the hospitals in the vicinity of the World Trade Center waited for an influx of injured victims that turned out to be disproportionately small compared with the number of fatalities. In the fourth event, the public health system was marshaled to screen thousands of people, because the full extent of the anthrax attack was unknown. In each case, the response was driven by the emergency as it evolved on a moment-to-moment basis. As was the case with the California fires, there were jurisdictional disputes following both the World Trade Center and the anthrax attacks.

There are other emergencies that have historically taxed local health care systems. Hurricanes, floods, forest fires, earthquakes, industrial accidents, and other natural or man-made disasters pose a threat either because of an overwhelming need for health care or the rebuilding or repair of infrastructure, or because health care facilities may be required to evacuate patients and close their doors. Whether an emergency is due to natural events or an act of man, the fundamental structure of the response plan must be the same. This has been termed the *all-hazards* concept. Someone must be in charge, and those who have training and experience in coping with the particular emergency should be called on to handle it.

In late summer 2005, as this chapter was being crafted, a tropical depression formed in the Caribbean and quickly became a tropical storm named Katrina. As Katrina was about to make landfall on the south east coast of Florida, it became a category 1 hurricane. Because of its size, Katrina caused more damage and deaths than anticipated from a category 1 storm. When Katrina entered the Gulf of Mexico, it encountered warmer-than-usual waters and rapidly developed into a category 2 hurricane. Within days, the storm became a category 3 hurricane and made a sharp turn to the north. As it neared the coasts of Alabama, Mississippi, and Louisiana, it encountered water temperatures that were about 90°F and became a category 5 storm that filled more than half of the Gulf of Mexico. Though Katrina lost some strength as it made landfall, the damage it caused was monumental. In New Orleans, Katrina caused a portion of a levee to fail, flooding 80 percent of that city. The most immediate consequences included the destruction of roads, the airport, and the power distribution system; the collapse of state and local emergency response plans; and the isolation of virtually every hospital in the city.

Chicken Little's emergency response plan was simple—run and tell the king. But in today's world much more is required if casualties are to be contained and the effects of an emergency are to be minimized.

Every health care facility must develop an emergency management plan that is simple, easy to activate, involves the appropriate departments, specifies clear lines of authority, and relies on the existing organization of the facility. The plan must also enable the facility to work with appropriate agencies and organizations within the local community or county and to be prepared to interact with federal authorities. The facility should follow the principles of the *all-hazards* concept, which requires the integration of individual departmental responses into a single coherent response and accommodates either the assistance or command of outside agencies. Furthermore, as Katrina has made clear, planning must accommodate the concept of a worst-case event.

Emergency management is a dynamic process. Planning, though critical, is not the only component. Other important functions are training; conducting drills; testing equipment; coordinating activities with the community, county, and state; and recovery. There are many positive aspects of preparedness:

☐ It helps facilities fulfill their moral responsibility to protect employees, patients, the community, and the environment.

☐ It facilitates compliance with regulatory requirements of federal, state, and local agencies.

☐ It enhances a facility's ability to recover from financial losses, regulatory fines, loss of market share, damages to equipment or products, or business interruption.

☐ It enhances the facility's image and credibility with employees, patients, suppliers and the community.

☐ It may reduce insurance premiums.

THE ROLE OF GOVERNMENT AND NONGOVERNMENTAL AGENCIES

An emergency action plan is known as an emergency management plan in many health care facilities. It describes the actions employees should take to ensure their safety if a fire or other emergency situation occurs. Well-developed emergency plans and proper employee training (such that employees understand their roles and responsibilities within the plan) will result in fewer and less severe employee injuries and less structural damage to the facility during an emergency. A poorly prepared plan likely will lead to a disorganized evacuation or other emergency response, resulting in confusion, injury, and property damage.

Planning for emergencies facilitates compliance with the requirements of federal, state, and local agencies. In addition, health care facility accreditation organizations require emergency planning to help protect patients and employees during emergencies. These requirements help health care facilities to address specific emergency management functions that might otherwise be a lower-priority activity for the given year.

OSHA

The Occupational Safety and Health Administration (OSHA) considers sound planning the first line of defense in all types of emergencies. By tailoring emergency plans to accommodate the reasonably predictable "worst-case" scenario, the health care facility can rely on these plans to guide decisions regarding personnel training and personal protective equipment (PPE). Worst-case scenarios take into account challenges associated with communication, resources, and victims. During mass-casualty emergencies, health care facilities may receive little or no warning before victims begin arriving.

The emergency management requirements of OSHA are addressed in several standards under 29 CFR 1910 Subpart E, Exit Routes, Emergency Action Plans, and Fire Prevention Plans, and Subpart L, Fire Protection. [Primary standards for health care facilities are on the CD-ROM.]

Emergency planning in health care facilities is subject to OSHA Standard 29 CFR 1910.38, Emergency action plans. [CD-ROM 12.1]

> 1910.38(a)
> *Application.* An employer must have an emergency action plan whenever an OSHA standard in this part requires one. The requirements in this section apply to each such emergency action plan.

> 1910.38(b)
> *Written and oral emergency action plans.* An emergency action plan must be in writing, kept in the workplace, and available to employees for review. However, an employer with 10 or fewer employees may communicate the plan orally to employees.

1910.38(c)
Minimum elements of an emergency action plan. An emergency action plan must include at a minimum:

☐ Procedures for reporting a fire or other emergency.
☐ Procedures for emergency evacuation, including type of evacuation and exit route assignments.
☐ Procedures to be followed by employees who remain to operate critical plant operations before they evacuate.
☐ Procedures to account for all employees after evacuation.
☐ Procedures to be followed by employees performing rescue or medical duties.
☐ The name or job title of every employee who may be contacted by employees who need more information about the plan or an explanation of their duties under the plan.

1910.38(d)
Employee alarm system. An employer must have and maintain an employee alarm system. The employee alarm system must use a distinctive signal for each purpose and comply with the requirements in Subpart L Fire Protection, 29 CFR 1910.165.

1910.38(e)
Training. An employer must designate and train employees to assist in a safe and orderly evacuation of other employees.

1910.38(f)
Review of emergency action plan. An employer must review the emergency action plan with each employee covered by the plan:

1910.38(f)(1)
When the plan is developed or the employee is assigned initially to a job

1910.38(f)(2)
When the employee's responsibilities under the plan change, and

1910.38(f)(3)
When the plan is changed.

National Fire Protection Association (NFPA)

The National Fire Protection Association has established criteria for disaster management, emergency management, and business continuity programs.

Standard 1600, *Standard on Disaster/Emergency Management and Business Continuity Programs: 2004 Edition*, provides criteria to assess current programs or to develop, implement, and maintain a program to mitigate, prepare for, respond to, and recover from disasters and emergencies. The Federal Emergency Management Administration (FEMA), the National

Emergency Management Association (NEMA), and the International Association of Emergency Managers (IAEM) have endorsed the NFPA program. [CD-ROM 12.2]

The standard *NFPA 99: Health Care Facilities* provides requirements minimizing the hazards of fire, explosion, and electricity in all types of health care environments and focuses on the total process of emergency management to maintain a facility's services and assist in its recovery from a disaster.

Accreditation Organizations

Health care accreditation organizations require emergency management plans, which are addressed in their accreditation guidelines for enhancing patient safety. As with OSHA, NFPA, and the Department of Homeland Security, accreditation organizations require an *all-hazards* approach to emergency management and outline specific elements that must be incorporated into planning.

Department of Homeland Security (DHS)

Following the attack on the World Trade Center in New York and the anthrax attack on the U.S. East Coast, Congress recognized the need for a unified emergency planning and response structure within the federal government. In 2002 it passed the Homeland Security Act, which established the Department of Homeland Security (DHS). [CD-ROM 12.3] Portions of the Homeland Security Act apply to health care facilities:

TITLE I—DEPARTMENT OF HOMELAND SECURITY
SEC. 101. EXECUTIVE DEPARTMENT; MISSION.

a) ESTABLISHMENT—There is established a Department of Homeland Security, as an executive department of the United States within the meaning of title 5, United States Code.

b) MISSION

1. IN GENERAL—The primary mission of the Department is to

(A) Prevent terrorist attacks within the United States.

(B) Reduce the vulnerability of the United States to terrorism.

(C) Minimize the damage, and assist in the recovery, from terrorist attacks that do occur within the United States.

(D) Carry out all functions of entities transferred to the Department, including by acting as a focal point regarding natural and manmade crises and emergency planning.

SEC. 505. CONDUCT OF CERTAIN PUBLIC HEALTH–RELATED ACTIVITIES.

a) IN GENERAL—With respect to all public health–related activities to improve State, local, and hospital preparedness and response to chemical, biological, radiological, and nuclear and other emerging terrorist threats carried out by the Department of Health and Human Services (including the Public Health Service), the Secretary of Health and Human Services shall set priorities and preparedness goals and further develop a coordinated strategy for such activities in collaboration with the Secretary.

b) EVALUATION OF PROGRESS—In carrying out subsection (a), the Secretary of Health and Human Services shall collaborate with the Secretary in developing specific benchmarks and outcome measurements for evaluating progress toward achieving the priorities and goals described in such subsection.

National Response Plan (NRP)

The purpose of the National Response Plan (NRP) is to establish a comprehensive, national, *all-hazards* approach to enhance the ability of the United States to manage domestic incidents across a spectrum of activities, including prevention, preparedness, response, and recovery. [CD-ROM 12.4]

President George W. Bush directed the development of the National Response Plan in Homeland Security Presidential Directive Number 5, in February 2003. [CD-ROM 12.5] The National Response Plan establishes a comprehensive *all-hazards* approach to enhance the ability of the United States to manage domestic incidents. The plan incorporates best practices and procedures from incident management disciplines—homeland security, emergency management, law enforcement, firefighting, public works, public health, responder and recovery worker health and safety, emergency medical services, and the private sector—and integrates them into a unified structure. It forms the basis of the federal government's coordination with state, local, and tribal governments and the private sector during incidents. It establishes protocols to:

□ Save lives and protect the health and safety of the public, responders, and recovery workers.

□ Ensure security of the homeland.

□ Prevent an imminent incident, including acts of terrorism.

□ Protect and restore critical infrastructure and key resources.

□ Conduct law enforcement investigations to resolve the incident, apprehend the perpetrators, and collect and preserve evidence for prosecution and/or attribution.

☐ Protect property and mitigate damage and impact on individuals, communities, and the environment.

☐ Facilitate recovery of individuals, families, businesses, governments, and the environment.

The NRP is built on the template of the National Incident Management System (NIMS), which provides a consistent doctrinal framework for incident management at all jurisdictional levels, regardless of the cause, size, or complexity of the incident.

The Department of Homeland Security/Emergency Preparedness and Response (EP&R)/Federal Emergency Management Agency (FEMA), in close coordination with the DHS Office of the Secretary, manages the National Response Plan. The NRP can be updated to incorporate new presidential directives, legislative changes, and procedural changes based on lessons learned from exercises and actual events. Congress expects that each health care facility in the United States will be prepared to participate in the National Response Plan for a national response to any man-made or natural disaster.

National Incident Management System (NIMS)

Homeland Security Presidential Directive 5 (HSPD-5) ordered the development of the National Incident Management System (NIMS) in addition to the National Response Plan. [CD-ROM 12.6] The NIMS brings together federal, state, local, and tribal emergency responders in a single system for managing incidents. Developed by the secretary of homeland security, the NIMS integrates effective practices in emergency preparedness and response into a comprehensive national framework for incident management. The NIMS enables responders at all levels to work together more effectively to manage domestic incidents, no matter what the cause, size, or complexity. The benefits of the NIMS system are significant:

☐ Standardized organizational structures, processes, and procedures

☐ Standards for planning, training, and exercising, and personnel qualification standards

☐ Equipment acquisition and certification standards

☐ Interoperable communications processes, procedures, and systems

☐ Information management systems

☐ Supporting technologies—voice and data communications systems, information systems, data display systems, and specialized technologies

The National Incident Management System was developed to provide a system that would help emergency managers and responders from different jurisdictions and disciplines work together more effectively to handle emergencies and disasters. Most incidents are handled on a daily basis by a single jurisdiction at the local level, often by fire, EMS, and local law enforcement personnel. But even for incidents that are limited in scope, coordination and cooperation among the responding organizations allows a more effective response.

When the NIMS is adopted and used nationwide, it will form a standardized, unified framework for incident management within which government and private entities at all levels can work together effectively. The NIMS provides a set of standardized organizational structures, such as the Incident Command System (ICS), and standardized processes, procedures, and systems. These processes and procedures are designed to improve interoperability among jurisdictions and disciplines in various areas—command and management, resource management, training, and communications.

THE INCIDENT COMMAND SYSTEM (ICS)

The modern Incident Command System (ICS) is a proven disaster management tool that facilitates disaster response and recovery with minimal business interruption, recovery time, and cost. Organization, rapid response, training, and knowledge are essential to any disaster or other emergency response. [CD-ROM 12.7]

The National Fire Protection Association (NFPA) adopted the Incident Command System, and in 1987 the International Association of Chiefs of Police (IACP) endorsed it. The ICS is also a required element under OSHA Standard 29 CFR 1910.120, Hazardous waste operations for emergency responders (HAZWOPER) [CD-ROM 12.8], and it is an integral part of the National Response Plan. The 1996 edition of the NFPA *Health Care Facilities Handbook* states in chapter 11-4.3, "The disaster planning committee shall model the disaster plan on the incident command system (ICS)."

The ICS is a well-organized and integrated team approach to managing both emergency and non-emergency situations. Span of control is predefined, each member of the response team has well-defined responsibilities, and standardized reporting and documentation procedures are utilized. Under ICS, responding agencies send representatives to the Incident Command Center, where they become part of a unified command system with standardized communications. Thus, if services or supplies are needed, the incident commander (IC) has direct access to the representative from the appropriate agency.

ICS Organization

Each event requires the performance of certain major management activities. Fires, bomb threats, mass-casualty events, and natural disasters all have the potential to negatively impact health care delivery and must be handled in the same fashion.

In the event of an emergency, the ICS provides an organized system of command, control, and coordination to deal with the confusion that develops.[1]

It is a management tool consisting of procedures for organizing personnel, facilities, equipment, and communications at the scene of an emergency. The ICS is built around major management functions. A basic tenet of ICS is that the person in charge of an incident is fully responsible for the response until being officially relieved, at which point either authority is delegated to another person or normal lines of authority are restored. The ICS requires the following seven management functions:

☐ *Command*. The incident commander has overall responsibility for managing the incident or event. In addition, the incident commander demobilizes when appropriate.

☐ *Public Information*. A designated individual is authorized to communicate with the media and the public and coordinates activities with local and government agencies.

☐ *Safety*. The safety officer oversees activities of the response team to ensure compliance with health and safety regulations and guidelines. The safety officer can halt operations if it is determined that the response cannot be conducted safely.

☐ *Operations*. The operations officer conducts response activities and organizes and directs all resources.

☐ *Planning/Intelligence*. The Planning/Intelligence group gathers information about the incident and develops the action plan for Operations. If Operations needs additional personnel, equipment, or materials, this group contacts Logistics.

☐ *Logistics*. The logistics officer provides resources and all other services needed to support the incident response, including transportation, equipment, and supplies.

☐ *Finance/Administration*. The finance/administrative officer monitors costs related to the incident. This individual also provides accounting, procurement, time recording, and cost analysis.

The typical ICS organizational structure is shown in figure 12-1.

Figure 12–1. Common Organizational Chart for an Incident Command System

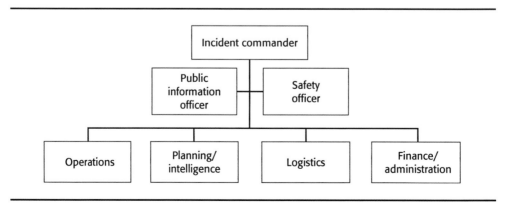

The Hospital Emergency Incident Command System (HEICS) is an emergency management system that employs a logical management structure, defined responsibilities, clear reporting channels, and a common nomenclature to help unify hospitals with other emergency responders. This system can prove valuable in helping hospitals to serve the community during a crisis and to resume normal operations as soon as possible. It was derived from the Incident Command System and, like the ICS, the HEICS employs an *all-hazards* approach for responding to an event or incident.

A hallmark of the ICS is that it can be customized to fit the particular needs of the organization and the event. But regardless of specific modifications, the basic ICS structure and functions always exist. In the case of a large, complex event that results in mass casualties, a fully staffed ICS organization will be required. It is also possible that in the event of mass casualties, local, state, and federal agencies may become involved. Each of those entities has its own comprehensive emergency management system, and one agency will have overall jurisdiction. In some cases, it will be necessary for the local Incident Commander to relinquish command to a higher authority.

For example, during the anthrax attacks of 2001, the Federal Bureau of Investigation assumed overall jurisdiction because it considered each site a crime scene. However, the U.S. Postal Service, the Capitol Police, the Department of Health and Human Services, the Environmental Protection Agency, the Occupational Safety and Health Administration, and a host of subordinate agencies all activated their own management structures controlling their actions.

In the event that a facility is involved in a fire or other incident requiring the local fire department, the response will be under the control of the local fire chief, who by law in most states will be the incident commander with overall jurisdiction and will coordinate with the principal facility incident commander.

The Incident Commander

The incident commander must be fully qualified through training and experience to manage the incident. Almost without exception, a senior official of the health care facility serves as the incident commander and makes the final management decisions concerning the facility's response. Personnel and operating officials are attuned to following senior administration's direction, and during critical conditions another chain of command would not elicit the leadership capabilities or the confidence necessary to meet the demands.

The incident commander must rely on the best available information, communications equipment, and resources to make critical judgments during the crisis. For example, deciding whether patients should be evacuated is a judgment that is sometimes difficult to make and that requires as much information as possible. The logistics and consequences of moving non-ambulatory and critically ill patients must be fully explored and understood. The incident commander must also work closely with the public information officer to ensure that the content and tone of messages disseminated throughout the facility and to the surrounding community are carefully chosen to avoid triggering fear or panic.

The incident commander also makes decisions concerning:

- ☐ Allocation of resources
- ☐ Requests for community assistance
- ☐ Controlling access to the environment
- ☐ Working with the press
- ☐ The need for outside medical aid and supplies
- ☐ Additional manpower requirements
- ☐ The condition of the facility and the extent of damage suffered
- ☐ The magnitude of the injuries
- ☐ The progress of the disaster management

These are judgments that can be made only on the basis of confirmed facts and in consultation with senior advisors on the incident command team. Consequently, a group made up of those responsible for key services of the organization must be available to the incident commander.

The incident commander typically assigns personnel to both command staff and general staff positions, and functions may be added as appropriate. For example, there may be a security officer function that reports to Operations or Logistics. In addition, the primary ICS organization sections are subdivided as needed. The ICS organization has the ability to expand to meet the requirements of the incident.

Since emergency situations may last for many hours or days, it is essential that there be redundancy at each position in the incident command team. If it becomes necessary to switch command during an incident, the incoming staff must receive a full briefing and all team members notified that a change in command is taking place.

Being educated on the Incident Command System is only one step in response preparation. A physical preparedness review of the facility, the development of a documented and tested plan, and the identification of critical resources in advance are also key elements of a complete emergency management program.

INTEGRATED EMERGENCY MANAGEMENT SYSTEM (IEMS)

Contemplation of each possible type of disaster or emergency situation that a health care facility may face will better position the facility to maintain operations in the event of mass casualties or another catastrophic event, and understand whom to notify and when to seek assistance. By considering the potential occurrence of a variety of hazards and relying on the skills and talents of its employees and the assets of the local community, the health care facility can develop an effective emergency management system, such as the Integrated Emergency Management System (IEMS).

The IEMS begins with the identification of universal activities needed in all types of emergency situations. The IEMS recognizes that emergency management activities occur in separate but related phases and are based on an analysis of potential hazards. As with the NRP, the IEMS requires hazard analysis, mitigation, preparation, response, and recovery:[2]

> **Hazard analysis** to evaluate what could happen, the likelihood of the event occurring and the magnitude of problems created because of the event. By identifying potential events that could occur, efforts can be directed towards mitigation activities and developing needed response plans.
>
> Although this is not a complex task, it does require a comprehensive review of the natural and technological (man-made) hazards of the region. Consideration must be given to the possibility of damage or failure of facilities, loss of basic utilities, and multiple casualty events, to name a few. The organization must also consider the effect of a loss of trust from the community as well as legal ramifications, if it fails to respond properly.
>
> Consulting with local emergency planners, public health, fire, police, public works, and utility company officials is essential to this process in identifying current hazards and historical events that have occurred in the region. Examples of this would be obtaining information on the region's 100-year flood plain record, hurricane or severe storm experience, earthquake potential, utility outage records, and hazardous materials concerns in the area.
>
> Also, while consulting with community officials, emergency planners can evaluate if community resources are adequate to meet the needs of the facility during these emergencies.
>
> A Hazards Scoring Worksheet [CD-ROM 12.9] should be used as a guide for the hazard analysis process. Potential hazards are scored on their likelihood of occurring, the magnitude of their effect, and the level of preparedness of the facility's operation. This scoring will assist the Environmental Health and Safety Department with establishing mitigation priorities and determining which events may need specific annexes in the emergency operations plan. While this scoring guideline serves as a tool in the hazard analysis process, it does not replace the judgment of the emergency management planners or senior management. It is through their evaluation that the final priorities are set.
>
> **Mitigation** refers to activities that actually eliminate or reduce the chance of occurrence or the effect of a disaster situation. Mitigation is the most cost-effective way to deal with disasters. However, senior management may be restricted in their use of limited resources to mitigate against hypothetical emergency losses given other immediate day-to-day concerns.

With this limitation in mind, it is important to set priorities based on the results of the Hazard Analysis, and establish a multi-year plan of improvement. Many healthcare mitigation efforts are required by local, state, and national codes and standards. Examples of these are building and fire codes, standards requiring emergency back-up systems, and hazardous materials regulations. Correction of deficiencies with these required facility features or systems must be a high priority. Whenever possible, mitigation projects should also serve an ongoing operational need (i.e., auxiliary water source).

Preparedness is planning how to respond in case an emergency or disaster occurs and working to increase resources available to respond effectively. These activities include the establishment of an effective emergency operations plan, training of personnel, and identification of back-up supply and service providers. The plan and supporting information must be current and consider the needs and capabilities of the health care facility and the community.

The emergency management planning process must be in-depth, but the emergency operations plan developed must be effectively simple. It will address the immediate response needs and recovery activity. The plan is based on identified capabilities; the "don't write it if you can't do it" principle is followed throughout the planning process.

Response is the phase of emergency management in which activities are taken to provide emergency assistance to the victims of the event and/or reduce the likelihood of secondary damage.

Depending on the suddenness and magnitude of the situation, the response may occur in three levels of activity: alert phase, onset of emergency conditions, and de-escalation of the event.

Response to an event will be based on the training received and the Emergency Operations Plan developed during the preparedness phase. The plan provides guidance for needed actions but is flexible within the structure established by the incident command system.

Activities during the response phase may include: monitoring of potential hazardous situations (i.e., hurricane, hazardous materials incident), activation of command center or incident command system, activation of alert phase procedures, activation of the Emergency Operation Plan, personnel call-back, activation of back-up systems, establishing contact with community emergency services and beginning emergency services and damage control.

As the situation subsides, the response activities will begin to de-escalate correspondingly. The severity and magnitude of the situation will, to a great degree, determine how quickly and to what extent recovery activity occur.

Recovery refers to activities taken to restore the organization or operations to pre-emergency condition. These activities may be short term (hours or days) or long term (weeks, months, or years). They include providing continuing care, addressing staff needs, obtaining extended services and supplies, performing facility repairs and construction, maintaining the financial viability of the organization, replenishing emergency kits and supplies, and evaluating the effectiveness of the emergency response. The magnitude and type of event will determine which of these activities will need attention and to what extent.

It is imperative that recovery tasks, responsibilities, and resources be identified during the preparedness phase of the emergency management process. Initial recovery planning activities must be included in the emergency operations plan the same as response activities.

Although recovery activities normally occur after the emergency event (response phase), planning for these may begin during the course of the emergency. Because of the diversity in the scope of possible recovery needs, only duties related to rapid damage assessment, continuing support of emergency needs and assignments for transitioning into recovery phase activities will be included in the emergency operations plans.

TYPES OF EMERGENCIES

During emergencies that result in a large number of injuries, the health care facility is the critical resource to which the community turns for help. In many cases, there is little opportunity for the normal deliberate and careful processing of patients, and medical, nursing, and support staff may be required to work irregular hours. When a disaster strikes a community, patients logically look to health care facilities for the treatment of their injuries. Having staff that is properly trained in emergency response and management can provide the health care facility with the opportunity to launch a proper response regardless of the nature of the event. Part of the training should include a vulnerability assessment to determine which types of emergencies are most likely to occur in the vicinity of the facility. If a facility is badly damaged, other health care facilities in the area will need to accept more casualties and possibly patients from the damaged facility.

If the health care facility has a solid program built on OSHA Standard 29 CFR 1919.38, Emergency action plans [CD-ROM 12.10], the Incident Command System, the Integrated Emergency Management System, NFPA 1600, and NFPA 99, then it will be well prepared to handle emergencies as they arise. Part of the preparation includes understanding the complete range of emergency situations that the health care facility may encounter. Table 12-1 presents a summary of types of disasters or emergencies and their characteristics.

Table 12–1. Types of Disasters or Emergencies and Their Characteristics

Disaster Type	Characteristics
Transportation accidents	Large numbers of casualties from transportation accidents are a potentially serious problem in urban areas where there is a large volume of traffic on high-speed roads. Airplane and railway disasters can also result in large numbers of casualties and can also create fires, chemical spills, and the possible loss of housing, community facilities, and infrastructure. Because normal transportation can be interrupted, transportation accidents may place an added burden on health care delivery.
Severe storms	Severe storms may occur at any time of the year. In the spring, summer, and fall the primary concerns are damaging thunderstorms, high winds, lightening, tornadoes, hurricanes, and flooding. Thunderstorms happen in every state, and every thunderstorm has lightning. Lightning can strike people and buildings and kills more people each year than tornadoes. Thunderstorms affect small areas compared with hurricanes and winter storms. Hurricanes are severe tropical storms that form in the southern Atlantic Ocean, the Caribbean Sea, the Gulf of Mexico, and in the eastern Pacific Ocean. Hurricanes gather heat and energy through contact with warm ocean waters. Evaporation from the seawater increases their power. Hurricanes rotate in a counterclockwise direction around an "eye." When they hit land, the heavy rain, strong winds and high waves can damage anything they come in contact with, including buildings, trees, roads, and cars. The heavy waves are called a storm surge and are very dangerous. Tornadoes are nature's most violent storms and can be deadly. They come from powerful thunderstorms and appear as rotating, funnel-shaped clouds. Tornado winds can reach 300 miles per hour. They cause damage when they touch down on the ground. Terms associated with tornadoes include *tornado watch* and *tornado warning*. Health care facility employees should know these terms and what they mean.
Winter storms and floods, snow, and ice	During the late fall, winter, and early spring, snow, floods, and ice storms result in electrical outages and fires associated with the use of alternative heating sources, and can isolate communities. Flooding may occur without warning and continue for extended periods. Water damage may also occur in health care facilities due to roof leaks, which may lead to fires, loss of electrical power, structural weakness, inaccessibility, and contamination from floodwaters or backed-up and overflowing sewers. Staffing may be affected due to poor road conditions or to staff members themselves being victims. In many areas of the country, winters bring heavy snowfall and very cold temperatures. Heavy snow can block roads and cause power lines to fall. The cold temperatures can be dangerous to individuals not dressed properly. Terms associated with floods are *flood watch* or *flash flood watch* and *flood warning* or *flash flood warning*.

(Continued on next page)

Table 12–1. *(Continued)*

Disaster Type	Characteristics
Earthquakes	Earthquakes are caused by sudden movement of the Earth's crust and occur along "fault lines." Earthquakes can have a direct impact on a health care facility by damaging it. Unlike other natural disasters, earthquakes provide no warning. The intensity varies widely, and aftershocks may occur for several days. The greatest number of casualties result from the collapse of buildings or from falling objects. The greatest number of injuries and most severe devastation usually occur in congested downtown urban areas. Earthquakes often cause gas leaks, fires, explosions, and severe damage to buildings and infrastructure. Communications and utilities are generally disrupted. As is the case with severe weather, health care staff may also be victims.
Tsunamis	A tsunami (Japanese for "harbor wave") is a series of huge waves that are produced by an undersea disturbance, such as an earthquake or volcano eruption. The waves travel in all directions from the area of disturbance, much like ripples after a rock is thrown into water. The waves may travel in the open sea as fast as 450 miles per hour. As they approach shallow coastal waters, they increase in size, perhaps growing as high as 100 feet, and cause catastrophic damage and loss of life.
Volcanoes	A volcano is the result of molten rock (lava) from the earth's core rising through a fissure in a mountain. Sometimes the lava simply flows out, but on occasion pressure can build and a violent eruption occurs. Toxic gases, rock, dust, and lava that can be hurled through the air accompany such eruptions. Eruptions can cause lateral blasts, lava flows, hot ash flows, mudslides, avalanches, falling ash, and floods. Volcanic eruptions have devastated forests and cities. Volcanic ash, made of pulverized rock, can be harsh, acidic, gritty, glassy, and smelly. The ash can cause lung damage.
Toxic Clouds	If the health care facility is near a major industrial area or transportation artery, it is possible that an accident may release a toxic cloud that directly affects the facility, posing a threat to both patients and staff. A nearby toxic release may also force the facility to shut down its ventilation system to prevent or limit the intake of toxic chemicals. If the facility is unaffected, then staff need to prepare to treat patients who may have been exposed to the chemical. Depending on the nature and the amount of the substance, patients may suffer skin, eye, or respiratory system damage, and in some cases death.
Fire	Unless quickly controlled, fire may destroy the entire facility and has the potential for widespread personal injury or death of patients and staff. Smoke transmitted through the ventilation system, stairwells, corridors, and false ceilings is the most significant hazard. Falling debris, burning materials, explosions, disruption of utilities, exposed wiring, and possible structural weaknesses add to the danger.

(Continued on next page)

Table 12–1. *(Continued)*

Disaster Type	Characteristics
Wildfires	Wildfires are a danger for people who live in the forest, prairies, or wooded areas and cities that are in their path. Fighting a wildfire places a burden on local health care delivery because of the number of people involved in the response.
Bomb Threats	Bomb threats are a significant concern in health care facilities. Each threat must be treated as if a bomb is in fact present. Bomb threats may lead to a partial or total evacuation, the disruption of services, the initiation of the facility's emergency response plan, and notification of local authorities. Bomb threats may also interrupt surgical procedures.
Demonstrations and Disruption	Health care facilities may become targets of demonstrations that are intended to express a particular viewpoint or provide information about the facility and its practices. Care must be exercised to ensure that the demonstration does not escalate and become violent. Demonstrations may also interrupt the flow of staff, patients, and visitors.
Technological Emergencies	Technological emergencies include any interruption or loss of a utility service, power source, life support system, information system, or equipment needed to keep the health care facility in operation.
	Power failures can affect elevator service, parking lot lighting, building operations, and temperature and humidity control. Medical air and suction devices may become inoperable. Water pressure may be lost. Interior rooms and areas may be dark, even during daylight hours.
	A telephone outage may be isolated or widespread. The facility may need to employ cellular, radio, or satellite phone capabilities, External communications may be disrupted.
	Loss of water supply affects patient bathing facilities, toilets, dietary services, and hydrotherapy.
Hazardous Materials	Hazardous materials are substances that can be flammable or combustible, explosive, toxic, noxious, corrosive, oxidizable, irritating, or radioactive. There are many hazardous materials used in health care facilities and in surrounding communities. External or internal incidents involving hazardous materials may require initiation of the facility's emergency response plan, or partial or total evacuation. If severe, hazardous materials incidents can produce casualties and may negatively impact the facility's normal health care delivery.
	Response to emergency, or potential emergency, releases of hazardous substances (whether internal or external) is covered by OSHA's HAZWOPER standard (29 CFR 1910.120).

(Continued on next page)

Table 12–1. *(Continued)*

Disaster Type	Characteristics

Terrorism	Terrorism is the use of force or violence against people or property for political purposes. Acts of terrorism include threats of violence, the use of biological or chemical weapons, assassinations, kidnappings, hijackings, bomb scares, and bombings.
	
	    The range of weapons a terrorist might use include biological, nuclear, incendiary, chemical, and explosive. These weapons may cause mass casualties and may disrupt the economy, resulting in mass hysteria and hardship.
	
	    Victims may self-report to the hospital and may use the first available entrance. Victims may display various signs and symptoms and may be infectious or contaminated with a hazardous chemical or radiation; or they may be injured from an explosive or incendiary device. The facility may or may not be notified in advance. An act of terrorism requires the initiation of the facility's emergency response plan and may easily overwhelm the facility's ability to provide care.

TERRORISM

Terrorists use a variety of methods to inflict harm and create fear. Threats of terrorism involving biological, chemical, nuclear or radiological, incendiary, or explosive weapons may be substantial.

Biological Weapons

Microbiology and infectious disease experts believe that the organisms of greatest concern at this time include those that cause anthrax, smallpox, plague, botulism, tularemia, and viral hemorrhagic fevers such as Ebola. Although not microorganisms, toxins such as ricin are also a concern.

    With the exception of botulism poisoning, days or weeks may elapse between the release of a biological organism and the realization that a release has occurred. Health care facility staff may be confronted with a patient who has entered the facility through an entrance other than that of the Emergency Department; therefore, staff should have basic knowledge of the nature of these diseases. Table 12-2 presents information on the biological organisms and other terrorism-related hazards of greatest concern at this time.[3] [CD-ROM 12.11]

Anthrax

Bacillus anthracis is a sporulating soil bacteria that is endemic (widespread) in many parts of the world. When the spores find a host and germinate, a

Table 12–2. Biological Agent Reference Chart

Agent	Dissemination	Person-to-Person Transmission	Incubation	Lethality
Anthrax	Spores in aerosol	No	1–5 days	High
Cholera	Ingestion and aerosol	Rare	12 hours to 6 days	Low with treatment
Plague	Aerosol	High	1–3 days	High if untreated
Tularemia	Aerosol	No	1–10 days	Moderate if untreated
Q fever	Ingestion and aerosol	Rare	14–16 days	Very low
Smallpox	Aerosol	High	10–12 days	Low
VEE (Venezuelan equine encephalitis)	Aerosol and infected vectors	Low	1–6 days	Low
Ebola	Contact and aerosol	Moderate	4–16 days	Moderate to high
Botulinum toxin	Ingestion and aerosol	No	Hours to days	High
T-2 mycotoxins	Ingestion and aerosol	No	2–4 hours	Moderate
Ricin	Ingestion and aerosol	No	Hours to days	High
Staphylococal enterotoxin B	Ingestion and aerosol	No	Hours	<1%

toxin is produced that can be fatal to humans and animals. Anthrax spores are microscopic, odorless, and tasteless. There is debate on how many spores are necessary to cause an infection; the estimates range between 1 and 10,000. During the anthrax attacks in 2001, spores treated to maximize distribution were spread throughout several mail handling facilities, infecting dozens of workers and killing five. [CD-ROM 12.12]

Smallpox

The threat of the variola virus as a biological weapon remains a concern. Known stocks of the virus exist only in two World Health Organization (WHO) labs, but it is not known whether other supplies exist and may be in the hands of terrorists or the arsenals of governments around the world. Signs and symptoms of smallpox include a high fever, fatigue, and aches, followed by a rash. The lesions resemble small pocks—tiny, pus-filled blisters most prominent on the face, arms, and legs. Smallpox released into a large population could potentially spread widely. There is no proven treatment for smallpox. The disease spreads by contact with the respiratory secretions of someone infected. A person could be exposed to smallpox but not develop signs and symptoms of infection for a week or longer, and therefore could spread the virus to others before seeking treatment. Smallpox can be fatal within weeks. However, not everyone with smallpox dies. In nonfatal cases, the disease runs its course in about a month; the lesions eventually crust over and disappear. Smallpox is fatal in about 30 percent of cases. There is documentation to support the theory that some tribes of American Indians were decimated after wearing blankets that were infected with the smallpox virus. One of the major concerns of public health officials is that the immunity of many who were vaccinated in the 1950s and 1960s has significantly diminished since. [CD-ROM 12.13]

Plague

In the Middle Ages, plague—also known as the Black Death or the pestilence—spread across Asia and Europe and killed between 20 million and 30 million people, representing about a third of the world's population. The plague was the first recorded agent used in biological warfare. In the fourteenth century, soldiers catapulted bodies of plague victims into the encampments of their enemies, and some who acquired it survived and traveled to Europe, spreading the plague as they went. This bacterium occurs in many areas of the world, including the United States.

Plague is an infectious disease that affects animals and humans. It is caused by the bacterium *Yersinia pestis*, found in rodents (rats, squirrels, and prairie dogs). It is transmitted by flea bites or by ingestion of contaminated animal tissues.

The bacterium is easily destroyed by sunlight and drying. Even so, when released into air, the bacterium will survive for up to one hour, although this could vary depending on conditions. There are three forms of plague: bubonic, pneumonic, and septicemic.

Bubonic plague is the most common form. It occurs when an infected flea bites a person or when materials contaminated with *Y. pestis* enter through a break in the skin. It is characterized by the sudden onset of fever, chills, weakness, and headache. After several hours, swelling of lymph nodes in the groin, armpit, or neck occurs. The swellings (called buboes) may be tender. Bubonic plague does not spread from person to person.

Pneumonic plague occurs when *Y. pestis* infects the lungs. This type of plague can spread from person to person through the air. Transmission can take place if someone breathes in aerosolized bacteria, which could happen in a bioterrorist attack. Pneumonic plague is also spread by breathing in *Y. pestis* suspended in respiratory droplets from a person (or animal) with pneumonic plague. Becoming infected in this way usually requires direct and close contact with the ill person or animal. Pneumonic plague may also occur if a person with bubonic or septicemic plague is untreated and the bacteria spread to the lungs. The pneumonia progresses for two to four days and may cause respiratory failure and shock. Without early treatment, patients may die.

Septicemic plague occurs when plague bacteria multiply in the blood. It can be a complication of pneumonic or bubonic plague, or it can occur by itself. When it occurs alone, it is caused in the same ways as bubonic plague; however, buboes do not develop. Patients experience fever, chills, prostration, abdominal pain, shock, and bleeding into skin and other organs. Septicemic plague does not spread from person to person. [CD-ROM 12.14]

Botulism

Botulism is a muscle-paralyzing disease caused by a toxin produced by *Clostridium botulinum*. Botulinum toxin is among the most lethal substances known. Botulism can kill within 24 hours.

Botulism can result from consuming improperly canned foods or from eating fish that contain the naturally occurring bacteria. There have been incidents in which the toxin was used to contaminate food at a restaurant. Botulism usually develops between 12 and 36 hours after ingestion of the organism and its toxin. Food-borne botulism may at first cause abdominal cramps, nausea, vomiting, and diarrhea. Other early signs and symptoms of botulism include double vision, drooping eyelids, dry mouth, slurred speech, and difficulty swallowing. Fever is usually absent. Botulism causes muscle weakness and eventual paralysis that starts at the top of the body and works its way down. The disease kills by paralyzing the muscles used in breathing. [CD-ROM 12.15, 12.16]

Tularemia

Tularemia is an illness that normally infects wild animals such as rabbits and squirrels. It is caused by the bacterium *Francisella tularensis*, which some experts fear may possibly be used in germ warfare. Humans can acquire the illness following contact with the blood or body fluids of infected animals, from the bite of a fly or tick that carries blood from an infected animal, or from contaminated food or water. As a biological weapon, tularemia could be dispersed through the air and inhaled. A potentially fatal disease, tularemia comes on suddenly and can cause fever, headache, chills, weakness, an ulcerated sore at the spot of the fly or tick bite, and enlarged and tender lymph nodes.

The signs and symptoms of tularemia vary. If contaminated meat or water is consumed, tularemia can result in sores in the mouth and throat, as well as vomiting and diarrhea. The infection may also affect the eyes or lungs, leading to pneumonia that can kill within two weeks. [CD-ROM 12.17]

Ebola

Ebola is a hemorrhagic disease characterized by high temperature, internal bleeding, and shock. The symptoms are severe and often fatal in humans and other primates. The disease is caused by an infection with Ebola virus, named after a river in the Democratic Republic of the Congo in Africa, where it was first recognized. Ebola is considered a possible bioterrorist threat because it is highly infectious, can be aerosolized, and causes death in a high percentage of those who develop symptoms. Once the virus is in humans, it spreads by direct contact with body fluids. It can also be spread by contact with contaminated objects, such as needles.

The infection is characterized by flu-like symptoms within a few days following exposure. In most patients, those symptoms include high fever, headache, muscle aches, stomach pain, fatigue, and diarrhea. Some patients exhibit a sore throat, hiccups, rash, red and itchy eyes, and bloody vomit and diarrhea. Within a week of the infection, symptoms include chest pain, massive hemorrhaging, and shock. There is no standard treatment for Ebola, other than supportive therapy. [CD-ROM 12.18]

Ricin

Ricin is a poison derived from the castor bean plant (*Ricinus communis*). These are the same beans that are used to make castor oil. Castor bean plants are grown worldwide. Ricin can be produced relatively easily and inexpensively in large quantities. Therefore, there is concern over its use as a "biological" weapon. In fact, ricin reportedly was used in the assassination of a government dissident in Bulgaria in 1978.

Ricin can be injected directly, or it can be aerosolized and released in an unsuspecting community. Ricin can also be ingested from poisoned food or a contaminated water supply. Ricin poisoning can be fatal. Inhaled, it causes weakness, fever, chest tightness, cough, and severe respiratory problems, including pulmonary edema. The poison can kill by damaging the lungs in as few as three days. Ingested, ricin can cause intestinal bleeding and organ damage. No antidote for ricin exists, which is why this agent poses a serious threat. [CD-ROM 12.19]

Nuclear or Radiological Weapons

According to the U.S. Federal Bureau of Investigation (FBI), bombings accounted for nearly 70 percent of all terrorist attacks in the United States and its territories between 1980 and 2001.[4] [CD-ROM 12.20]

There are two different types of radiological weapons that could be used by terrorists: nuclear explosives (bombs) and radiological dispersal devices (RDDs). Nuclear bombs use the splitting of atoms to create an explosion. Radiological dispersal devices use a conventional explosive device to disperse radioactive material; these are commonly called dirty bombs. A dirty bomb is a mix of an explosive, such as dynamite, with radioactive powder or pellets. When the dynamite or other explosive is set off, the blast carries radioactive material into the surrounding area. [CD-ROM 12.21] Table 12-3 compares nuclear explosives and RDDs.

Table 12–3. Comparison of Nuclear Explosives and RDDs

Nuclear Explosive	RDD
Explosion caused by sudden release of energy during uncontrolled nuclear fission	Conventional explosive device that disperses radioactive material
Blast zone and area of radiation spread may be tens of miles	Blast zone is limited, as is the resulting area of radioactive contamination
Significant number of fatalities and casualties related to the blast; burn casualties many miles from blast area	Immediate casualties are significantly fewer and localized to immediate blast area
Produces ionizing radiation that can cause burns and long-term health effects, such as birth defects and cancer	Non-ionizing radiation rarely causes illnesses but requires extensive decontamination

There are many symptoms of radiation sickness, and their severity varies greatly depending on the dosage. The initial symptoms may include nausea, vomiting, diarrhea, and fatigue. Symptoms resemble many of those of common illnesses, including influenza and the common cold. Symptoms appear shortly after exposure and then disappear for a few days, only to reappear in a much more serious form in a week or so.

If individuals report to or are brought to the health care facility, physicians will treat them depending on the nature and seriousness of the exposure. Medical assistance may include controlling bleeding, treating shock, tending to burns, caring for injuries to muscles and bones and joints, and administering CPR.

Chemical Weapons

Chemical agents are poisonous chemical compounds that injure or kill individuals through contact, inhalation, or ingestion. Chemical agents have been used on the battlefield to kill or injure enemy combatants. During World War I phosgene, chlorine, and mustard agents were all used with deadly effect.

As with biological agents, it is possible that victims may self-report to the facility and use the first available entrance. The first line of defense is not to panic—but to be armed with information.

Chemical weapons include the following categories: nerve agents, blister agents, blood agents, choking agents, and irritant agents. Table 12-4 provides basic information about each of these types of chemical weapons along with their military classification codes.[5] [CD-ROM 12.22]

The results of a chemical attack are apparent within minutes or hours and may have a direct impact on all health care facilities in the area. The most recent experience with a chemical attack is the 1995 sarin attack on the Tokyo

Table 12–4. Chemical Agent Reference Chart

Group	Name (Code)	Rate of Action	Route of Entry	Symptoms	Decontamination Methods
Nerve agents	Tabun (GA) Sarin (GB) Soman (GD) VX	Rapid Rapid Rapid Rapid	Respiratory and skin	Headache, runny nose, salivation, pinpointing of pupils, difficulty breathing, tight chest, seizures or convulsions	Remove the agent by flushing with warm water and soap
Blister agents	Mustard (H) Lewisite (L) Phosgene oxime (CX)	Delayed Rapid Rapid	Skin, inhalation, and eyes	Red, burning skin, blisters, sore throat, dry cough, pulmonary edema, memory loss, coma/seizures. Some symptoms may be delayed from 2 to 24 hours	Remove the victim from area and flush with warm water and soap
Blood agents	Hydrogen cyanide (AC) Cyanogen chloride (CK) Arsine (SA)	Rapid Rapid Rapid	Inhalation, skin, and eyes	Cherry red skin/lips, rapid breathing, dizziness, nausea, vomiting, convulsions, dilated pupils, excessive salivation, gastrointestinal hemorrhage, pulmonary edema, and respiratory arrest	Remove the victim from area, remove wet clothing, flush with soap and water, and aerate
Choking agents	Chlorine (CL) Phosgene (CG) Diphosgene (DP)	Rapid in high concentrations; up to 3 hours in low concentrations	Respiratory and skin	Eye and airway irritation, dizziness, tightness in chest, pulmonary edema, painful cough, nausea, and headache	Wash with copious amounts of water and aerate
Irritant agents/Riot control	Tear gas (CS, CR) Mace (CN) Pepper spray (OC)	20–60 seconds Rapid Rapid	Respiration and skin	Tearing eyes, nose and throat irritation, coughing, shortness of breath, vomiting	Brush off materials, use decon wipes and water, remove contaminated clothing

subway. The U.S. Department of Health and Human Services offered this summary:

> Victims came to the hospital by taxi, ambulance, car, walked, etc.; widespread panic; Sarin identified 3 hours post attack and later determined to have been diluted; 5,510 casualties; 12 deaths, 17 critical casualties, 37 severe casualties, 984 moderate casualties; roughly 4,000+ casualties showed no signs of intoxication— psychological 278 hospitals and clinics received casualties.[6] [CD-ROM 12.23]

This report has implications for the health care facility first-receiver security officer. Most important, the first-receiver security officer must avoid direct victim contact unless trained to respond to a chemical weapons incident and must wear personal protective equipment and clothing.

The following caution is also based on the Tokyo sarin incident:

> During the Sarin incident on the Tokyo subway, for example, the Tokyo Fire Department sent a total of 1,364 personnel to the 16 affected subway stations and other locations. Of these first responders, 135 (about 10%) were themselves injured by direct or indirect exposure to the poison gas.[7]

Injuries to the first responders came about as a direct result of their failure to respect the nature of the event and to wear appropriate personal protective clothing and equipment while attempting to assist victims.

Nerve Agents

Following the release of a nerve agent into the air, people can be exposed through skin or eye contact. They can also be exposed by breathing air that contains the nerve agent.

Some nerve agents (e.g., sarin, soman, and tabun) mix easily with water, so they could be used to poison a water supply. Following the release of one of these agents into water, touching or drinking water that contains the agent can cause exposure. Although VX does not mix with water as easily as other nerve agents do, it could be released into water. Following such a release, drinking contaminated water or getting it on the skin can expose people.

Following contamination of food with sarin, soman, tabun, or VX, people can be exposed by eating the contaminated food. A person's clothing can release the agent for about 30 minutes after contact with the vapor, which can expose others. These agents break down slowly in the body, meaning that repeated exposures can have a cumulative effect (i.e., build up in the body). Because the agents are heavier than air, they will sink to low-lying areas and create a greater exposure hazard there. [CD-ROM 12.24–12.26]

Blister Agents

Blister agents do not occur naturally in the environment; some were produced to be used in World War I as chemical warfare agents. If blister agents are released into the air as a vapor, people can be exposed through skin contact, eye contact, or breathing. Sulfur mustard vapor can be carried long distances by wind. If blister agents are released into water, people who drink the contaminated water or get it on their skin can become exposed. Phosgene oxime does not last very long in the environment; it breaks down in soil within two hours under normal temperatures, and it breaks down in water within a few days. Sulfur mustard can last in the environment from one to two days under average weather conditions and from weeks to months under very cold conditions. Lewisite, on the other hand, remains a liquid under a wide range of environmental conditions, from below freezing to very high temperatures. Therefore, it could persist for a long time in the environment. [CD-ROM 12.27, 12.28]

Blood Agents

The Germans in World War II used hydrogen cyanide, under the name Zyklon B, as a genocidal agent. Reports indicate that during the Iran-Iraq War in the 1980s, hydrogen cyanide gas may have been used along with other chemical agents against the inhabitants of the Kurdish city of Halabja in northern Iraq. Although arsine was investigated as a warfare agent during World War II, it was never used on the battlefield. The extent of poisoning caused by arsine or cyanide depends on the amount to which a person has been exposed, the route of exposure, and the length of time of the exposure. Arsine is a colorless, nonirritating toxic gas with a mild garlic odor. The odor can be detected only at levels greater than those necessary to cause poisoning. Cyanide sometimes is described as having a "bitter almond" smell, but it does not always give off an odor, and not everyone can detect this odor. [CD-ROM 12.29, 12.30]

Choking Agents

Some choking (pulmonary) agents were used extensively during World War I. Chlorine is one of the most commonly manufactured chemicals in the United States. Its most important use is as a bleach in the manufacture of paper and cloth, but it is also used to make pesticides (insect killers), rubber, and solvents. Phosgene gas may be colorless or appear as a white to pale yellow cloud. At low concentrations, it has a pleasant odor similar to that of newly mown hay or green corn, but its odor may not be detected by all people exposed. At high concentrations, the odor may be strong and unpleasant. People's risk of exposure to choking agents depends on how close they are to the place where the agent was released. [CD-ROM 12.31, 12.32]

Irritant Agents (Riot Control)

Riot control agents are chemical compounds that temporarily make people unable to function by causing irritation to the eyes, mouth, throat, lungs, and skin. Several different compounds are considered to be riot control agents. The most common compounds are chloroacetophenone (CN) and chlorobenzylidenemalononitrile (CS). Other examples are chloropicrin (PS), which is also used as a fumigant (a substance that uses fumes to disinfect an area); bromobenzylcyanide (CA); dibenzoxazepine (CR); and combinations of various agents.

Riot control agents are used by law enforcement officials for crowd control and by individuals and the general public for personal protection (e.g., pepper spray). Chlorobenzylidenemalononitrile is also used in military settings in testing the speed and ability of military personnel to apply their gas masks.

Because they are liquids or solids (i.e., powder), riot control agents such as CN and CS could be released in the air as fine droplets or particles. If these agents are released into the air, people may be exposed to them through skin contact, eye contact, or breathing.

The extent of poisoning caused by riot control agents depends on the amount of the agent to which a person is exposed, the location of exposure (indoors versus outdoors), how the person is exposed, and the length of time of the exposure. Riot control agents work by causing irritation to the area of contact (e.g., eyes, skin, nose) within seconds of exposure. The effects of exposure to a riot control agent are usually short-lived (15–30 minutes) after the person has been removed from the source and decontaminated (cleaned off). [CD-ROM 12.33]

Incendiary Devices

Other weapons a terrorist might use include incendiary devices, such as firebombs. These devices range from the simple Molotov cocktail (made of a bottle, gasoline, rag, and match) to much larger and more sophisticated bombs, including napalm or any large container filled with flammable fluid that is ignited by some sort of fuse. Incendiary devices are capable of causing loss of life and property damage from fire. They are also used to generate panic. These devices can be used in terrorist attacks; however, the use of incendiary devices is difficult to classify as terrorism. Incidents are often misidentified as arson, insurance fraud, or some other non-terrorist criminal activity.

Explosives

Terrorists choose explosives because they are simple to use. A terrorist does not need to construct an elaborate device to cause havoc and mass destruction. A pipe bomb attached to a propane storage container can be just as destructive as a complex explosive device.

Terrorists use an assortment of dangerous materials to fabricate bombs of various sizes—from a pipe bomb weighing several pounds to a truck bomb weighing several tons. Explosives used by terrorists are often classified according to the following categories:

- □ *Unconventional use:* A conventional object used in an unconventional way to create mass destruction. In the September 11, 2001, attack on the World Trade Center and the Pentagon, hijackers flew passenger planes into their intended targets, relying on the impact of the planes and their full fuel tanks to create havoc and devastation.
- □ *Vehicle bomb:* Usually a large, powerful device that consists of a large quantity of explosives fitted with a timed or remotely triggered detonator and packed in a car or truck.
- □ *Pipe bomb:* A quantity of explosives sealed in a length of metal or plastic pipe. A timing fuse usually controls detonation, but other methods can be used, including electronic timers, remote triggers, and motion sensors. These are the most common explosive devices, and are at the opposite end of the scale from vehicle bombs in terms of size and power.
- □ *Satchel charge:* An old military term for an explosive device in a canvas carrying bag. In recent history, "daypacks" or knapsacks have been used as the carrying device, and the explosives have been combined with materials such as nails and glass to cause more casualties.
- □ *Package or letter bomb:* The explosive material is contained in a package or letter that is usually triggered when opened.

Bomb making materials are readily available. Most communities keep enough propane and common hazardous materials in storage to produce a significant explosion. Access to these materials often requires little effort from the terrorist.

HAZARDOUS SUBSTANCES INCIDENTS

In mass-casualty incidents involving the release of hazardous substances, OSHA believes that health care facility employees in most circumstances will be "first receivers" rather than "first responders." This distinction is based on the belief that health care facilities will likely be receiving the victims of a mass-casualty event rather than sending teams to the site of the event to decontaminate and transport victims. However, the roles of first responder and first receiver overlap to some degree.

Health care workers risk occupational exposure to chemical, biological, or radiological materials when a hospital receives contaminated patients, particularly during mass-casualty incidents. These employees, who may be termed first receivers, work at a site remote from the location where the hazardous substance release occurred. This means that their exposures are limited to the substances transported to the hospital on victims' skin, hair, clothing, or personal effects. The location and limited presence of contaminant distinguishes first receivers from other first responders (e.g., firefighters, law enforcement, ambulance service personnel), who typically respond to the incident.

The Occupational Safety and Health Administration has published *Best Practices for Hospital-Based First Receivers of Victims from Mass Casualty Incidents Involving the Release of Hazardous Substances*. [CD-ROM 12.34] These guidelines explain the differing roles of first responders and first receivers. According to OSHA, first receivers are most likely to include clinicians and other hospital staff who have a role in receiving and treating contaminated victims (e.g., triage, decontamination, medical treatment, and security) and those whose roles support these functions (e.g., setup and patient tracking). "Clinician" is further defined by OSHA as meaning physicians, nurses, nurse practitioners, physicians' assistants, and others.

First responders include those individuals who have a responsibility to initially respond to emergencies and take action to save lives, protect property, and meet basic human needs; examples are firefighters, emergency medical personnel, and law enforcement officers. First responders must comply with OSHA Standard 29 CFR 1910.120, Hazardous waste operations and emergency response (HAZWOPER). [CD-ROM 12.35] Those instances not covered by federal OSHA are covered by a parallel rule under the U.S. Environmental Protection Agency (EPA). By agreement, OSHA interprets the EPA HAZWOPER rule.

First receivers, on the other hand, must comply only with certain portions of the HAZWOPER standard. In its best-practices guidelines, OSHA clarified the crucial requirements for the selection and use of respirators.

If a health care facility is required to receive casualties from a biological or chemical weapons attack, it must be prepared to handle patients as if they were still contaminated, even though they may have undergone some level of decontamination at the site of the incident.

Table 12-5 summarizes OSHA's current guidance on training first receivers for mass-casualty emergencies.[8] Employees are categorized according to zone (namely, Hospital Decontamination Zone and Post-decontamination Zone); whether they have designated roles in the zone; and their likelihood of contact with contaminated victims, their belongings, equipment, or waste. Hospitals should note that the training levels presented are the minimum levels and can be increased or augmented, as appropriate, to better protect employees, other patients, and the facility in general.

OSHA makes it clear that when health care facilities receive patients from mass-casualty incidents involving hazardous substances, they must also comply with certain parts of 29 CFR 1910.120 (HAZWOPER), 29 CFR 1910.132 (Personal protective equipment) [CD-ROM 12.36], 29 CFR 1910.134 (Respiratory protection) [CD-ROM 12.37], 29 CFR 1910.1030 (Bloodborne pathogens), and 29 CFR 1910.1200 (Hazard communication) [CD-ROM 12.38]. It is not sufficient simply to have respiratory equipment on hand in the event that it might be needed. Training must be proactive, and compliance with these standards is mandatory, including the development and management of a respiratory protection program by a qualified program administrator. Further, PPE selection must be based on a hazard assessment that carefully considers employees' roles and the hazards that they might encounter, along with the steps taken to minimize the extent of employees' contact with hazardous substances.

CORE PLANNING CONSIDERATIONS

The Environmental Health and Safety Department should establish and direct a planning team. The size of the planning team will depend on the facility's operations, requirements, and resources. Involving a group of people encourages participation and invests more people in the process. It increases the amount of time and energy that participants are able to give. In addition, it enhances the visibility and stature of the planning process. A team also provides for a broad perspective on the issues.

Table 12–5. Training for First Receivers

Mandatory Training	First Receivers Covered
First Responder, Operations Level[A] Initial training Annual refresher (both initial and refresher training may be satisfied by demonstration of competence)	All employees with designated roles in the Hospital Decontamination Zone.[B] This group includes, but is not limited to, decontamination staff, including decontamination victim inspectors; clinicians who will triage and/or stabilize victims prior to decontamination[C]; security staff (e.g., crowd control and controlling access to the emergency department [ED]); setup crew; and patient tracking clerks.
Briefing at the time of the incident[D,E]	Other employees whose role in the Hospital Decontamination Zone was not previously anticipated (i.e., who are called in incidentally), such as a medical specialist, or a trade person, such as an electrician.
First Responder, Awareness Level Initial training Annual refresher (both initial and refresher training may be satisfied by demonstration of competence)	Security personnel, setup crew, and patient-tracking clerks assigned only to patient-receiving areas proximate to the Decontamination Zone, where they might encounter, but are not expected to have contact with, contaminated victims, their belongings, equipment, or waste. ED clinicians, clerks, triage staff, and other employees associated with emergency departments, who might encounter self-referred contaminated victims (and their belongings, equipment, or waste) without receiving prior notification that such victims have been contaminated.

(Continued on next page)

Table 12–5. *(Continued)*

Recommended Training	Personnel Covered
Training similar to that outlined in the Hazard communication standard[F]	Other personnel in the Hospital Post-decontamination Zone who reasonably would not be expected to encounter or come in contact with unannounced contaminated victims, their belongings, equipment, or waste (e.g., other ED staff, such as housekeepers).[G,H]

[A]The employer must certify that personnel trained at the "First Responder Operations Level" have received at least eight hours of specific training (which can include awareness level training, PPE training, and training exercises/drills) or have had sufficient experience to objectively demonstrate competency in specific key areas. Refresher training must be provided annually and must be of sufficient content and duration to maintain competencies. Alternatively, the employee may demonstrate competence (i.e., skills) in OSHA HAZWOPER 29 CFR 1910.120(q)(6)(ii). Participation in training exercises/drills is recommended to ensure competency during initial and refresher training.

[B]The *Hospital Decontamination Zone* includes any areas where the type and quantity of hazardous substance is unknown and where contaminated victims, contaminated equipment, or contaminated waste may be present. It is reasonably anticipated that employees in this zone might have exposure to contaminated victims, their belongings, equipment, or waste. This zone includes, but is not limited to: places where initial triage and/or medical stabilization of possibly contaminated victims occur, pre-decontamination waiting (staging) areas for victims, the actual decontamination area, and the post-decontamination victim inspection area. This area will typically end at the ED door.

[C]The term *clinician* includes physicians, nurses, nurse practitioners, physicians' assistants, and others.

[D]The briefing must include (at a minimum) instruction on wearing the appropriate PPE, the nature of the hazard, expected duties, and the safety and health precautions the individual should take (29 CFR 1910(q)(4)).

[E]Note that the individual must be medically qualified (29 CFR 1910.134), fitted (1910.132 and .134), and trained (1910.132 and .134) to use the required PPE. These qualifications are difficult to achieve at the time of the incident and, whenever possible, should be satisfied prior to an incident.

[F]While HAZCOM training is not required pursuant to the OSH Act for most of the scenarios contemplated in this document, a prudent employer may consider adopting and appropriately modifying the training provisions in the HAZCOM standard to provide information to personnel who would not be expected to come in contact with unannounced contaminated victims, their belongings, equipment, or waste.

[G]The *Hospital Post-decontamination Zone* is an area considered uncontaminated. Equipment and personnel are not expected to become contaminated in this area. At a hospital receiving contaminated victims, the Hospital Post-decontamination Zone includes the ED (unless contaminated).

[H]If the ED becomes contaminated, the hospital's decontamination procedures must be activated by the properly trained and equipped employees (refer to Hospital Decontamination Zone in this table and table 3 in *Best Practices for Hospital-Based First Receivers* [CD-ROM 12.34]).

Adapted from *Best Practices for Hospital-Based First Receivers of Victims from Mass Casualty Incidents Involving the Release of Hazardous Substances*. OSHA 3249-08N, 2005, p. 28.

The needs assessment and worksite analysis must include the emergency management program. These steps entail gathering information about current capabilities and about possible hazards and emergencies, and then conducting a hazard vulnerability analysis to determine the facility's capabilities for handling emergencies. Internal documents will be reviewed and meetings will take place with government agencies, community organizations, and utilities. Ask about potential emergencies and about plans and available resources for responding to them.

Implementing the plan means more than simply exercising the plan during an emergency. It means acting on recommendations made during the vulnerability analysis, integrating the plan into facility operations, training employees, and evaluating the plan. Emergency planning must become part of the corporate culture.

The team should look for opportunities to build awareness, to educate and train personnel, to test procedures, to involve all levels of management and all departments and the community in the planning process, and to make emergency management part of what employees do on a day-to-day basis. Are there opportunities for distributing emergency preparedness information through corporate newsletters, employee manuals, or employee mailings? What kinds of safety posters or other visible reminders would be helpful? Do employees know what they should do in an emergency? How can all levels of the organization be involved in evaluating and updating the plan? How well does senior management support the responsibilities outlined in the plan?

Steps Involved in Planning

Developing the plan includes briefly describing the facility's approach to the core elements of emergency management, which are command and control, communications, life safety, mitigation, property protection, community outreach, recovery and restoration, and administration and logistics. These elements are the foundation for the emergency procedures the facility will follow to protect personnel, patients, and equipment and to resume operations.

Following is a summary of the core elements of emergency management, which are a part of a facility's comprehensive plan.

Command and Control

Someone must be in charge in an emergency and be responsible for managing resources, analyzing information, and making decisions.

Communications

A communications failure can prevent an effective response. Communications are necessary to report emergencies, to warn personnel of the danger, to keep families and off-duty employees informed about what's happening at the facility, to coordinate response actions, and to maintain contact with patients, their families, and suppliers.

Life Safety

Protecting the health and safety of everyone in the facility is the first priority during an emergency. Life safety measures include sheltering in place, evacuation planning, evacuation routes and exits, assembly areas and accountability, training and information, and family preparedness.

Mitigation

Mitigation refers to activities that actually eliminate or reduce the possibility or the effect of a disaster situation. Mitigation is the most cost-effective way to deal with disasters.

Property Protection

Protecting facilities, equipment, and vital records is essential to restoring operations once an emergency has occurred. Procedures must be established for fighting fires, containing material spills, closing doors, preserving vital records, and shutting down and securing equipment and the facility.

Personnel must be designated to authorize, supervise, and perform a facility shutdown and trained to recognize when to abandon the effort. Facility shutdown is generally a last resort but always a possibility. An improper or disorganized shutdown can result in confusion, injury, and property damage.

Community Outreach

The health care facility's relationship with the community will influence its ability to protect personnel, patients, and property and to return to normal operations. There are many ways to involve outside organizations in the emergency management plan, including maintaining a dialogue with community leaders and government agencies, establishing mutual aid agreements with local response agencies and businesses, taking part in community service activities, public information, and media relations.

The Joint Commission publication *Standing Together: An Emergency Planning Guide for America's Communities* provides expert guidance on the emergency management planning process that is applicable to small, rural, and suburban communities. The guide emphasizes two planning strategies that are of particular significance to small, rural, and suburban communities. The first is to enable people to care for themselves, and the second is to build on existing relationships. Its goal is to remove readiness barriers by providing all communities with strategies, processes, and tools for coordinated emergency management planning. The guide is offered as a multi-functional tool or template. It outlines 13 essential components of an effective community-based emergency management planning process and provides multiple planning strategies addressing each component. [CD-ROM 12.39]

Recovery and Restoration

Recovery and restoration of service is the goal of the emergency management plan. Continuity of management procedures preserves the chain of command and lines of succession for key personnel. An alternative headquarters site should be identified. Planning considerations include contractual arrangements with vendors for such post-emergency services as records preservation, equipment repair, earth moving, or engineering.

There should be discussions with insurance carriers regarding property and business resumption policies. Lack of appropriate insurance can be financially devastating. Topics that should be discussed with the facility's insurance advisor include property value, cost of required upgrades to code, perils or causes of loss covered, deductibles, records and documentation, and procedures to follow in the event of a loss.

Employees are the facility's most valuable asset, and there are a range of services that should be considered for employees. These include cash advances, salary continuation, flexible work hours, reduced work hours, crisis counseling, care packages, and day care.

Immediately after an emergency, take steps to resume operations. Establish priorities for resuming operations. Continue to ensure the safety of personnel on the property. Assess remaining hazards. Maintain security at the incident scene. Account for all damage-related costs. Follow notification procedures. Protect undamaged property and segregate damaged from undamaged property.

Administration and Logistics

Maintain complete and accurate records at all times to ensure a more efficient emergency response and recovery. Certain records may also be required by regulation or by the facility's insurance carriers, and they may prove invaluable in case there is legal action after an incident.

Surge Hospitals

Surge capacity is a health care facility's ability to expand quickly beyond its normal services to meet an increased demand for medical care. Surge hospitals have been defined as facilities designed to supplement existing facilities in the case of an emergency.

Because many health care organizations have a limited ability to expand the surge capacity of a functioning health care facility, the facility's plans for increasing surge capacity should include the establishment of temporary surge facilities. It is critical that health care organizations (in concert with community leadership) initiate relationships and agreements with other organizations such as medical centers, schools, hotels, veterinary hospitals, and/or convention centers to establish locations for the off-site triage of patients as well as for acute care during an emergency. Health care facilities must develop community-wide response plans that integrate their capacities into a single, organized response. Communications and data sharing that link health care organizations to local and state public health agencies are critical to this process.

The Joint Commission publication *Surge Hospitals: Providing Safe Care in Emergencies* provides information to health care planners at the community, state, and federal levels about what surge hospitals are, the kind of planning they require, how they can be set up, and who should be responsible for their establishment and operation. Case studies describe how surge hospitals along the Gulf Coast were established and operated in response to Hurricane Katrina, providing a real-life perspective on the importance of creating safe surge hospitals after a disaster strikes, as well as on the challenges that come with providing care under these makeshift conditions. [CD-ROM 12.40]

OSHA EMERGENCY ACTION PLAN EXPERT SYSTEM

The Occupational Safety and Health Administration's Internet-based planning software may be helpful for small health care facilities. Users should consider the special characteristics of their workplaces and supplement OSHA's plan to address any situations that require special attention.

The OSHA Expert System provides only information based on federal OSHA Emergency Action Plan requirements. If the facility is covered by a state OSHA plan, that office should be contacted for assistance in using the OSHA Expert System.[9]

TAKING CARE OF WORKERS AND THEIR FAMILIES

The process of planning for emergencies incorporates many elements included in the Environmental Health and Safety program, such as stress management, infection control, electrical safety, slips and falls, personal protective equipment, working in temperature extremes, data collection, medical surveillance, training, physical fitness, and family preparedness.

Natural or human-caused disasters such as earthquakes, health emergencies, terrorist attacks, or acts of war can engage caregivers in long hours spent helping people of all ages to understand and manage the many reactions, feelings, and challenges triggered by these stressful circumstances.

The massive effort put forth by caregivers in response to the psychosocial effects of catastrophic events is a critical contribution to their community's recovery. However, caregivers sometimes need to be reminded that a sustained response can also lead to physical and emotional wear and tear. Without conscious attention to self-care, caregivers' effectiveness (and ultimately their health) will suffer.

One of the most difficult challenges for caregivers is to maintain some kind of balance between the demands of the emergency work and the needs of their own families. Lines of communication must be kept open. The Public Health Agency of Canada has published a series of documents that may be helpful to caregivers and their families. *Responding to Stressful Events: Taking Care of Ourselves, Our Families and Our Communities* is one pamphlet in the series that may be especially helpful to caregivers. [CD-ROM 12.41]

In addition to families preparing for emergencies that impact their community, employers need to be sensitive to the needs of caregivers and their families in ways that help families reduce their fears. Employees and their families will be impacted in different ways depending on the disaster situation. Following a disaster, people may develop post-traumatic stress disorder (PTSD), which is psychological damage that can result from experiencing, witnessing, or participating in an overwhelming traumatic (frightening) event. The symptoms of PTSD rarely appear during the trauma itself. Though its symptoms can occur soon after the event, the disorder often surfaces several months or even years later. Employers should be alert to these possibilities regarding their employees and families. Children in particular experience a variety of reactions and feelings in response to a disaster based on their age, and need special attention to meet their needs. *Crisis Counseling Guide to Children and Families in Disasters* is a helpful guide for families in planning for disasters. [CD-ROM 12.42]

Stress Management

The Center for the Study of Traumatic Stress, Uniformed Services University School of Medicine, released a document addressing stress management for health care providers. [CD-ROM 12.43] The information in the document is summarized below.

The magnitude of death and destruction in disasters and the extent of the response demand special attention to the needs of health care providers. The psychological challenges that health care providers face after disasters are related to exposure to patients and their families, who are traumatized by suffering nearly unbearable losses. These psychological challenges combine with long hours of work, decreased sleep, and fatigue. Seeing the effects of disaster on others and hearing their stories increase the stress on providers. Self-care, self-monitoring, and peer monitoring are as important as caring for patients. The following management plan for staff may help minimize later difficulties:

- ☐ Communicate clearly and in an optimistic manner.
- ☐ Encourage health care providers to monitor themselves and each other with regard to basic needs such as food, drink, and sleep.
- ☐ Make sure people take regular breaks from tending to patients.
- ☐ Help people recognize that normal life events are an important respite from the horrors of a disaster.
- ☐ Establish a place for providers to talk to their colleagues and receive support from one another.
- ☐ Encourage contact with loved ones as well as activities for relaxation and enjoyment.
- ☐ Remember that not all people are the same. Some need to talk whereas others need to be alone.
- ☐ Hold department or facility-wide meetings to keep people informed of plans and events.
- ☐ Use facility newsletters or newspapers as ways to recognize successes and to transmit information.
- ☐ Consider establishing awards or other recognition for dedicated service during a disaster.
- ☐ Establish family support programs for staff that provide information about the status of loved ones who are not able to return home on a regular basis.

Additional help for staff include the Center for Mental Health Services' *Self-Care Tips for Emergency and Disaster Response Workers* [CD-ROM 12.44] and NIOSH's *Traumatic Incident Stress: Information for Emergency Response Workers* [CD-ROM 12.45].

Preventing Illnesses and Injuries

The Centers for Disease Control and Prevention (CDC) provides numerous guidelines and fact sheets on preventing injuries and illnesses during disasters:

Key Facts About Hurricane Recovery provides guidance on food safety, water safety, preventing musculoskeletal injuries, hazardous materials, staying cool, washing hands, preventing illness from sewage, and wearing protective gear for cleanup work. [CD-ROM 12.46]

How to Protect Yourself and Others from Electrical Hazards Following a Natural Disaster advises about being careful to avoid electrical hazards in the home and elsewhere. It also outlines steps to take if it appears someone has been electrocuted. [CD-ROM 12.47]

Protect Yourself from Mold provides direction regarding how excess moisture and standing water after natural disasters contribute to the growth of mold. Mold may be a health risk to employees and their families. [CD-ROM 12.48]

Numerous guidelines and fact sheets on working safely during and after disasters are also available from OSHA:

Working Safely with Chain Saws provides guidance for avoiding injury when using a chain saw. [CD-ROM 12.49]

Tree Trimming Tips advises about accidents that can happen with the clearing of trees. [CD-ROM 12.50]

Working Safely with Electricity explains the dangers of electricity and provides safety guidance to prevent electrical incidents. [CD-ROM 12.51]

Preventing Skin Cancer highlights the importance of blocking UV rays. [CD-ROM 12.52]

Heat Stress offers guidance on avoiding heat stress, heat exhaustion, and heat stroke and tips for treating heat-related illness. [CD-ROM 12.53]

Preventing Falls is an informational fact sheet that emphasizes fall prevention measures. [CD-ROM 12.54]

THE JOINT COMMISSION'S EMERGENCY ACTION PROGRAM

The Joint Commission defines an emergency as:[10]

A natural or manmade event that significantly disrupts the environment of care (for example, damage to the organization's building[s] and grounds due to severe winds, storms, or earthquakes); that significantly disrupts care, treatment, and services (for example, loss of utilities such as power, water, or telephones due to floods, civil disturbances, accidents, or emergencies within the organization or in its community); or that results in sudden, significantly changed or increased demands for the organization's services (for example, bioterrorist attack, building collapse, plane crash in the organization's community).

Although Joint Commission's standard on safety management (EC.1.10) sets the stage for its approach to dealing with emergencies, its standard on emergency management (EC.4.10) is the primary standard governing health care facility emergencies. Standard EC.4.10, Element of Performance (EP) 2 requires that health care facilities establish an *all-hazards* command structure within the facility that links with the community's command structure. Other pertinent standards include emergency drills (EC.4.20), initial job training (HR.2.10), and ongoing education (HR.2.20).

THE ROLE OF THE SECURITY DEPARTMENT

Because of the unique service health care facilities provide, and the Security Department's relationship to the Environmental Health and Safety Department in the model program presented in this book, this section provides information on the primary duties of security officers during emergencies. The capability of response depends entirely upon the level of planning that has gone into the emergency preparedness effort of the health care facility. Security officers must be trained to maintain an environment where tranquility and order prevail without resorting to authoritarian conduct and appearance. Security officers have specific roles in the protection of the facility during emergencies, and they must understand their duties and responsibilities. Although they must demonstrate flexibility, they should not become messengers, porters, couriers, or jacks-of-all-trades. Moreover, security officers must be careful not to become victims by engaging in action for which they are not trained or responsible. The security officer's duties and range of responsibilities depend on the circumstances and scope of the incident. However, there are a number of common responsibilities, including:

- Interacting with and providing security for the Incident Command Center
- Maintaining crowd control
- Patrolling to check for and report safety hazards
- Controlling access to areas in the facility and on the grounds
- Controlling the traffic flow
- Assisting in evacuation and accounting for people
- Coordinating with outside law enforcement and directing response agencies to appropriate locations

In some cases, security officers receive the same training as other staff who are first receivers in the hospital decontamination zone. If security officers are assigned to any of the roles outlined in OSHA's best-practices guideline presented earlier in this chapter, they must be trained for that role according to OSHA requirements. Security officers need to be trained to respond quickly to mass-casualty events and to control incoming vehicular traffic flow to minimize interruptions and chaos. If traffic is not properly monitored, vehicles carrying victims, the media, and the curious can quickly block entrances required by emergency vehicles.

Security officers may be assigned to the entrance of the Emergency Department to assist with incoming patients or to ensure that only staff with appropriate identification can enter. They may also be assigned to other entrances to control traffic and escort family members to a waiting location. Officers may be called upon to act as liaisons with local law enforcement, fire, and other local emergency services. Officers may also be asked to deliver communications to and from the command center.

THE ROLE OF THE ENVIRONMENTAL HEALTH AND SAFETY DEPARTMENT

The model Environmental Health and Safety Department plays a significant role in the facility's emergency planning and response. With the Environmental Monitoring, Safety (both general and fire), Training, and Employee Health functions, the department staff are uniquely qualified to coordinate the various elements of planning, response, and recovery, including training and the required elements of the hazard communication, bloodborne pathogens, personal protective equipment, and respirator programs. The Environmental Health and Safety Department has a significant role in managing a disaster or disaster response.

The Environmental Health and Safety Department and department liaisons and their representatives should receive comprehensive training in emergency management. The Federal Emergency Management Agency (FEMA) Emergency Management Institute (EMI) offers educational resources and serves as the national focal point for the development and delivery of emergency management training. EMI curricula are structured to meet the needs of diverse audiences, including health care facilities, with an emphasis on how the various elements work together in emergencies to save lives and protect property.

Instruction focuses on the four phases of emergency management: mitigation, preparedness, response, and recovery. EMI develops courses and administers resident and non-resident training programs in areas such as natural hazards (earthquakes, hurricanes, floods, dam safety), technological hazards (hazardous materials, terrorism, radiological incidents, chemical stockpile emergency preparedness), professional development, leadership, instructional methodology, exercise design and evaluation, information technology, public information, integrated emergency management, and "training the trainers."

The EMI provides numerous courses beneficial to health care facilities, including:

- □ IS-700 National Incident Management System, an Introduction
- □ Integrated Emergency Management Course (IEMC)
- □ Introduction to Incident Command System (I-100)
- □ Principles of Emergency Management—Professional Development Series (IS-230)

References

1. Reciprocal of America. *Emergency Operations Plan* (adapted).
2. Reciprocal of America. *Emergency Management Program* (adapted).
3. *Emergency Response to Terrorism Job Aid—Edition 2.0.* Joint Publication of the Department of Homeland Security, Federal Emergency Management Agency, U.S. Fire Administration, Department of Homeland Security Office for Domestic Preparedness (ODP), and U.S. Department of Justice Office of Justice

Programs. February 2003. Available at http://www.usfa.fema.gov/downloads/ pdf/publications/ert-ja.pdf (accessed 3/21/2006).

4. U.S. Department of Justice, Federal Bureau of Investigation. *Terrorism 1980–2001.* Available at http://www.fbi.gov/publications/terror/terror2000_2001.pdf (accessed 3/21/2006).

5. *Emergency Response to Terrorism Job Aid—Edition 2.0.* Joint Publication of the Department of Homeland Security, Federal Emergency Management Agency, U.S. Fire Administration, Department of Homeland Security Office for Domestic Preparedness (ODP), and U.S. Department of Justice Office of Justice Programs. February 2003. Available at http://www.usfa.fema.gov/downloads/pdf/publications/ ert-ja.pdf (accessed 3/21/2006).

6. USASBCCOM. *Guidelines for Mass Casualty Decontamination During a Terrorist Chemical Agent Incident.* January 2000; Revision 1, August 2003, p. 48.

7. *JAMA* 278 (5) (August 6, 1997), pp. 362–368.

8. OSHA. *Best Practices for Hospital-Based First Receivers of Victims from Mass Casualty Incidents Involving the Release of Hazardous Substances.* OSHA 3249-08N, 2005, p. 28.

9. OSHA. *Emergency Action Plan Expert System.* Available at http://www.osha.gov/ SLTC/etools/evacuation/expertsystem/default.htm (accessed 3/21/2006).

10. Joint Commission on Accreditation of Healthcare Organizations. *Management of the Environment of Care, Standard EC.4.10.* Oakbrook Terrace, IL: Joint Commission.

CHAPTER 13

FIRE PREVENTION AND CONTROL

St. Joseph County, MI—Investigators are blaming a construction crew for an electrical fire at Sturgis Hospital last night, which led to the evacuation of the building's patients. Officials were called to the scene just after 7 PM Tuesday night. When they arrived on the scene, smoke could be seen throughout the hospital. Officials say they believe construction crews working in the basement struck an electrical cable, which sparked the fire. There were no injuries reported from the blaze and there's no word yet on how much damage was done to the building. All the patients were transferred to other area hospitals.

Posted: 05/23/2005 09:36 PM
Last Updated: 05/24/2005 09:28 AM
www.wndu.com

In March 2002 the U.S. Fire Administration reported that each year from 1996 to 1998 there were approximately 2,500 fires totaling $8.7 million in property losses in medical facilities. Those fires were associated with an injury rate per facility that was four times greater than the injury rate for all U.S. fires. Two-thirds of those injuries were due to smoke inhalation. The leading cause of those fires was listed as cooking, which occurred in the facilities' kitchens. Other major sources of such fires were appliances and air conditioning systems, followed by "other equipment," "electrical distribution," and "incendiary/suspicious."[1]

The most remarkable thing about those fires is that they resulted in only five deaths (four of which occurred in one facility) and 125 injuries. The reason for the small number of casualties is most certainly the fire prevention programs that are a feature of health care facilities.[2]

Despite the relatively small number of casualties that resulted, those fires caused a significant disruption of patient care. The U.S. Fire Administration highlighted four hospital fires that occurred between 1994 and 2001.

Although they were relatively minor, they resulted in 122 patient transfers to other hospitals and four patient deaths.[3]

Fire is an ever-present danger in every health care facility. Health care facility fires are especially dangerous because workers must protect patients as well as themselves. The risk is increased because work conducted in health care facilities may involve flammable liquids and other hazardous substances. In addition, the use of specialized equipment, such as lasers and other ignition sources utilized in oxygen-enriched atmospheres, increases the threat of fire. Further, the threat is far more critical in patient care areas since patients are often incapable of taking care of themselves in the event of a fire.

As with other health and safety functions, hazard analysis is the basis for the development of a fire safety program. The program evaluates what could happen, the likelihood of a fire event occurring, and the magnitude of problems created by a fire. Identifying potential events that could occur allows efforts to be directed toward prevention activities. Fire prevention measures are aimed at reducing the incidence of fires by eliminating opportunities for the ignition of flammable materials.

FIRE PREVENTION STANDARDS

The Occupational Safety and Health Administration (OSHA), the National Fire Protection Association (NFPA), and the Social Security Act all provide codes and standards that are intended to minimize the possibility and the effects of fire in health care facilities and to enhance the facility's ability to keep its employees and patients safe.

The Social Security Act mandates the establishment of minimum health and safety standards as well as Clinical Laboratory Improvement Amendments (CLIA) standards that must be met by providers and suppliers participating in the Medicare and Medicaid programs. These standards are found in Part 42 of the Code of Federal Regulations. "Providers," according to Medicare, include patient care institutions such as hospitals, critical access hospitals, hospices, nursing homes, and home health agencies.

Health care facilities also must follow standards established by OSHA, NFPA, and local authorities having jurisdiction. In addition, health care facilities must implement accreditation standards relating to fire and life safety.

Centers for Medicare & Medicaid Services

Unless waivers or provisions are approved, the basic life safety code requirement for health care facilities participating in Centers for Medicare & Medicaid Services (CMS) programs is compliance with the *NFPA 101®: Life Safety Code®* (*LSC*). The January 10, 2003, *Federal Register* published a CMS final rule mandating that health care facilities follow the regulations in the 2000 edition of the *LSC*. In announcing the rule, an agency press release stated, "In the past, the government issued its own rules for fire safety, which sometimes contradicted the widely used *LSC* and did not add any benefits to the facilities' fire protection programs."

The final rule adopts the 2000 edition of the *LSC* for long-term care facilities, inpatient hospice services, Intermediate Care Facilities for the Mentally Retarded (ICF/MRs), hospitals, ambulatory surgery centers, Program of All-Inclusive Care for the Elderly (PACE), critical access hospitals, and religious nonmedical health care institutions. It eliminates references in relevant regulations to all earlier editions.

The final rule became effective March 11, 2003. New provisions are listed in figure 13-1.[4]

Figure 13–1. CMS Fire Safety Requirements: New Provisions

☐ **Performance-Based Option.** In the October 2001 proposed rule, CMS solicited comments on whether to adopt this provision. Although CMS does not expect many providers to choose this option, they decided to include the performance-based design provision.

☐ **19.3.6.3.2. Roller Latch Exception Provision.** CMS has proposed non-adoption of section 2 of this provision, which would allow the use of roller latches if the latch can withstand a specific level of applied force. CMS did not adopt this exception, stating that roller latches constitute one of the top three cited deficiencies for life safety and the number 1 cited *LSC* deficiency in skilled nursing facilities (SNFs). In "protect in place" facilities such as health care, it is imperative that door hardware function properly to confine fire and smoke to specified areas. Fire investigations have shown that roller latches have been an unreliable means, partially due to the fact that the extensive maintenance required is often neglected, rendering the device nonfunctional. This poses a danger to the health and safety of the patients and staff. Because of this danger, CMS has required all roller latches to be replaced before March 13, 2006.

☐ **19.1.1.4.5. Renovations, Alterations, and Modernization.** Existing facilities that are being extensively renovated must be retrofitted with sprinkler systems as required in Chapter 18 for New Healthcare Occupancies, including the installation of sprinkler systems to non-sprinklered buildings. Determinations of what constitutes "major or minor" renovations, when questionable, will be made on a case-by-case basis by the authority having jurisdiction.

☐ **19.2.9. Emergency Lighting.** Emergency lighting must be provided for a period of 1½ hours in health care facilities in the event of failure of normal lighting. Emergency lighting is important to help staff and patients move safely in an emergency. Most emergency lighting systems meet this requirement when the emergency lighting is powered by the emergency generator; however, some facilities still rely on battery-powered emergency lights. Battery-powered units that do not provide the mandatory 1½ hours of lighting must be replaced with units complying with the rules before March 10, 2006.

(Continued on next page)

Figure 13–1. *(Continued)*

☐ **19.3.1. Protection of Vertical Openings.** Unprotected vertical openings, such as open stairwells, must be enclosed or protected to prevent the spread of fire and toxic gases from floor to floor. According to CMS estimates, there are approximately 5,573 vertical openings in 1,115 facilities that do not comply with the provisions of this section.

Vertical openings between floors are often installed in facilities as "convenience stairs." These stairways are typically used by staff who often travel between floors, such as in medical libraries, file storage areas, or administrative office areas. Open stairways are prohibited in patient sleeping and treatment areas.

☐ **19.3.4.3.2. Emergency Forces Notification.** The fire alarm system must provide automatic notification of a fire to emergency forces (i.e., a fire alarm transmission system). It is estimated that 2,358 facilities in the United States do not have a fire alarm retransmission system and would have to be brought into compliance. An independent study by the National Institute of Standards and Technology (NIST) indicates a high rate of nuisance alarms related to smoke detectors installed in health care facilities.* For every actual alarm, there are approximately 14 nuisance alarms. Smoke detection devices or systems are allowed to confirm an alarm for up to 120 seconds without transmitting the alarm to the fire department.

☐ **19.3.6.1. Corridors.** All areas in non-sprinklered buildings or smoke compartments are required to be separated from the corridor by fire-rated corridor walls. Rated corridors provide a protected passageway during an emergency and provide a higher level of patient safety.

Corridor walls are often compromised during the installation of cabling, piping, and other systems after the initial construction is completed. The holes in these barriers must be repaired to maintain the integrity of the fire-rated wall. In other instances, it has been found that walls that were intended to extend completely to the underside of the structure above were not completed at the time of construction. Sometimes this has been a result of poor coordination of the construction documents.

☐ **19.7.5.2/19.7.5.3. Upholstered Furniture.** Patient-provided upholstered furniture is allowed in the patient sleeping rooms of nursing homes only when a smoke detector is installed in the rooms. It is very common for nursing homes to allow patient-owned furnishings. In order to maintain patient rights, the required smoke detection must be provided. In this instance, the code allows single-station smoke detectors to be installed. Smoke detectors are required by CMS to be installed on or before September 11, 2003.

---

* Beebe, Chad E. *Am I Ready For My CMS Survey?* (adapted). Available at http://www.wsshe.org/CMSSurvey.htm (accessed 12/20/2005).

Figure 13–2. Self-Assessment Questions for *Life Safety Code* Compliance Regarding Exceptions to CMS Final Rule

1. Have all roller latches been removed? (Roller Latch Exception Provision, Section 19.3.6.3.2)
2. Is the sprinkler system upgraded? (Renovations, Alterations, and Modernization, Section 19.1.1.4.5)
3. Has emergency lighting been upgraded? (Emergency Lighting, Section 19.2.9)
4. Does the facility have any vertical openings that do not comply with the *Life Safety Code*? (Protection of Vertical Openings, Section 19.3.1)
5. Are systems are in place to notify emergency responders in case of a fire alarm? (Emergency Forces Notification, Section 19.3.4.3.2)
6. Has the facility ensured that corridor walls are fire rated? (Corridors, Section 19.3.6.1)
7. Has the facility installed a fire alarm where resident-provided upholstered furnishing is located? (Upholstered Furniture, Section 19.7.5.2/19.7.5.3)

All referenced health care facilities were required to be in compliance with the requirements of this rule by September 11, 2003, with certain exceptions. For those listed exceptions, the effective date was March 13, 2006. For those health care facilities that received an exception, figure 13-2 lists considerations for achieving compliance with the rule.

The final rule allows the Secretary of the Department of Health and Human Services (DHHS) to continue to grant waivers on a case-by-case basis if specific provisions would result in unreasonable hardship for the provider and if the safety of patients would not be compromised. Also, CMS may continue to accept a state's fire safety code in lieu of the *LSC* if the state code adequately protects patients. In addition, CMS would be given the authority to allow facilities to choose the Fire Safety Evaluation System (FSES) as an alternative equivalency system to meet the requirements of the *LSC*.[5]

Accreditation Organizations

Centers for Medicare & Medicaid Services mandates that accreditation organizations require health care facilities to develop and implement a fire response plan that complies with NFPA *Life Safety Code* requirements. If a national accreditation organization has and enforces standards that meet the federal Conditions of Participation, CMS may grant the accrediting organization "deeming" authority and "deem" each accredited health care organization as meeting the Medicare and Medicaid certification requirements. The health care organization would have "deemed status" and would not be subject to the Medicare survey and certification process.

Accreditation organizations are automatically "deemed" to meet the CMS *Life Safety Code* requirements, and CMS "deems" each accredited health care organization as meeting the Medicare and Medicaid *LSC* requirements.

NFPA

The National Fire Protection Association develops, publishes, and disseminates more than 300 consensus codes and standards, of which more than 60 apply to health care facilities. Two of NFPA's fire safety codes relating to health care facilities are *NFPA 101®: Life Safety Code®* and *NFPA 99: Standard for Health Care Facilities.* The *LSC* includes requirements for construction, protection, and operational features designed to provide safety from fire, smoke, and panic.

NFPA 101®: Life Safety Code®

The NFPA's *Life Safety Code* covers a host of topics related to reducing the spread of fire in buildings and providing means of egress from buildings when necessary. The code includes different requirements for different types of buildings, including health care facilities.

The *LSC*, which is used in every state, and adopted statewide in 34 states, sets minimum building design, construction, operation, and maintenance requirements necessary to protect building occupants from dangers caused by fire, smoke, and toxic fumes. The *LSC* also provides prompt-escape requirements for new and existing buildings, including health care occupancies.

A number of regulatory and compliance organizations and many state and local "authorities having jurisdiction" (AHJs) enforce the *LSC*. Standard 1910 Subpart E of OSHA is derived from the *NFPA 101®-1970 Life Safety Code®*.

Applying the LSC to the Joint Commission Statement of Conditions® for Interim Life Safety Measures

The Joint Commission requires health care facilities to develop a comprehensive, written Statement of Conditions® (SOC) for each building in which patients are housed or treated. The document identifies structural features for fire protection required under the *Life Safety Code*, details code deficiencies or construction activities, and, when necessary, includes a plan for improvement. The SOC is designed to be a "living, ongoing" management tool that facilities should use to continuously assess, identify, and resolve code deficiencies.

Knowledge needed to comply with the SOC includes the elements listed in figure 13-3.

NFPA 99: Health Care Facilities

The idea for the standard for health care facilities, *NFPA 99: Health Care Facilities*, came about as an effort to coordinate and correlate the information con-

Figure 13–3. Knowledge Needed to Comply with the Joint Commission Statement of Conditions

☐ What to include in the facility's management plans for safety, security, hazardous materials, emergency preparedness, life safety, medical equipment, and utility systems

☐ How to measure and assess the effectiveness of the facility's Environment of Care management plan and risk assessment activities

☐ Identification of key standards and how to implement them

☐ The chapters of *NFPA 101* that are specific to health care occupancies

tained in 12 existing documents on various subjects. Eleven of the 12 documents directly addressed fire-related problems in and about health care facilities.

The intent of *NFPA 99* is to establish criteria to minimize the hazards of fire, explosion, and electricity in health care facilities providing services to patients. These criteria include performance, maintenance, testing, and safe practices for all facilities, material, equipment, and appliances, as well as other hazards associated with the primary hazards.

The criteria of *NFPA 99* apply to all health care facilities. The standard is intended for use by those persons involved in the design, construction, inspection, and operation of health care facilities and in the design, manufacture, and testing of appliances and equipment used in patient care areas of health care facilities. Depending on the edition, *NFPA 99* includes topics listed in figure 13-4.

Figure 13–4. Sample Entries from the *NFPA 99* Table of Contents

☐ Electrical Systems
☐ Gas and Vacuum Systems
☐ Environmental Systems
☐ Electrical Equipment
☐ Gas Equipment
☐ Manufacturer Requirements
☐ Laboratories
☐ Health Care Emergency Management
☐ Other Health Care Facilities
☐ Nursing Home Requirements
☐ Limited Care Facility Requirements
☐ Electrical and Gas Equipment for Home Care
☐ Hyperbaric Facilities
☐ Freestanding Birthing Centers

OSHA

Although OSHA standards pertain to employees, it is assumed that in health care facilities employees will be trained to take care of patients during fires and other emergencies. Standards for fire prevention and fire protection include the standards in OSHA 29 CFR 1910, Subpart E, Exit Routes, Emergency Action Plans, and Fire Prevention Plans, and Subpart L, Fire Protection.[6] [CD-ROM 13.1] Some states may have their own OSHA-approved plans and different enforcement policies. Primary OSHA Subpart E fire safety requirements related to health care facilities include:

- □ Design and construction requirements for exit routes. [1910.36] [CD-ROM 13.2]
  - An exit route must be permanent. [1910.36(a)(1)]
  - An exit route must be separated by fire-resistant materials. [1910.36(a)(2)]
  - The number of exit routes must be adequate. [1910.36(b)]
  - An exit door must be unlocked. [1910.36(d)]
  - The capacity of an exit route must be adequate. [1910.36(f)]
- □ Maintenance, safeguards, and operational features for exit routes. [1910.37] [CD-ROM 13.3]
  - The danger to employees must be minimized. [1910.37(a)]
  - Exit routes must be free and unobstructed. No materials or equipment may be placed, either permanently or temporarily, within the exit route. [1910.37(a)(3)]
  - Safeguards designed to protect employees during an emergency (e.g., sprinkler systems, alarm systems, fire doors, exit lighting) must be in proper working order at all times. [1910.37(a)(4)]
  - Lighting and marking must be adequate and appropriate. [1910.37(b)]
  - The fire-retardant properties of paints or solutions must be maintained. [1910.37(c)]
  - Exit routes must be maintained during construction, repairs, or alterations. [1910.37(d)]
  - Employees must not be exposed to hazards of flammable or explosive substances or equipment used during construction, repairs, or alterations, that are beyond the normal permissible conditions in the workplace, or that would impede exiting the workplace. [1910.37(d)(3)]
  - An employee alarm system must be operable. [1910.37(e)]
- □ Emergency action plans. [1910.38] [CD-ROM 13.4]
  - An emergency action plan must have:
    - ○ Procedures for reporting a fire. [1910.38(c)(1)]
    - ○ Procedures for emergency evacuation. [1910.38(c)(2)]

- Procedures to be followed by employees who remain to perform critical plant operations before they evacuate. [1910.38(c)(3)]
- An employer must designate and train employees to assist in the safe and orderly evacuation of other employees. [1910.38(e)]
- An employer must review the emergency action plan with each employee covered by the plan: [1910.38(f)]
  - When the plan is developed or the employee is assigned initially to a job. [1910.38(f)(1)]
  - When the employee's responsibilities under the plan change. [1910.38(f)(2)]
  - When the plan is changed. [1910.38(f)(3)]
- ☐ Fire prevention plans. [1910.39] [CD-ROM 13.5]
  - A fire prevention plan must be in writing, be kept in the workplace, and be made available to employees for review. [1910.39(b)]
  - A fire prevention plan must include:
    - A list of all major fire hazards, proper handling and storage procedures for hazardous materials, potential ignition sources and their control, and the type of fire protection equipment necessary to control each major hazard. [1910.39(c)(1)]
    - Procedures to control accumulations of flammable and combustible waste materials. [1910.39(c)(2)]
    - Procedures for regular maintenance of safeguards installed on heat-producing equipment to prevent the accidental ignition of combustible materials. [1910.39(c)(3)]
    - The names or job titles of employees responsible for maintaining equipment to prevent or control sources of ignition or fires. [1910.39(c)(4)]
    - The names or job titles of employees responsible for the control of fuel source hazards. [1910.39(c)(5)]
  - Employee information. An employer must inform employees upon initial assignment to a job of the fire hazards to which they are exposed. An employer must also review with each employee those parts of the fire prevention plan necessary for self-protection. [1910.39(d)]

Requirements listed under OSHA Subpart L, Fire Protection, include:

☐ Fire brigades. A fire brigade represents an organized group of employees who are knowledgeable, trained, and skilled in at least basic firefighting operations. [1910.156] [CD-ROM 13.6]

☐ Portable fire extinguishers. The requirements of this section apply to the placement, use, maintenance, and testing of portable fire extinguishers provided for the use of employees. [1910.157] [CD-ROM 13.7]

□ Standpipe and hose systems. This section applies to all small hose, and Class II and Class III standpipe systems installed to meet the requirements of a particular OSHA standard. [1910.158] [CD-ROM 13.8]

□ Employee alarm systems. The requirements in this section that pertain to maintenance, testing, and inspection apply to all local fire alarm signaling systems used for alerting employees regardless of the other functions of the system. [1910.165] [CD-ROM 13.9]

Additional OSHA fire protection standards in Subpart L, Subpart S (Electrical), and Subpart Z (Toxic and Hazardous Substances) include standards for automatic sprinkler systems, fixed extinguishing systems, fire detection systems, wiring methods, components, and equipment for general use and hazard communication.

Fire Prevention Responsibilities

Fire safety incorporates several topics that health and safety professionals need to be knowledgeable about, which are divided into two primary areas:

Administration of building and systems management functions
Administration of the fire prevention plan

Administration of Building and Systems Management Functions

Many codes that apply to health care facilities address built-in fire protection systems. These codes concern building design, structural features for fire protection required under *NFPA 101®: Life Safety Code®*, fire alarm and detection equipment, automatic extinguishing equipment, standpipe systems, and equipment such as fire dampers and automatic smoke detectors.

Several areas and structures that pose a fire hazard can be found around many health care facilities. They may or may not be physically attached to the main or central medical portion of the facility. These include parking garages, outdoor storage facilities, hydrants and external water supplies, and fire lanes.

The Engineering Department directs the functions involved in building protection. However, many of these areas overlap with the facility's Environmental Health and Safety program, and the Environmental Health and Safety Department must work closely with the Engineering Department to ensure maximum protection.

Examples of OSHA standards that apply to the responsibilities of the Engineering Department but that the Environmental Health and Safety Department should be familiar with include:

1. 1910.35, Compliance with *NFPA 101®: Life Safety Code®–2000 edition*

An employer who demonstrates compliance with the exit route provisions of *NFPA 101®: Life Safety Code®–2000 edition*, will be deemed to be in compliance with the corresponding requirements in 1910.34, Coverage and definitions; 1910.36, Design and construction requirements for exit routes; and 1910.37, Maintenance, safeguards, and operational features for exit routes. [CD-ROM 13.10]

Those who manage today's health care facilities are aware of the enormous benefits of a fast and thorough emergency building evacuation.

OSHA has revised its standards for means of egress, concluding that NFPA's 2000 edition of the *LSC* provides comparable safety to the OSHA Exit routes standard. The OSHA final rule became effective December 7, 2002, and permits employers to comply with *NFPA 101–2000 edition* in order to meet means-of-egress standards.

2. 1910.37, Maintenance, safeguards, and operational features for exit routes

This section is devoted to the "components" of the means of egress, which must be constructed as an integral part of the health care facility buildings or must be permanently affixed thereto. For example, if a door to an exit or to a means of exit access is not of the side-hinged, swinging type, it is not approved.

Although Subpart E is devoted to the provisions for ensuring that personnel can egress from a building under emergency conditions, it also contains several provisions for preventing or reducing the risk of such an emergency.

One of the most frequently cited OSHA violations in Subpart E in health care facilities is failure to satisfy the requirement that means of egress be continuously maintained free of all obstructions or impediments to full instant use in the case of fire or other emergencies. Signs and other identification are important elements of this requirement.

3. 1910.37, Signs

Exit signs must clearly identify how to leave a building or facility. Exit signs must be adequately lighted. [1910.37(b)(1)] Each exit must be clearly visible and marked by a sign reading "Exit." [1910.37(b)(2)] Each exit route door must be free of decorations or signs that obscure the visibility of the exit route door. [1910.37(b)(3)]

4. 1910.157(c)(1), Portable fire extinguisher signs

Portable fire extinguisher signs are used to identify extinguishers so that they are readily accessible without subjecting individuals to possible injury.

Administration of the Fire Prevention Plan

The fire prevention plan should be part of the facility's comprehensive emergency management plan, as detailed in OSHA 3088, *How To Plan For Workplace Emergencies and Evacuations*. [CD-ROM 13.11] Quick response, confidence, understanding, and organization are important in dealing with a fire, as they are in any disaster recovery situation. Fire prevention management should be one of the responsibilities of the Environmental Health and Safety Department and includes the following components.

FIRE PREVENTION PLAN (29 CFR 1910.39)

An effective fire prevention plan counteracts panic and indecision and replaces it with purposeful acting during an emergency. Further, an effective fire prevention plan includes measures to control fire hazards in a building on a daily basis.

The dual objectives of such a plan should be:

☐ *Fire prevention:* To prevent the incident of fire by the control of fire hazards in the building and the maintenance of the building facilities provided for the safety of the occupants

☐ *Emergency evacuation:* To establish a systematic method for a safe and orderly evacuation of an area or building, by and of its occupants, in case of fire or other emergency

The plan should be divided into two basic sections with a table of contents and/or index, and the fire prevention plan and diagrams should identify evacuation routes and the location of alarms:

The fire prevention plan should contain both measures to control fire hazards and procedures for responding to fire emergencies:

☐ General measures, which include emergency procedures in case of fire:
  ▪ The designation and organization of staff to carry out fire safety duties
  ▪ The preparation of diagrams showing the type, location, and operation of the building fire emergency systems
  ▪ The holding of fire drills
  ▪ The control of fire hazards in the building
  ▪ The inspection and maintenance of building facilities provided for the safety of occupants
☐ Maintenance of the plan
☐ Distribution
☐ Posting of instructions

□ A general description of the building(s), with safety systems described in a clear and concise manner:

- Fire alarm system, which includes locations of pull stations and instructions for authorized persons for silencing the alarm
- Exit system
- Communications, including instructions for use of the public address system
- Emergency power, including instructions for the use and maintenance of the emergency power system
- Elevators, including the location and instructions for operation during emergency conditions
- Fire-extinguishing equipment
- Smoke control equipment
- Keys provided for firefighters and where they are located
- Boilers and furnace rooms, including drawings to show locations and control of utilities, gas, water, and steam
- Special hazards, such as chemicals, compressed-gas areas, special fire-extinguishing systems, and areas such as computer rooms, libraries, and file storage

The team involved in the development of the plan should ask the questions listed in figure 13-5, along with other "what if" questions.

As with other health and safety plans and policies, the required codes and standards must be referenced in the plan.

FIRE AND EXPLOSION PLANNING

Because of the threat of terrorism, OSHA developed the Fire and Explosion Planning Matrix to provide employers with planning considerations and online

Figure 13–5. Questions to Consider in Developing a Fire Plan

□ Who will meet the arriving fire trucks?

□ Where will the command center be?

□ What if the command center is on fire?

□ Where are phone numbers, e-mail addresses, and fax numbers?

□ What happens if the Environmental Health and Safety Director is not on duty?

□ How will patients be kept calm during an emergency?

□ How will people be fed if the cafeteria is damaged or destroyed?

□ How will the media be managed?

□ How will people communicate if telephones and cellular telephones do not work?

resources to reduce their vulnerability to, or the consequences of, an explosive or incendiary device or act of arson.[7] While OSHA does not assume that an employer can reasonably be expected to identify and attempt to control explosive or incendiary devices or to protect against arson, an effective fire prevention plan that addresses these possible threats may increase workplace safety and security and ensure that employees know how to respond to such events.

To provide accurate, current information on this rapidly developing area of occupational safety and health, OSHA continues to work with other federal response agencies, including the Federal Emergency Management Agency (FEMA), the Environmental Protection Agency (EPA), the U.S. Army Soldier and Biological Chemical Command (SBCCOM), the Centers for Disease Control and Prevention (CDC), and, within CDC, the National Institute for Occupational Safety and Health (NIOSH).

Assessing the Risk of a Terrorist Incident

To use this fire prevention guidance effectively, an employer must first assess the risk of a terrorist incident in the workplace. The level of risk is based on the social and political importance of the facility, its vulnerabilities, and anticipated consequences of the event. This kind of assessment is not a typical safety and health evaluation. However, guidance on conducting an assessment involving a terrorist incident is becoming more widely available. *Best Practices in Workplace Security* can offer valuable assistance.[8] [CD-ROM 13.12]

Using OSHA's Fire and Explosion Planning Matrix

The Fire and Explosion Planning Matrix is not a tool for conducting a comprehensive compliance evaluation of a fire prevention plan developed to meet the requirements of OSHA Standard 29 CFR 1910.39, Fire prevention. Rather, it addresses general aspects of fire prevention planning and includes broad questions to help an employer review the plan as it relates to a terrorist act. Each broad question is followed by planning considerations and suggested preparedness measures appropriate for workplaces in each of the three risk areas.

The facility's fire prevention plan should work in conjunction with the procedures identified in existing emergency action plans. Therefore, any modification to the fire prevention plan can affect the facility's emergency action plan.

FIRE DRILLS

Fire drills are an opportunity to familiarize staff members with proper fire plan procedures. The NFPA and accreditation organizations require fire drills. The Environmental Health and Safety Department and department liaisons should lead the drills and document successes, failures, and corrective actions. The information should be shared with other departments and the Environmental Health and Safety Committee.

Patient relocation and/or evacuation may be a critical responsibility for fire brigade members. Although health care facilities are designed for a "shelter in place" strategy for fire emergencies, health care personnel should be trained and prepared to relocate or evacuate patients when hazardous conditions are present. The NFPA *Life Safety Code* recommends that fire drills include provisions for moving patients to adjacent smoke compartments. The *Life Safety Code* further recommends practicing patient relocation using simulated patients or empty wheelchairs.[9]

EMPLOYEE TRAINING

Fire safety is everyone's job in the workplace. Employers should train employees about fire hazards in the workplace and what to do in a fire emergency. This plan should outline the assignments of key personnel in the event of a fire and provide an evacuation plan for workers. The major sources of employee fire safety training requirements are OSHA, accreditation organizations, and local authorities having jurisdiction regarding fire safety.

Organizations have separate requirements and guidelines, although there is some overlap. The primary fire safety training requirements for OSHA can be found in standards 29 CFR 1910.38, Emergency action plans; 29 CFR 1910.39, Fire prevention plans; 29 CFR 1910.156, Fire brigades; 29 CFR 1910.164, Fire detection systems [CD-ROM 13.13]; 29 CFR 1910.157, Portable fire extinguishers; and 29 CFR 1910.160, Fixed extinguishing systems [CD-ROM 13.14].

FIRE BRIGADES (29 CFR 1910.156)

Many health care facilities choose to maintain a group of employees whose responsibilities include responding to fire alarms and fire-related emergencies throughout the facility. Such groups are often designated as fire brigades or fire response teams; these are synonymous terms.[10] According to OSHA, a fire brigade represents an organized group of employees who are knowledgeable, trained, and skilled in at least basic firefighting operations.[11] Fire brigades vary widely in responsibility, function, and size. Some facilities choose to maintain a fire brigade capable of interior structural firefighting; however, most health care facilities maintain a fire brigade capable of only incipient-stage firefighting. Either designation requires compliance with OSHA standards, including specific sections of 29 CFR 1910.156, Fire brigades, depending on the level of responsibility.

Standard 1910.156 outlines levels of responsibility. An incipient-stage fire is defined by OSHA as follows:

> 29 CFR 1910.155, Scope, application and definitions applicable to this subpart.
> (c)(26) "Incipient stage fire" means a fire which is in the initial or beginning stage and can be controlled or extinguished by portable fire extinguishers, Class II standpipe or small hose systems without the need for protective clothing or breathing apparatus.[12] [CD-ROM 13.15]

Figure 13-6 lists the actions included in incipient-stage firefighting according to *NFPA 600: Standard on Industrial Fire Brigades*, 2000 edition.[13]

In health care facilities, incipient-stage fire brigade or fire response team responsibilities often include removing patients and personnel from danger, using fire extinguishers or other firefighting techniques (such as smothering the fire), and working with the fire department on arrival.

Interior-structural fires are large fires and must also be fought by fire brigades trained per OSHA Standard 29 CFR 1910.156.[14] Fire brigades fighting interior-structural fires must receive additional training, including proper use of protective clothing and respiratory protection, and administering first aid (1910.156(c)(3)).

Regardless of their level of responsibility, function, or size, employers are required to follow standards established by OSHA, accreditation organizations, and local authorities having jurisdiction regarding fire brigades.

Policies and Procedures

If a health care facility chooses to utilize a fire brigade, written policies and procedures regarding its program must be developed and maintained. The program must be part of an overall institutional fire safety program.

An important part of a fire brigade program is the preparation and maintenance of an OSHA-compliant organizational statement that establishes the existence of the fire brigade. The organizational statement must include the elements listed in figure 13-7.

Figure 13–6. Actions of Incipient-Stage Firefighting

- ☐ Able to fight the fire in normal work clothing
- ☐ Not required to crawl or take evasive action to avoid heat or smoke
- ☐ Not required to wear thermal protective clothing (including coats, trousers, gloves, and head, eye, and face protection) or self-contained breathing apparatus (SCBA)
- ☐ Able to fight the fire effectively with portable fire extinguishers or handlines flowing up to 125 gallons per minute of water (i.e., Class II standpipe systems).

Figure 13–7. OSHA-Required Elements of an Organizational Statement for a Fire Brigade

---

☐ Basic organizational structure of the fire brigade

☐ Type, amount, and frequency of training for the fire brigade members

☐ Expected number of members of the fire brigade

☐ Functions that the fire brigade will perform at the workplace

---

In addition to the information required in the organizational statement, paragraph 1910.156(b)(1), it is suggested that the organizational statement also contain the information in 29 CFR 1910 Subpart L, Appendix A, Fire Protection, which are listed in figure 13-8. [CD-ROM 13.16]

The organizational statement must be available for inspection by OSHA and by employees or their designated representatives.

Training

Because of the inherent dangers in responding to fire emergencies, health care fire response teams should be adequately trained and prepared to deal with such situations. Both OSHA and accreditation organizations require fire brigade members to receive training.

The frequency and content of the training depends on the duties of the fire response team. At a minimum, fire brigade members who perform incipient-stage firefighting must receive hands-on training annually.[15] Although it does not specify required content for fire brigade training and education, as it expects organizations to develop site-specific, performance-oriented training programs, OSHA strongly recommends that fire brigade training include the topics listed in figure 13-9.[16]

Accreditation organizations also require periodic implementation of the plan through fire drills and annual evaluations to determine the effectiveness of training.

Figure 13–8. Additional Information Recommended for the Organizational Statement

---

☐ A description of the duties that the fire brigade members are expected to perform

☐ The line authority of each fire brigade officer

☐ The number of fire brigade officers and the number of training instructors

☐ A list and description of the types of awards or recognition that brigade members may be eligible to receive

---

Figure 13–9. Fire Brigade Training Topics

□ Emergency action procedures

□ Pre-fire planning

□ Special hazards in the workplace to which brigade members may be exposed during a fire or other emergency (i.e., flammable liquids, flammable gases, toxic chemicals, radioactive sources, and water-reactive substances)

□ Procedures for actions involving exposure to special hazards

□ Locations of exits and egress routes

□ Use of fire equipment, such as fire extinguishers and standpipes

---

Fire brigade leaders and instructors must be provided training that is more comprehensive than that provided to other members of the fire brigade. Although OSHA and accreditation organizations provide no performance requirements, fire brigade instructors should be knowledgeable about site-specific hazards and the functions of the brigade and able to demonstrate skills in communication, teaching methods, and motivation.

Fire brigade training should not be confused with fire extinguisher training for other employees. As an additional standard, OSHA requires annual fire extinguisher training for employees (including those not on the fire brigade) who have access to portable fire extinguishers for use in the workplace.[17]

PORTABLE FIRE EXTINGUISHERS (29 CFR 1910.157)

The Occupational Safety and Health Administration does not require that portable fire extinguishers be placed and used in workplaces. However, in facilities where portable fire extinguishers are placed and provided for the use of employees, OSHA Standard 29 CFR 1910.157, Portable fire extinguishers, applies. The standard includes general requirements (1910.157(c)); selection and distribution (1910.157(d)); inspection, maintenance, and testing (1910.157(e)); hydrostatic testing (1910.157(f)); and training and education (1910.157(g)).

The *Life Safety Code* requires that portable fire extinguishers be provided in all health care and ambulatory health care occupancies. Fire extinguishers must also be installed, inspected, and maintained in accordance with *NFPA 10: Standard for Portable Fire Extinguishers*.[18] Fire extinguishers must be strategically located throughout health care facilities and placed in visible, well-traveled locations. Travel distances for different classes of fire extinguishers are also specified in *NFPA 10*.

Employees using portable fire extinguishers can often put out small fires or control a fire until additional help arrives. Portable extinguishers are not designed to fight large or spreading fires. However, even against small fires, they are useful only under certain conditions:

☐ The location of the extinguisher must be known beforehand. Taking time to locate a fire extinguisher will only allow the fire to grow beyond the extinguisher's firefighting limits.

☐ The proper type of extinguisher must be used for the fire that is to be extinguished.

☐ The operator must know how to use the extinguisher. There is no time to read directions during an emergency. According to OSHA requirements, employees who are required to use portable fire extinguishers be trained at initial employment and at least annually thereafter.

☐ The extinguisher must be in working order and fully charged.

Although the great majority of fire extinguishers placed in health care facilities are classified as ABC, some facilities may have other types of extinguishers that are intended to be used on specific types of fires. Water Mist portable fire extinguishers are an alternative that can be used for Class A fires, especially where a potential Class C (electrical) hazard exists. The unique misting nozzle not only provides safety from electrical shock but greatly enhances the cooling and soaking characteristics of the agent. Potential applications for Water Mist fire extinguishers in health care facilities include operating rooms, endoscopic suites, areas where lasers and cautery devices are used, and locations where there is direct contact with patients. Instruction on the proper use of fire extinguishers must be included in each employee's safety training program.

Accreditation organizations and OSHA[19] require portable fire extinguishers to be given monthly visual inspections. Portable fire extinguishers must also receive annual maintenance checks.

Labels on portable fire extinguishers indicate the class and relative size of fire that they can be expected to handle. Classes of fire extinguishers most often used in health care facilities are listed in figure 13-10.

Figure 13–10. Classes of Fire Extinguishers Most Often Used in Health Care Facilities

☐ Class A extinguishers are used on fires involving ordinary combustibles, such as wood, cloth, and paper.

☐ Class B extinguishers are used on fires involving liquids, greases, and gases. Appropriate places for Class B fire extinguishers include laboratories, boiler rooms, hazardous material storage areas, and kitchens.

☐ Class C extinguishers are used on fires involving energized electrical equipment.

The recommended system to indicate extinguisher suitability according to class of fire is pictorial and combines the approved and non-approved uses of extinguishers on a single label. In most areas of the health care facility, Class ABC, or all-purpose, fire extinguishers are used.

Employees must know how to use an extinguisher before attempting to do so. A fire doubles in size about every minute. Time wasted on trying to figure out how to use the extinguisher will allow the fire to grow beyond control.

Employees should be taught that they may fight a fire if:

- Everyone is safe.
- The fire alarm has been activated.
- The fire is small and contained.
- There is a way to escape.
- The employee is trained.

RESPONDING TO A FIRE

Being prepared has saved many lives. Practicing what to do in the event of a fire can help employees think and act quickly and safely, potentially saving the lives of employees and patients. A code, such as "code red," may be used to announce the presence of a fire so that the staff can be alerted without frightening patients and visitors and risking a panicked rush to escape.

Acronyms, such as RACE, are often used to help teach employees critical responses and steps to take in the event of a fire:

Rescue anyone in immediate danger. This step requires teamwork. Someone else may activate the alarm.

Activate the alarm or call the facility's emergency number or 911 immediately. If necessary, continue to evacuate staff, patients, and visitors while awaiting the fire department.

Confine the fire. Be sure all windows and doors are tightly closed to prevent the spread of smoke and flames.

Extinguish the fire or Evacuate patients and others to adjacent smoke compartments, if necessary. Attempts to extinguish the fire should be made only if the fire is small and easily doused, such as a fire in a wastebasket. Although smothering it—with a blanket or raincoat, perhaps—is one way to extinguish a fire, it presents the possibility of the fabric catching fire as well. The most preferable way to put out a fire is with a fire extinguisher.

Whether the procedural rules are for small or large facilities, they must be consistently observed and practiced. In an emergency, it is easy to become disoriented or even briefly immobilized. Memorizing the procedure can make an enormous difference to the safety of employees and patients.

Preventing Fires

Throughout the health care facility, fires can be prevented. The worksite analysis and periodic hazard surveillance activities should include observations of safety and housekeeping issues and should address proper storage of chemicals and supplies, unobstructed access to fire extinguishers, and emergency evacuation routes. In addition, employees should be questioned as to their familiarity with the plan. During fire inspections, the Environmental Health and Safety Department and the department liaison for each department in the facility should look for any items that could cause accidental fires or limit the ability of the facility's occupants to safely escape if a fire were to occur.

Potential fire hazards found in health care facilities include:

- ☐ Blocked exits
- ☐ Material storage in hallway
- ☐ Blocked corridors
- ☐ Unsafe storage of chemicals
- ☐ Improper storage of gas cylinders
- ☐ Using extension cords for permanent wiring
- ☐ Using door chocks or fire extinguishers to hold open a fire door
- ☐ Poor housekeeping (offices)
- ☐ Open electrical panel
- ☐ Inoperable exit sign
- ☐ No fire stopping in open penetration
- ☐ Storage in stairwells

Electricity

Electricity can be a potent fire source. Many fires have started from old or defective wiring. Overloaded wiring can be very dangerous. Potential electrical fire hazards are everywhere. A build-up of dust, trash, and spider webs is an invitation for fire to start in the electrical system. Electrical wiring can be hit when workers are drilling holes or driving nails in walls, possibly causing a fire.

Power Delivery System

Many fires result from defects in, or misuse of, the power delivery system. Wiring often fails due to faulty installation, overloading, physical damage, aging, and deterioration by chemical action, heat, moisture, and weather. Such wiring should be replaced and new circuits installed.

Overloading circuits by hooking up more electrical devices than they are designed to handle is a typical problem. It is hazardous to overload electrical circuits by using extension cords and multi-plug outlets. Use extension cords only when necessary, and make sure they are heavy enough for the job. Avoid creating an octopus by inserting several plugs into a multi-plug outlet connected to a single wall outlet.

Motor and Power Tool Fire Hazards

Motor troubles can trigger a fire. Overheating due to excessive dirt, overloading, poor ventilation, arcing or sparking could ignite combustible materials (chaff, grease, trash) on or near a motor. Keep the area around motors and heaters free of flammable or combustible materials. Provide plenty of ventilation for motors, and keep them clean. Internal failures or shorts could cause a motor to burst into flames.

Most electrical devices are subject to internal wiring failures, worn power cords, and faulty switches, all of which add to fire risk. Inspect all electrical devices and their cords. Repair frayed insulation on wiring at once. If an electrical device does not work or works poorly, makes unusual noises, smokes or has a burnt smell, or issues sparks or a pop, unplug it immediately and have the problem fixed.

Equipment Maintenance

Preventive maintenance (PM) is a major consideration in health care facilities. When equipment malfunctions, it is not only expensive to repair but can be a disaster in terms of fire loss as well. Without a properly planned and implemented PM program, facilities run a greater risk of experiencing unscheduled outages and downtime from fires that can prove costly to the facility.

Alcohol-Based Hand Sanitizers

Alcohol-based hand sanitizers are useful for improving health care personnel hand hygiene, reducing health care–associated infection, and improving overall patient safety. Alcohol-based hand rubs have been used safely for more than 30 years in European hospitals. However, local fire marshals in several states have considered the placement of alcohol-based hand rub dispensers in hallways a potential fire hazard. Based on their interpretation of local or regional fire codes, some fire marshals have demanded that dispensers located in hallways that serve as egress corridors be removed. As a result, until recently, existing national fire codes have permitted hand rub dispensers in patient rooms but prohibited their installation in exit corridors.

Effective May 2004, the NFPA amended its 2000 and 2003 *Life Safety Code* to specifically recognize and permit the use of alcohol-based hand rub solutions in patient rooms, corridors, and suites of health care facilities. On March 25, 2005, the Centers for Medicare & Medicaid Services (CMS) issued an "Amendment to Fire Safety Requirements for Certain Health Care Facilities"— File code CMS-3145-IFC, in the Federal Register. This final rule, effective March 24, 2005 (following a public comment period), adopts the substance of the April 15, 2004, temporary interim amendment (TIA) 00-1 (101), Alcohol Based Hand

Rub Solutions, an amendment to the 2000 edition of the *Life Safety Code*, published by the National Fire Protection Association (NFPA). This amendment will allow certain health care facilities to place alcohol-based hand rub dispensers in egress corridors under specific conditions. The NFPA and CMS should be consulted for current requirements. Local or state fire code requirements may differ from the national codes. Health care facilities should work with local fire marshals to ensure that such installations are consistent with local fire codes.

Hospital Beds

Under certain conditions, electrically powered hospital beds may be fire hazards. In response to reports of fires involving such beds, the U.S. Food and Drug Administration (FDA) developed *FDA Public Health Notification: Safety Tips for Preventing Hospital Bed Fires* to help reduce the risk of fires caused by these types of beds. [CD-ROM 13.17]

Following is a summary of the items listed in the document that clinical staff can incorporate into their department's hazard surveillance program:

1. Connect the bed's power cord directly to a wall-mounted outlet.
2. Do not connect the bed's power cord to an extension cord or to a multiple-outlet strip.
3. Visually inspect the bed's power cord for damage.
4. Do not cover the bed's power cord or any other power cord with a rug or carpet.
5. Ensure that appropriate staff inspect all parts of the bed frame, motor and hardware, mattress, and the floor beneath and near the bed for build-up of dust and lint.
6. Test the bed to ensure that it moves freely to its full limit in both directions.
7. Test the bed's hand and panel controls, including the patient lockout features, to ensure that the bed is working properly.
8. Inspect the covering of the bed's control panel and the patient control panel to ensure that the covering is not cracked or damaged.
9. Check patient bed occupancy monitors and all other equipment in the patient's room with plug-in power supplies for indications of overheating or physical damage.
10. Report to the bed maintenance personnel any unusual sounds, burning odors, or movement deviations observed in the controls, motors, or the limit switch functions.
11. Ensure that all manufacturer's recalls, urgent safety notices, and other product alerts have been followed.

The document also lists tips for the staff responsible for bed maintenance, which include checking electrical power cable connectors, reviewing the manufacturer's recommended service plan regarding the bed's motors, and ensuring that heavy-duty or hospital-grade plugs are used on power cords.

Table 13–1. Examples of Flammable and Combustible Liquids and Their Flash Points

Liquid	Flash Point (°F)
Flammable liquids	
Xylene	81
Most alcohols	50–60
Toluene	40
Benzene	12
Acetone	1.4
Combustible liquids	
Lubricating oils	250–475
Ethylene glycol	232
Phenol	175
Some cleaning solvents	140
Most oil-based paints	105–140

Flammable and Combustible Liquids (29 CFR 1910.106)

Flammable and combustible liquids are liquids that can burn. They are classified, or grouped, as either flammable or combustible by their flashpoints. Generally speaking, flammable liquids will burn easily, usually at normal (ambient) working temperatures. Combustible liquids have the ability to burn at temperatures that are usually above ambient temperatures.

The widespread use and storage of flammable and combustible liquids presents a major fire hazard in health care facilities. Employees should be aware of important facts about flammable and combustible liquids (particularly requirements for their storage) that can help to prevent fires.

Flammable liquids produce ignitable vapors, and in most workplaces there are many ignition sources. In addition, nearly all flammable liquid vapors are heavier than air and may accumulate in areas of poor ventilation. This may pose a risk of fire if they come in contact with an ignition source such as a sparking hand tool, a cutting torch, an operating motor, or an open flame.

In order to prevent these hazards, OSHA Standard 29 CFR 1910.106, Flammable and combustible liquids, addresses the primary concerns of design and construction, ventilation, ignition sources, and storage. [CD-ROM 13.18] The primary basis of OSHA's standard is *NFPA 30: Flammable and Combustible Liquids Code*. This standard applies to the handling, storage, and use of flammable and combustible liquids with a flash point below 200°F.

Because a flammable liquid can reach its flash point even at room temperature, any unrecognized leak can pose a particular hazard. If escaping vapors are heavier than air, they can move for some distance along the ground in an invisible cloud and settle in low areas.

Examples of flammable and combustible liquids and their flash points are listed in table 13-1.

Piping systems (including the pipe, tubing, flanges, bolting, gaskets, valves, fittings, and the pressure-containing parts of other components) that contain flammable and combustible liquids must meet the requirements of *NFPA 30*.

Following are some of the precautions that must be taken for flammable and combustible liquids:

☐ Spills of flammable and combustible liquids must be cleaned up promptly and properly and in accordance with relevant OSHA and EPA regulations, including OSHA Standard 29 CFR 1910.120, Hazardous waste and emergency response (HAZWOPER), and OSHA Standard 29 CFR 1910.1200, Hazard communication. The material safety data sheet (MSDS) should be consulted for response options for the specific chemical. Cleanup personnel must use the appropriate types and amounts of spill cleanup materials and personal protective equipment appropriate to the hazard. If a major spill occurs, remove all ignition sources and ventilate the area. Such liquids should never be allowed to enter a confined space, such as a sewer, because explosion is possible.

☐ Flammable or combustible liquids must be used from and stored in approved containers according to *NFPA 30*.

☐ Flammable liquids must be kept in closed containers (29 CFR 1910.106).

☐ Combustible waste material such as oily shop rags and paint rags must be stored in covered metal containers and disposed of daily (29 CFR 1910.106).

☐ Storage areas must be posted as NO SMOKING areas (29 CFR 1910.106).

The material safety data sheet and the supplier's labels on the containers should advise about the hazards for the flammable and combustible liquids used by the facility.

Questions often arise as to how flammable and combustible liquids should be stored in the workplace. Storage requirements are detailed in 29 CFR 1910.106. Categories and standards for safe storage are listed in figure 13-11.

Figure 13–11. Categories for Storage

☐ Container and portable tank storage (29 CFR 1910.106(d))

☐ Design, construction, and capacity of storage cabinets (29 CFR 1910.106(d)(3))

☐ Design and construction of inside storage rooms (29 CFR 1910.106(d)(4))

☐ Storage inside building (29 CFR 1910.106(d)(5))

☐ Storage outside buildings (29 CFR 1910.106(d)(6))

☐ Fire control (29 CFR 1910.106(d)(7))

The OSHA standard limits the amount of flammable liquids that can be placed in each form of storage, the construction requirements for different types of containers, and requirements for types of facilities.

Arson

The most serious fire risk health care facilities face today is from deliberate fire. Arson is an ever-present threat to health care facilities. No building is immune. Much arson is associated with vandalism and burglaries.

It is estimated that at least 40 percent of all fires in Europe are started deliberately. Every day the future of nearly 50 businesses in the United Kingdom is put at risk as a result of arson. The proportion of fires in hospitals is currently running at about 24 percent of all reported fires. Arson is now recognized in most countries as the major fire problem and as such needs to be treated with "zero tolerance."[20]

Each year, juvenile fire setting accounts for a significant number of injuries and property damages. One study found that 49 percent of fires involved a motive of curiosity. According to a 2001 report by NFPA, 8.8 percent of all civilian fire deaths are caused by a "child playing."

Children playing with fire (intentional fire setting not included) between 1994 and 1998 were responsible for 428,100 reported fires in the United States, resulting in $1.38 billion in property damages, 1,514 civilian deaths, and 11,795 injuries. Statistics compiled by the Federal Bureau of Investigation (FBI) for the uniform crime reports show that in 1999 juveniles (under age 18) accounted for 54 percent of all arson arrests and 48 percent of all arson offenses solved by arrest, both historically high values. No other FBI index crime (serious felony) has such a high rate of juvenile involvement.[21]

Task forces have been set up to fight arson. There is no simple solution to the problem, and a plan can be formulated only after a proper risk assessment has been carried out. Then by taking a few positive steps, such as alerting staff to dangers and ways of preventing arson, health care facilities can frustrate the arsonist. Health care facilities can greatly reduce the risk of arson by adopting the safeguards spelled out in figure 13-12.[22]

Different approaches have been effective in reducing crime generally, as opposed to arson specifically. Approaches such as closed-circuit television (CCTV) and Secure by Design are recommended as possible tactics for reducing arson. However, favorable findings do not mean that an approach will work in every situation. The appraisal tools listed in table 13-2 can help facilities assess whether a particular approach meets their needs.[23]

OSHA FIRE SAFETY ADVISOR 1.0A

The Fire Safety Advisor software by OSHA is in development.[24] It gives users interactive expert help in applying OSHA's fire safety standards. It addresses OSHA general industry standards for fire safety and emergency evacuation

Figure 13–12. Examples of Safeguards for Reducing Arson Risk

☐ Responsibility
- A named individual of senior grade must be made responsible for fire safety, including protection from arson attack. (In the model presented in this book, the Environmental Health and Safety director has overall responsibility.)
- Think about the ease with which intruders/arsonists could break into the premises. Take immediate steps to strengthen the facility's defenses.
- If there have been any small fires on the premises or neighboring premises, inform the police immediately. A small fire could be a warning of something worse to come.

☐ Security
- Man entrances, when possible.
- Doors and windows must be in good repair and locked when not in use.
- Gaps under doors should be as small as possible.
- Know who holds keys; chase down any that are missing.
- Stored material of any kind should not be stacked adjacent to fences or walls where it could be set alight from outside.

☐ Employees
- Warn employees of the threat from arson fires.
- Ask employees to challenge anyone who should not be on the premises and to report any suspicious activities.
- Investigate new employees.
- Keep an eye on outside contractors.

☐ Visitors
- The movement of visitors within the building should be controlled as much as possible.

☐ Fire protection
- Ensure that equipment the facility has installed—extinguishers, hose reels, alarms, detectors, sprinklers—is in good working order and protected against sabotage attempts.

☐ Periodic checks
- No combustible materials should be left lying around when not in use.
- Alarms should be switched on.
- Outside illumination should be kept on at night.
- Flammable liquids should be locked away in secure storage when not in use.

Table 13–2. Tackling Arson: Evaluated Options

Approach	Reasoning/Mechanism	Summary of Research Findings
Increase CCTV coverage	Cameras can: ☐ Deter offenders ☐ Aid detection ☐ Support successful prosecutions	Can be effective where it is clear what impact the scheme is meant to have, and where the right conditions are in place for the cameras to have the intended effect. Works best as part of an integrated and evolving package of measures.
Secure by Design	Crime can be reduced by making it harder and riskier to commit.	Target premises are less vulnerable in well-lit, open areas.

Improved lighting	Better lighting will deter antisocial behavior and make detection more likely.	Small-scale studies suggest that better lighting may reduce crime and incivilities in localized areas, at least in the short term.
		   An evaluation of area-wide lighting improvements found that these were popular and reassuring to the public but did not reduce crime to a great extent.
		   A recent study, "A Review of Street Lighting Evaluations: Crime Reduction Effects" (Pease 1999), argues that "precisely targeted increases in street lighting generally have crime reduction effects."

Targeted policing of hotspots	The more precisely patrol presence is concentrated at the "hotspots," the less crime/disorder/antisocial behavior there will be at those places and times.	U.S. evidence indicates that this is an effective strategy for dealing with local problems.

(Continued on next page)

Table 13–2. *(Continued)*

Approach	Reasoning/Mechanism	Summary of Research Findings
Targeting known offenders	Disrupting offenders' methods/routines can reduce crime. The higher the police arrest rate for high-risk offenders, the lower the rates of crime/disorder/antisocial behavior.	Targeting repeat offenders appears to be worthwhile.

(29 CFR, Subpart E, 1910.36–38). It also addresses OSHA standards for fire-fighting, fire suppression, and fire detection systems and equipment (29 CFR, Subpart L, 1910.156–165). The Advisor can be used online or it can be downloaded and run in the Windows environment.

This software interviews the user about the building, work practices, and policies at the facility to determine whether and how OSHA's fire safety standards may apply. The Fire Safety Advisor Version 1.0a analyzes answers with expert decision logic, alerts the user to fire safety hazards, points out applicable OSHA standards, and helps the user write customized emergency action plans and fire prevention plans.

THE JOINT COMMISSION'S LIFE SAFETY REQUIREMENTS

Joint Commission Environment of Care standard EC.5.20 specifies that newly constructed and existing environments must be designed and maintained to comply with the *Life Safety Code* of the National Fire Protection Association (*NFPA 101*). To assist health care facilities, the Joint Commission has developed a self-assessment tool called a Statement of Conditions™, which allows a health care facility to determine its current state of compliance with *NFPA 101* and determine how to remedy any deficiencies.

The Environment of Care standards are part of the Joint Commission's effort to ensure compliance with the NFPA rules. In particular, the following standards address NFPA rules:

- ☐ EC.5.10, The health care facility manages fire safety risks
- ☐ EC.5.30, The health care facility conducts fire drills regularly
- ☐ EC.5.40, The health care facility maintains fire-safety equipment and building features
- ☐ EC.5.50, The health care facility develops and implements activities to protect occupants during periods when a building does not meet the applicable provisions of the *Life Safety Code*

Additional applicable Joint Commission standards regarding life safety include the following:

□ EC.3.10, The health care facility manages its hazardous materials and waste risks

□ EC.7.30, The health care facility maintains, tests, and inspects its utility systems

□ HR 2.10, HR.2.20, and HR.2.30, which require orientation and on-going education about safety

Achieving Joint Commission accreditation is not equivalent to OSHA compliance. By the same token, compliance with OSHA regulations alone does not ensure that the requirements of the Joint Commission have been met.

THE ROLE OF THE ENVIRONMENTAL HEALTH AND SAFETY DEPARTMENT

The role of the Environmental Health and Safety Department is to support the health care facility in maintaining a safe atmosphere for employees and other personnel, patients, and visitors. This is accomplished through:

□ Identifying existing fire and life safety hazards within the buildings and correcting them

□ Reviewing incidents and forming plans and policies to prevent them from happening again

□ Working with the Engineering Department to assist with extra safety measures in construction sites

□ Developing a fire prevention plan

□ Training employees in fire and life safety

□ Conducting fire drills

□ Interacting with the local fire authority

As is known from some of the tragedies that have occurred over the years, inadequate egress provisions are often responsible for more deaths and injuries than the original emergency.

The Engineering department liaison is an integral team member of the fire prevention program. Experience has demonstrated that the more input that is received from others on risk management projects, such as a fire prevention plan, the better and more comprehensive the result.

Start with the list of fire hazards and risks identified in the worksite analysis. Share this information with department liaisons. Ask them to review the list and add to it from their own perspective and experience. The objectives of this process are to:

□ Expand everyone's awareness.

□ Focus on the goal of protecting the health care facility's assets through an aggressive plan of prevention.

□ Protect the employees, patients, and visitors from injuries from a fire or other emergency.

The Environmental Health and Safety Department should get to know local fire department personnel who are assigned to respond to the health care facility's fire alarm. The local fire department should participate in pre-fire planning with the facility's fire brigade. Pre-fire planning will familiarize local fire department members with workplace and process hazards within a health care facility. Involvement with the local fire department may promote coordination and communication between the fire brigade and the local fire department.

References

1. U.S. Fire Administration. *Topical Fire Research Series*, Vol. 2, No. 8 (October 2001) (rev. March 2002). Available at http://www.usfa.fema.gov/downloads/pdf/tfrs/v2i8-508.pdf (accessed 3/23/2006).

2. U.S. Fire Administration. *Topical Fire Research Series*, Vol. 2, No. 8 (October 2001) (rev. March 2002). Available at http://www.usfa.fema.gov/downloads/pdf/tfrs/v2i8-508.pdf (accessed 3/23/2006).

3. U.S. Fire Administration. *Topical Fire Research Series*, Vol. 2, No. 8 (October 2001) (rev. March 2002). Available at http://www.usfa.fema.gov/downloads/pdf/tfrs/v2i8-508.pdf (accessed 3/23/2006).

4. Beebe, Chad E. *Am I Ready For My CMS Survey?* (adapted). Available at http://www.wsshe.org/CMSSurvey.htm. (accessed 12/20/2005).

5. "CMS Issues Final Rule on Fire Safety Requirements," *NJANPHA News* (2003), Issue 2. Available at http://www.njanpha.org/pdf/ns2003_i2.pdf (accessed 3/23/2006).

6. OSHA Standard 29 CFR 1910 Subpart E, *Exit Routes, Emergency Action Plans, and Fire Prevention Plans.* Available at http://www.osha.gov/pls/oshaweb/owastand.display_standard_group?p_toc_level=1&p_part_number=1910 (accessed 3/23/2006); and OSHA Standard 29 CFR 1910, Subpart L, *Fire Protection.* Available at http://www.osha.gov/pls/oshaweb/owadisp.show_document?p_table=STANDARDS&p_id=10123 (accessed 3/24/06).

7. OSHA Fire and Explosion Planning Matrix. Available at http://www.osha.gov/dep/fire-expmatrix/index.html (accessed 3/23/2006).

8. South Carolina Department of Labor. *Best Practices in Workplace Security.* A homeland security guide developed by the South Carolina Department of Labor, Licensing and Regulation (which operates an OSHA-approved state plan). Available at http://www.llr.state.sc.us/workplace/workplacesecurity.htm (accessed 3/23/2006).

9. *NFPA 101®: Life Safety Code®–2000 edition.* Section A.19.7.1.2. Quincy, MA.

10. Old, Leo P.E. "Is Your Fire Brigade Up to Snuff?" *Hospital Engineering Trends*, Smith Seckman Reid, Inc. August 2005. Portions of this article adapted in this section.

11. OSHA Standard 29 CFR 1910.155(c)(18), *Scope, Application and Definitions Applicable to This Subpart*. Available at http://www.osha.gov/pls/oshaweb/owadisp.show_document?p_table=STANDARDS&p_id=9809 (accessed 3/24/2006).

12. OSHA Standard 29 CFR 1910.155(c)(18), *Scope, Application and Definitions Applicable to This Subpart*. Available at http://www.osha.gov/pls/oshaweb/owadisp.show_document?p_table=STANDARDS&p_id=9809 (accessed 3/24/2006).

13. *NFPA 600: Standard on Industrial Fire Brigades*, 2000 edition. Section 1.4.3.1. Quincy, MA.

14. OSHA Standard 29 CFR 1910.156, *Fire Brigades*. Available at http://www.osha.gov/pls/oshaweb/owadisp.show_document?p_table=STANDARDS&p_id=9810 (accessed 3/24/2006).

15. OSHA Standard 29 CFR 1910.156, *Fire Brigades*. Available at http://www.osha.gov/pls/oshaweb/owadisp.show_document?p_table=STANDARDS&p_id=9810 (accessed 3/24/2006).

16. OSHA Standard 29 CFR 1910.156, *Fire Brigades*. Available at http://www.osha.gov/pls/oshaweb/owadisp.show_document?p_table=STANDARDS&p_id=9810 (accessed 3/24/2006); and OSHA Standard 29 CFR 1910, Subpart L, Appendix A, *Fire Protection*. Available at http://www.osha.gov/pls/oshaweb/owadisp.show_document?p_table=STANDARDS&p_id=10124 (accessed 3/24/2006).

17. OSHA Standard 29 CFR 1910.157(g), *Portable Fire Extinguishers*. Available at http://www.osha.gov/pls/oshaweb/owadisp.show_document?p_table=STANDARDS&p_id=9811 (accessed 3/24/2006).

18. *NFPA 101®: Life Safety Code®–2000 edition*. Sections 19.3.5.6 and 21.3.5.2. Quincy, MA.

19. OSHA Standard 29 CFR 1910.157(e), *Portable Fire Extinguishers*. Available at http://www.osha.gov/pls/oshaweb/owadisp.show_document?p_table=STANDARDS&p_id=9811 (accessed 3/24/2006).

20. *Arson Prevention Advice*. Available at http://www.afs-firewise.co.uk/arson_prevention.html (accessed March 24, 2006).

21. *U-M Health System Implements Straight Talk at Hurley Medical Center in National Crusade to Prevent Burn Injuries: Fire Safety Program Extinguishes the Desire for Kids to Set Fires*. Available at http://www.med.umich.edu/opm/newspage/2003/hurley.htm (accessed 3/24/2006).

22. Fire Net International. *Arson Alert! 24 Ways to Stop Your Building Becoming an Arson Statistic* (adapted). Available at http://www.fire.org.uk/advice/alert.htm (accessed 3/24/2006).

23. *Tackling Arson: Evaluated Options*. Available at http://www.crimereduction.gov.uk/toolkits/an0402.htm (accessed 3/24/2006).

24. OSHA. *Fire Safety Advisor—Version 1.0a*. Available at http://www.osha.gov/dts/osta/oshasoft/softfirex.html (accessed 3/24/2006).

CHAPTER 14

IMPROVING PATIENT SAFETY THROUGH IMPROVED EMPLOYEE HEALTH AND SAFETY

Humpty Dumpty sat on a wall,
Humpty Dumpty had a great fall.
All the King's horses, And all the King's men
Couldn't put Humpty together again!

Between 1642 and 1649, the people of England were engaged in a civil war. The opposing sides were the Royalists and the Parliamentarians. The Parliamentarian stronghold was in Colchester, where they had erected an unusually large cannon on the wall of St. Mary's at the Wall Church to protect them from the Royalists. Because of its size, the cannon was dubbed Humpty Dumpty. However, the Royalists managed to gain temporary control of St. Mary's and the cannon. In an effort to regain control, the temporarily ousted Parliamentarians concentrated their cannon fire on the wall where Humpty was mounted. The cannon fire damaged the wall, and poor old Humpty fell to the ground.

The Royalists understood the importance of Humpty's well-being to their mission, and so they made a valiant effort to relocate Humpty to another part of the wall. For days and days, the Royalists tried to restore Humpty to good health, and even with the aid of "All the King's horses, And all the King's men," they failed. Despite their best efforts, the Royalists had failed to maintain the health and well-being of Humpty. Eleven weeks later, the Parliamentarians regained control of Colchester.

It was clear that the Parliamentarians and the Royalists both failed to protect Humpty Dumpty. Perhaps they were a bit cavalier in their assumption that the sheer strength of Humpty Dumpty would be sufficient protection in and of itself. Perhaps they had not considered the importance of the foundation that was holding Humpty up. Had they realized that the health and well-being of Humpty Dumpty was dependent on their constant vigilance, the outcome might have been different.

Now consider this. What if during their dispute, the neighboring Aardvarkians decided it would be a perfect time to invade and conquer merry old England? Perhaps the Parliamentarians and the Royalists would have put their differences aside and worked together to put Humpty Dumpty back together again. Things always seem to work better when all parties understand the goal and work together to achieve it.

Patient safety is no different; it requires that management and staff work together to find solutions to patient safety problems and that the patients themselves take an active role in ensuring their own safety. Further, the theories and practices of patient safety and health and the theories and practices of employee safety and health are interchangeable. The best explanation of this interrelationship is found in the examination of the goals of regulatory standards and similar goals of accreditation organizations.

A BRIDGE BETWEEN PATIENT SAFETY AND EMPLOYEE HEALTH AND SAFETY

Patient health and safety and employee health and safety should not be viewed as distinct and isolated programs, nor should they be separated from family health and safety. Accreditation organizations were established to enhance patient safety and have come to realize that patient safety relies on a safe and healthy workforce. This recognition has led to a partnership between the Occupational Safety and Health Administration (OSHA) and the Joint Commission.

The bridge between patient safety and employee health and safety derives from an understanding that the theories and practices of health and safety are universal in their application.

The mission of OSHA is to ensure the safety and health of America's workers by setting and enforcing standards; providing training, outreach, and education; establishing partnerships; and encouraging continual improvement in workplace safety and health. Accreditation organizations apply these same methods to enhance patient safety.

Ensuring patient and employee safety is a process that is independent of the type of facility. Whether the facility provides primary care or specialty services, such as dialysis, mental health treatment, diagnostic imaging, or acute care, the process of ensuring patient and employee safety is the same. The first step in that process is to conduct a hazard assessment. Once the hazard assessment has been completed, it can be used to create an Environmental Health and Safety plan or a patient safety plan, either of which can be tailored to a facility's particular needs but still accommodate the others' goals. This chapter explores the interrelationship between worker health and safety and patient safety by briefly revisiting some of the topics presented in previous chapters.

In addition to OSHA and the accreditation organizations, a number of other agencies and organizations develop standards, guidelines, and recommendations that have an impact on patients and employees alike. For example, the National Fire Protection Association (NFPA) provides recommendations and requirements designed to protect all building occupants as well as the building itself. The Centers for Disease Control and Prevention (CDC) issues guidelines and recommendations that are intended to prevent the spread of infectious and communicable diseases among both patients and staff. The National Institute for Occupational Safety and Health (NIOSH) makes recommendations that are intended to protect employees, and an unintended consequence of adopting those recommendations is enhanced patient safety. The regulations of the Environmental Protection Agency (EPA), while primarily designed to protect the community, also have a positive impact on the health and well-being of patients and facility employees.

REQUIREMENTS FOR COMMUNICATION

Despite the efforts of these groups, there remains a significant rate of morbidity and mortality due to medication and other errors within health care facilities. Recent data demonstrates the magnitude of the patient safety problem. Medical errors are a leading cause of death in the United States, killing between 44,000 and 98,000 Americans each year, according to various studies.[1] Medication errors are among a health care facility's most common and lethal errors. A significant number of medication errors result from neglecting to label medications or mislabeling them. Another source of medication errors is poor communication between staff. In a recent review of 16,000 hospital deaths due to error, twice as many deaths were caused by communication errors as by clinical inadequacy.[2] Embedded in each OSHA standard are instructions for communicating information to workers. Similar requirements for communications can be found in the recommendations offered by other agencies and organizations, and they can be applied to protect patients from harm.

In a document developed as a result of a National Science Foundation grant, the Association of Operating Room Nurses (AORN) lists coordination of care for surgical patients as the first item in their outline of the responsibilities of perioperative nursing practice. The document specifically mentions communication skills as a key component of coordination. [CD-ROM 14.1] The OSHA Standard 29 CFR 1910.1200, Hazard communication, is intended to protect employees who work with hazardous chemicals. [CD-ROM 14.2] Among the requirements of the Hazard communication standard is a mandate that containers of hazardous chemicals be labeled, tagged, or marked with the identity of the material and appropriate hazard warnings. Other requirements of 1910.1200 are that all employees who work with hazardous chemicals be trained in their safe handling and learn how to understand the information provided on material safety data sheets (MSDSs).

In response to numerous inquiries related to the mishandling of cytotoxic drugs, OSHA published guidelines for the management of cytotoxic (antineoplastic) drugs in the workplace in 1986. Those recommendations were revised in 1999.[3] The guidelines now provide recommendations consistent with current scientific knowledge and have been expanded to cover hazardous drugs (HDs). In addition, some of the agents covered in OSHA's guidelines are also covered under the Hazard communication standard. Incorrect labeling or failure to label cytotoxic or other hazardous drugs may expose pharmacists, nurses, physicians, and patients to adverse effects from improper use of medication.

In addition to standard pharmacy labeling practices, all syringes and IV bags containing HDs must be labeled with a distinctive warning label, such as:

SPECIAL HANDLING/DISPOSAL PRECAUTIONS

If HDs are used in the facility, sound practice dictates that a written hazardous drug safety and health plan be developed. Such a plan assists in protecting employees from health hazards associated with HDs and can protect patients from the same hazards. The American Society of Health-System Pharmacists (ASHP) recommends that the facility's plan include specific elements and indicate specific measures that the employer is taking to ensure employee protection. Section VI, Chapter 2 of the OSHA technical manual *Controlling Occupational Exposure to Hazardous Drugs* presents the elements recommended by ASHP. [CD-ROM 14.3] The ASHP also recommends the assignment of a hazardous drug officer (who is an industrial hygienist, nurse, or pharmacist health and safety representative). In the model presented in this book, the Pharmacy Department Liaison may be the facility's hazardous drug officer.

In addition to OSHA's Hazard communication standard and technical manual, resources available to assist in reducing medication errors include:

- ☐ *NIOSH Alert: Preventing Occupational Exposures to Antineoplastic and Other Hazardous Drugs in Health Care Settings*[4] [CD-ROM 14.4]
- ☐ NIH, *Recommendations for the Safe Handling of Cytotoxic Drugs* (2002), which includes recommendations for the safe preparation and administration of cytotoxic drugs[5] [CD-ROM 14.5.1, 14.5.2, 14.5.3, 14.5a]
- ☐ ASHP, *Technical Assistance Bulletin on Handling Cytotoxic and Hazardous Drugs* (1990), an informed discussion of the dangers of and safe handling procedures for hazardous drugs[6] [CD-ROM 14.6]

INFECTIOUS AND COMMUNICABLE DISEASE PREVENTION

Over the last 30 years, a considerable effort has been made to reduce the incidence of nosocomial infections in U.S. hospitals. Controlling health and safety risks in the facility is necessary to prevent infections among patients, staff and their families, and visitors. Both public health and occupational safety and health authorities recommend a hierarchy of controls for workplace hazards, and this same process can be used to prevent the transmission of infectious diseases in health care facilities. The hierarchy is the preferred order of control measures for health and safety risks and for the prevention of infectious diseases and includes administrative controls, engineering controls, and personal protective equipment. This hierarchy of controls is both cost-effective—since administrative controls can cost very little—and critical for minimizing the exposure of employees and patients to infectious diseases. Health and safety resources available to assist in protecting patients and employees from infectious diseases include:

- OSHA Standard 1910.1030, Bloodborne pathogens[7] [CD-ROM 14.7]
- CDC, *Guidelines for Environmental Infection Control in Health-Care Facilities* (2003)[8] [CD-ROM 14.8, 14.8a]
- AIA's Infection Control Risk Assessment (ICRA)[9]
- The Centers for Disease Control and Prevention (CDC)

Clearly, those actions that are successful in preventing nosocomial infections among patients are the same ones that have been shown to be effective in preventing the transmission of bloodborne pathogens and infectious diseases among workers.

FIRE PREVENTION

An unexpected fire in the health care facility is terrifying for patients, staff, and visitors. Despite the many precautions taken in a health care facility to prevent fires, they do occur with regularity. There are an estimated 100 fires involving surgical patients nationally each year.[10] While the risk of injury or death is relatively small, the cost of repairs and equipment replacement is significant. The principal organization responsible for ensuring that facilities are safe from fires is the NFPA. Many NFPA standards have been incorporated by reference into OSHA standards and are required by the Joint Commission's Environment of Care standards.[11]

As is the case with an Environmental Health and Safety plan, the development of a fire prevention plan should begin with a hazard assessment that identifies high-risk situations. For example, areas that store or use flammable gases deserve special attention, as do devices such as lasers and electrocautery equipment that generate significant heat. The fire prevention plan must include information on evacuation of patients and staff, and it should be rehearsed in a manner that does not interfere with routine health care delivery.

The same concepts of fire prevention that are applied in health care facilities are also applied to the construction of housing, the buildings in which we do business, and the schools that our children attend.

Figure 14–1. OSHA Standards for 29 CFR 1910 Subpart S, Electrical

---

- ☐ Protective equipment
  - ■ 1910.137, Electrical protective devices
- ☐ Electric power
  - ■ 1910.269, Electric power generation, transmission, and distribution
- ☐ Design safety standards for electrical systems
  - ■ 1910.302, Electric utilization systems
  - ■ 1910.303, General requirements
  - ■ 1910.304, Wiring design and protection
  - ■ 1910.305, Wiring methods, components, and equipment for general use
  - ■ 1910.306, Specific-purpose equipment and installations
  - ■ 1910.307, Hazardous (classified) locations
  - ■ 1910.308, Special systems
- ☐ Safety-related work practices
  - ■ 1910.331, Scope
  - ■ 1910.332, Training
  - ■ 1910.333, Selection and use of work practices
  - ■ 1910.334, Use of equipment
  - ■ 1910.335, Safeguards for personnel protection

ELECTRICAL HAZARDS

Electricity has long been recognized as a serious workplace hazard. The electrical safety standards issued by OSHA are numerous and are designed to protect employees exposed to dangers such as electric shock, exposed wiring, electrical fires, and explosions. These standards can also protect patients.

Figure 14-1 lists OSHA's general industry electrical safety standards that relate to health care facilities. Electrical safety standards are among the top standards cited by OSHA in health care facilities. Selected standards in figure 14-1 are included on the CD-ROM accompanying this book.

For contractors working at health care facilities or for facilities undertaking construction work, OSHA's construction industry standards in 29 CFR 1926 Subpart K, Electrical (1926.400–1926.449), are designed to protect employees and contractors exposed to electrical dangers, which will also protect patients. Selected standards are provided on the CD-ROM accompanying this book.

The National Fire Protection Association has several codes, including *NFPA 70: National Electrical Code*® and *NFPA 70E: Standard for Electrical Safety in the Workplace*, which covers the full spectrum of electrical safety issues, from safety-related work practices to maintenance, special equipment requirements, and installation.[12]

The standard *NFPA 70E* includes the following chapters and annexes that can be of particular assistance to health care facilities:

- Chapter 1, Safety-Related Work Practices
- Chapter 1, Safety-Related Maintenance Requirements
- Chapter 3, Safety Requirements for Special Equipment
- Chapter 4, Installation Safety Requirements
- Annex E, Electrical Safety Program
- Annex F, Hazard Risk Evaluation Procedure
- Annex G, Sample Lockout/Tagout Procedure
- Annex I, Job Briefing and Planning Checklist
- Annex J, Energized Electrical Work Permit
- Annex K, General Categories of Electrical Hazards
- Annex M, Cross-Reference Tables

Compliance with its electrical safety mandates—1910 Subpart S, Electrical, and 1926 Subpart K, Electrical—is evaluated by OSHA using the requirements of *NFPA 70* and *70E*.

As is the case with standards and regulations for fire prevention, standards and regulations for electrical safety are embedded in Joint Commission standards and in the specifications for our homes, schools, and businesses.

SLIPS, TRIPS, AND FALLS

Protecting patients from falls is no different from protecting workers from falls. Injuries to workers as a result of slips, trips, and falls account for a significant portion of work-related injuries in the health care facility. In addition to the normal steps taken to prevent patients from falling out of beds, when getting in and out of bed, or when using walkers or canes, there are a number of other actions that will prevent patients, employees, and visitors from being injured as a result of a slip, trip, or fall. Figure 14-2 lists examples of measures that can be taken to prevent falls, whether they are falls by patients, staff, or

Figure 14-2. Examples of Measures That Can Prevent Falls

- Do not allow power cords to cross walking surfaces.
- Do mopping at night, when there are fewer people in the facility.
- Post warning signs in areas that are being mopped.
- Inspect all walking surfaces for cracks or other defects that present a tripping hazard.
- Inspect stairs routinely to ensure that handrails and steps are in sound condition.

visitors. Additional attention needs to be given to those patients who may be at particular risk for falls.

Violent Acts

Violent acts in workplaces, whether intentional or unintentional, have become a matter of significant concern. Although OSHA has no specific standard that is designed to prevent workplace violence, it has developed guidelines for preventing intentional violence in the workplace. The Joint Commission has a number of standards designed to prevent both intentional and unintentional violent acts between patients, staff, and visitors.

Intentional violent acts seldom occur in the absence of anger. Employees should know that anger progresses through more or less recognizable stages, so being alert to body language or other clues can often give them a head start in dealing with an agitated patient. The first manifestation often is irritation or jumpy behavior. The patient may do something unusual, such as snapping at other patients or staff. The patient may withdraw, mutter, or fidget. Often, this early stage of anger is characterized by tense posture and restlessness. At this time, the employee should try to understand the patient's situation. Many times, the patient is reacting to a legitimate source of stress. The employee should talk in a soothing (although not a condescending) manner.

The stages of anger culminate in actual rage, where physical violence is possible. This is the point at which appropriate physical management by staff may be necessary. It is crucial that staff members be taught established methods of physically restraining or transporting violent or potentially destructive patients. The Joint Commission Restraint and Seclusion standards (PC.11.10–11.100) must be followed when patient restraint and/or seclusion is necessary.

Several groups have suggested measures for helping to reduce intentional and unintentional workplace violence. In 1999 the American Nurses Association (ANA) provided testimony to the Joint Commission's Task Force on Behavioral Health Care Restraint. In that testimony the ANA suggested a number of alternatives to patient restraint.[13] The importance of health care facility design in helping to curb workplace violence has been recognized by both the National Association of Psychiatric Health Systems (NAPHS) and the American Institute of Architects (AIA). The NAPHS has developed *Guidelines for the Built Environment of Behavioral Health Facilities*. [CD-ROM 14.9]

Whether we are concerned about intentional or unintentional violent acts in the workplace or in our daily lives, it is important to understand situations that can lead to them and how to manage these situations.

Data Collection and Investigation

Just as it is necessary to keep records of worker injuries and illnesses, it is important to do the same for patient injuries and illnesses. Analyses required to identify trends in worker injuries and illnesses are also required for patient injuries and illnesses to determine the proper course of corrective action. When an employee accident occurs in the facility, the process of determining what happened, why it happened, and how it can be prevented from happening again must be undertaken. Patient incidents require the same process. In health care facilities, accreditation organizations require data collection and investigation for patients and employees, and OSHA requires these measures for employees.

Using the concepts and requirements provided in OSHA Standard 1904 Subpart C, Recordingkeeping forms and recording criteria, will assist in the accurate recording and reporting of patient injuries and illnesses. [CD-ROM 14.10] The AORN article "Incident Reports—Correcting Processes and Reducing Errors" describes systems approaches to assessing the ways in which an organization operates and explains the types of failures that cause errors. Steps to guide managers in adopting an incident reporting system that incorporates continuous quality improvement are identified. [CD-ROM 14.11]

MANAGING RISK

Just as health care facilities are obligated to provide a safe environment for employees, they are also required to provide the best quality of care possible, as well as the continuous assessment and improvement of the quality of care and services rendered to patients. A risk management program plays a crucial role in fulfilling these commitments. Risk management is a planned and systematic process to reduce and/or eliminate the possibility that losses will occur in the health care facility. As with employee health and safety, for maximum effectiveness in the health care setting, risk management involves a multidisciplinary, proactive approach and it begins with a risk assessment.

As is the case with the Environmental Health and Safety hazard assessment, the risk assessment and management program are intended to identify areas of actual or potential risk; prevent, to the extent possible, injuries to patients, visitors, and employees; and prevent or limit financial loss to the facility and its staff. Financial loss can occur in a number of ways. From a risk management perspective, the primary concern is financial losses associated with the inherent risks in providing health care services, which can result in a patient's instituting a medical malpractice claim or lawsuit against the facility and/or a health care provider. The key element in the success of the risk management program in preventing or reducing these particular claims and associated financial losses is the participation of physicians, nurses, other health care providers, and health care employees in implementing effective risk management strategies. Each individual must be committed to reducing risks. Having a well-formulated Environmental Health and Safety program is essential to risk reduction.

Effective risk management relies on a clear understanding of the infrastructure, programs, experience, and issues and the identification of early risk reduction opportunities in the organization. The net result of these efforts will be a reduction in the overall cost of risk and safer care systems for patients and providers.

When patient safety incidents occur, an analysis must be conducted to identify the underlying causes of the event, to determine why the process failed, and to develop risk reduction strategies and corrective action plans to prevent future occurrences of the same incident. As with employee health and safety, this analysis is commonly referred to as a root cause analysis (RCA). The Joint Commission requires a root cause analysis for sentinel events in health care facilities.

Risk management also involves prevention strategies. A "fault tree analysis" (FTA) or "failure mode and effect analysis" (FMEA) should be performed in health care facilities, as in other industries. FTA and FMEA are analyses that are generally undertaken system wide to identify and prevent multiple control failures that could lead to a catastrophic event.

JOINT COMMISSION: THE DRIVER FOR IMPROVING PATIENT AND EMPLOYEE HEALTH AND SAFETY

The Joint Commission and its affiliated organization, Joint Commission Resources, are uniquely positioned to help elevate the status of the health and safety of patients and employees. Using their expertise and unique understanding of health care facilities, these two organizations can use the tools and techniques developed to enhance patient safety and apply them to the health and safety of health care workers. By working in concert with the Environmental Health and Safety professional, the Joint Commission and Joint Commission Resources can be the catalysts for putting Humpty Dumpty together again.

THE ROLE OF THE ENVIRONMENTAL HEALTH AND SAFETY DEPARTMENT

The organizational structure of the Environmental Health and Safety Department model presented in this book includes fire safety, general safety, emergency management, data collection and recordkeeping, hazard assessment, epidemiology, industrial hygiene, training, and employee health expertise. Furthermore, the structure includes trained liaisons in every department. Using the techniques and the assets of the Environmental Health and Safety Department in conjunction with the facility's patient safety coordinator and risk manager will work to the benefit of patients, employees, visitors, and employee and patient families.

In a very real sense, the members of the Environmental Health and Safety Department are involved in patient safety and risk reduction activities every day. The hazard assessments and routine inspections performed by the department's staff identify potential worker hazards that also may be patient hazards. In many instances, remedial action taken to protect workers will necessarily protect patients.

For example, ergonomics training in lifting techniques that is intended to protect workers from being injured while lifting or moving patients will protect the patient from being dropped or injured as well.

The communication requirements of OSHA's Hazard communication standard, when applied to cytotoxic and other hazardous drugs, may help prevent medication errors. The techniques of assessing hazards are no different from those of the risk analysis or the fire safety inspection. Moreover, standards, such as OSHA's Bloodborne pathogens standard, protect workers and patients equally.

In short, the concepts and techniques of worker safety and health are no different from those of patient safety and health; it is only their application that differs.

The Parliamentarians, the Royalists, and the Aardvarkians discovered that none of them alone could put Humpty Dumpty together again. But imagine what they might have accomplished had they worked together.

References

1. "Heal Thyself: Once Seen as Risky, One Group of Doctors Changes Its Ways," *Wall Street Journal*, June 21, 2005.

2. Moss, Jacqueline. "Technological System Solutions to Clinical Communication Error," *Journal of Nursing Administration* 35 (2) (February 2005), pp. 51–53.

3. OSHA. *Controlling Occupational Exposure to Hazardous Drugs*. OSHA technical manual, Section VI, Chapter 2. Available at http://www.osha.gov/dts/osta/otm/otm_vi/otm_vi_2.html (accessed 3/29/2006).

4. NIOSH. *NIOSH Alert: Preventing Occupational Exposures to Antineoplastic and Other Hazardous Drugs in Health Care Sett*ings. DHHS (NIOSH) Publication No. 2004-165. Available at http://www.cdc.gov/niosh/docs/2004-165/pdfs/2004-165.pdf (accessed 3/29/2006).

5. NIH. *Recommendations for the Safe Handling of Cytotoxic Drugs* (2002). Available at http://www.nih.gov/od/ors/ds/pubs/cyto/(accessed 3/24/2006).

6. ASHP. *ASHP Technical Assistance Bulletin on Handling Cytotoxic and Hazardous Drugs*. Available at http://www.ashp.org/bestpractices/drugdistribution/Prep_TAB_Cytotoxic.pdf (accessed 3/23/2006).

7. OSHA 29 CFR 1910.1030, *Bloodborne Pathogens*. Available at http://www.osha.gov/pls/oshaweb/owadisp.show_document?p_table=STANDARDS&p_id=10051 (accessed 3/27/2006).

8. Sehulster, L., and R.Y.W. Chinn. "Guidelines for Environmental Infection Control in Health-Care Facilities," *MMWR* 52, RR-10 (June 6, 2003). Available at http://www.cdc.gov/mmwr/preview/mmwrhtml/rr5210a1.htm (accessed 3/27/2006).

9. American Institute of Architects and the Facility Guidelines Institute. *The Guidelines for Design and Construction of Hospital and Health Care Facilities*. New York: AIA, 2001. Available at www.aia.org (accessed 2/21/2006).

10. ECRI (formerly the Emergency Care Research Institute). Available at http://www.ecri.org/Education_and_Conferences/Audio_Conferences_Archive.aspx (accessed 4/7/2006).

11. OSHA 29 CFR 1910.6, *Incorporation by Reference*. Available at http://www.osha.gov/pls/oshaweb/owadisp.show_document?p_table=STANDARDS&p_id=9702 (accessed 3/29/2006).

12. *NFPA 70: National Electrical Code*, and *NFPA 70E: Handbook for Electrical Safety in the Workplace*. Quincy, MA.

13. Broan, Elissa, Beatrice A. Yorker, and Catherine F. Kane. *Testimony Presented to: Joint Commission on the Accreditation of Healthcare Organizations Behavioral Healthcare Restraint Task Force*. Executive Summary. 1999. Available at http://www.nursingworld.org/readroom/bhcres.htm (accessed 3/30/2006).

CHAPTER 15

SURVEILLANCE, DATA ANALYSIS, AND INCIDENT MANAGEMENT

They knew it was coming. But when, how, where? Those were the mysteries, the pieces of the puzzle that needed to be found. It had to be stopped, because the price of allowing it to happen unchallenged was simply too great. If it succeeded, the best that could be hoped for was the loss of the promised future. If it succeeded, lives would be changed forever, and perhaps many would be lost. How to find out was the problem. When will it happen, how will it happen, where will it happen, and perhaps they even asked why will it happen?

Listen my children and you shall hear
Of the midnight ride of Paul Revere,
On the eighteenth of April, in Seventy-five;
Hardly a man is now alive
Who remembers that famous day and year.
He said to his friend, "If the British march
By land or sea from the town to-night,
Hang a lantern aloft in the belfry arch
Of the North Church tower as a signal light,—
One if by land, and two if by sea;
And I on the opposite shore will be,
Ready to ride and spread the alarm
Through every Middlesex village and farm,
For the country folk to be up and to arm."

That was the plan, elegant in its simplicity: watch for the event, warn of its beginning, explain how it will occur, and then the warning will be given so that people can prepare themselves. A church tower, two lanterns, a man with sharp eyes and an "eager ear," and a man on horseback with a very loud voice were all the tools that were needed.

Meanwhile, his friend through alley and street
Wanders and watches, with eager ears,
Till in the silence around him he hears
The muster of men at the barrack door,
The sound of arms, and the tramp of feet,
And the measured tread of the grenadiers,
Marching down to their boats on the shore.

His friend saw the event unfold before him. He saw the forces being mustered. He saw them go to their boats on the shore. Now he could give the first warning: *It will come by sea.*

So through the night rode Paul Revere;
And so through the night went his cry of alarm
To every Middlesex village and farm,—
A cry of defiance, and not of fear,
A voice in the darkness, a knock at the door,
And a word that shall echo for evermore!
For, borne on the night-wind of the Past,
Through all our history, to the last,
In the hour of darkness and peril and need,
The people will waken and listen to hear
The hurrying hoof-beats of that steed,
And the midnight message of Paul Revere.

Henry Wadsworth Longfellow (1807–1882)

Surveillance (n)   Close observation of a person or group, especially of one under suspicion.

The American Heritage Dictionary

Observation is the key to understanding circumstances, whether they involve spying on British troops preparing an attack or the astute eighteenth-century Italian physician, Bernardino Ramazzini, watching how men and women of different trades perform their work and the illness and injuries that they incur. Chicken Little observed a sentinel event and rushed to warn the king that the sky was falling. The Three Little Pigs kept a suspicious eye on the wolf. All of them were practicing surveillance. Sometimes the analysis was faulty; it is, of course difficult to imagine the sky falling. But sometimes, as in the case of Ramazzini, the observation and analysis were so thorough that what he wrote of occupational injuries and illnesses remains accurate more than 300 years later.

Longfellow, Ramazzini, Alice Hamilton, and Studs Terkel all made careful observations and chronicled them. Because of their surveillance, a wealth of information was made available for analysis and for the development of solutions to correct problems and then observe whether the solutions were working. That is one of the reasons for the inclusion of medical surveillance in each Occupational Safety and Health Administration (OSHA) standard. By collecting baseline health data on all employees who are potentially at risk of a chronic adverse health effect and looking for changes in their health status, employers can tell if their efforts to reduce exposures and improve health have been successful.

In the health care facility, the Environmental Health and Safety Department is tasked with the responsibility of protecting the health and safety of employees, patients, and visitors. To do that successfully, department staff must know what to look for. Most of the time they are watching events within the facility, but on occasion they must also be cognizant of events outside the facility. Surveillance, data collection, incident investigation, and analysis form the thread that stitches the quilt of Environmental Health and Safety.

OSHA Surveillance and Recordkeeping Requirements

Congress recognized the importance of surveillance and data analysis when it crafted the Occupational Safety and Health Act (OSH Act). [CD-ROM 15.1] Section 6(C)(7) requires that when OSHA promulgates a standard, the standard:

> shall prescribe the type and frequency of medical examinations or other tests which shall be made available, by the employer or at his cost, to employees exposed to such hazards in order to most effectively determine whether the health of such employees is adversely affected by such exposure.

Medical surveillance is the fundamental strategy for protecting workers. Medical surveillance is a planned program of physical examination and biological testing that tracks and monitors employee health so that workers are protected from illnesses caused by on-the-job exposures. Medical surveillance programs can be used to achieve many objectives, including the prevention, detection, and treatment of disease; verification of the effectiveness of an employer's hazard control program; and measurement of the adequacy of OSHA's permissible exposure limit (PEL).

Early detection, before the development of symptoms, will improve a person's prognosis. In addition, OSHA recommends a medical evaluation for employees, and certain OSHA standards include specific medical requirements. Information from the facility's program may also be used to conduct epidemiological studies, settle claims, provide evidence in litigation, and report workers' medical conditions to federal, state, and local agencies, as required by law.

Medical surveillance does not require a physician to perform all examinations. An examination may be provided by a nurse acting under a physician's direction (e.g., standing orders). However, certain OSHA standards or sound medical judgment may require a physician's expertise.

At a minimum, workplace medical surveillance should include the elements listed in figure 15-1.[1]

Figure 15–1. Elements of a Comprehensive Medical Surveillance Program

- □ Pre-placement examinations
- □ Periodic physical medical examinations required by some OSHA standards or the facility's policies
- □ An ongoing employee health program
- □ Recordkeeping of work-related injuries and illnesses
- □ Exit examinations

Pre-placement Examinations

The pre-placement examination has two major functions: (1) determination of an individual's fitness for duty, including the ability to work while wearing protective equipment; and (2) provision of baseline medical surveillance data for comparison with future medical data.

The pre-placement screening will depend on the potential health hazards of the job. This examination should be repeated if the employee is assigned to a different job that poses different potential adverse health effects. Newly hired workers should be afforded every opportunity to resolve any health issues that are revealed during their pre-placement examinations before being disqualified from work.

Periodic Physical Examinations Required by Some OSHA Standards or Facility Policies

Periodic physical examinations are conducted for the early recognition of illnesses resulting from a workplace exposure. The examination should be tailored to the specific hazards located in the workers' occupational environment. Periodic examinations are required under some regulatory standards, such as OSHA 29 CFR 1910.1047, Ethylene oxide [CD-ROM 15.2], and OSHA 29 CFR 1910.1048, Formaldehyde [CD-ROM 15.3].

Routine physical examinations are given at least annually. Annual medical examinations are used in conjunction with pre-placement screening examinations for the purpose of comparing subsequent medical findings with those from the pre-placement examinations. It is essential to identify trends that may be early signs of changes in an employee's health status and to provide employees with information for protecting their health. The examining health care provider should have information about the worker's exposure history, including exposure monitoring at the job site, supplemented by worker-reported exposure history and general information on possible exposures at previous worksites. Linking pre-placement and annual physical examination results will provide the physician and employee with a more accurate picture of the effects of work and lifestyle on the employee's health and sets the stage for the Total Health and Safety™ program.

Return-to-Work Physical Examinations

Return-to-work examinations are performed when the worker has been absent from work for a significant period of time. Employer policies vary on the number of days or reasons for the absence that requires the completion of a physical examination. The period may vary from three days to weeks or months. The purpose of the return-to-work examination is to determine the worker's physical ability to perform the job. In some cases, if an employee has become ill as a consequence of a chemical exposure, OSHA requires that certain medical examinations be performed before the worker can be allowed to return to normal duties. In those cases in which an employee is assigned other duties until the return-to-work medical requirements are satisfied, OSHA requires that the employee's wages be maintained at the level paid for the job from which the employee was removed.

Medical Records

Medical screening and surveillance requirements, as well as requirements for exposure monitoring, are specified in a number of OSHA standards for general industry (29 CFR 1910). But none is more important to understanding the origin of occupational injuries and illness than 29 CFR 1904.0, Recording and reporting occupational injuries and illnesses: [CD-ROM 15.4]

> 1904.0 Purpose.
> The purpose of this rule (Part 1904) is to require employers to record and report work-related fatalities, injuries and illnesses. Note to 1904.0: Recording or reporting a work-related injury, illness, or fatality does not mean that the employer or employee was at fault, that an OSHA rule has been violated, or that the employee is eligible for workers' compensation or other benefits.

Just as Ramazzini chronicled the events he observed, health care facilities as well as other workplaces must chronicle work-related injuries and illnesses. According to OSHA, those injuries and illnesses must be recorded on a specific form:

> 1904.29(a)
> Basic requirement. You must use OSHA 300, 300-A, and 301 forms, or equivalent forms, for recordable injuries and illnesses. The OSHA 300 Form is called the Log of Work-Related Injuries and Illnesses, the 300-A is the Summary of Work-Related Injuries and Illnesses, and the OSHA 301 Form is called the Injury and Illness Incident Report. [CD-ROM 15.5]

In Standard 29 CFR 1904.5, OSHA explains what a work-related injury or illness is:

> You must consider an injury or illness to be work-related if an event or exposure in the work environment either caused or contributed to the resulting condition or significantly aggravated a pre-existing injury or illness. Work-relatedness is presumed for injuries and illnesses resulting from events or exposures occurring in the work environment, unless an exception in 1904.5(b)(2) specifically applies. [CD-ROM 15.6]

Also, OSHA recognizes that knowing what is not an occupational injury or illness is as important as recognizing what is:

> 1904.5(b)(2) Are there situations where an injury or illness occurs in the work environment and is not considered work-related? Yes, an injury or illness occurring in the work environment that falls under one of the following exceptions is not work-related, and therefore is not recordable:
>
> You are not required to record injuries and illnesses if . . .
>
> i. At the time of the injury or illness, the employee was present in the work environment as a member of the general public rather than as an employee.
> ii. The injury or illness involves signs or symptoms that surface at work but result solely from a non-work-related event or exposure that occurs outside the work environment.
> iii. The injury or illness results solely from voluntary participation in a wellness program or in a medical, fitness, or recreational activity such as blood donation, physical examination, flu shot, exercise class, racquetball, or baseball.
> iv. The injury or illness is solely the result of an employee eating, drinking, or preparing food or drink for personal consumption (whether bought on the employer's premises or brought in). For example, if choking on a sandwich while in the employer's establishment injured the employee, the case would not be considered work-related.
> **Note:** If the employee is made ill by ingesting food contaminated by workplace contaminants (such as lead), or gets food poisoning from food supplied by the employer, the case would be considered work-related.
> v. The injury or illness is solely the result of an employee doing personal tasks (unrelated to their employment) at the establishment outside of the employee's assigned working hours.
> vi. The injury or illness is solely the result of personal grooming, self-medication for a non-work-related condition, or is intentionally self-inflicted.

vii. The injury or illness is caused by a motor vehicle accident and occurs on a company parking lot or company access road while the employee is commuting to or from work.

viii. The illness is the common cold or flu (Note: contagious diseases such as tuberculosis, brucellosis, hepatitis A, or plague are considered work-related if the employee is infected at work).

ix. The illness is a mental illness. Mental illness will not be considered work-related unless the employee voluntarily provides the employer with an opinion from a physician or other licensed health care professional with appropriate training and experience (psychiatrist, psychologist, psychiatric nurse practitioner, etc.) stating that the employee has a mental illness that is work-related.

It is also important to know what must be recorded:

1904.7(a)

Basic requirement. You must consider an injury or illness to meet the general recording criteria, and therefore to be recordable, if it results in any of the following: death, days away from work, restricted work or transfer to another job, medical treatment beyond first aid, or loss of consciousness. You must also consider a case to meet the general recording criteria if it involves a significant injury or illness diagnosed by a physician or other licensed health care professional, even if it does not result in death, days away from work, restricted work or job transfer, medical treatment beyond first aid, or loss of consciousness. [CD-ROM 15.7]

Of particular importance to the health care facility are the requirements of 1904.8 and 1904.11:

1904.8(a)

Basic requirement. You must record all work-related needlestick injuries and cuts from sharp objects that are contaminated with another person's blood or other potentially infectious material (as defined by 29 CFR 1910.1030). You must enter the case on the OSHA 300 Log as an injury. To protect the employee's privacy, you may not enter the employee's name on the OSHA 300 Log (see the requirements for privacy cases in paragraphs 1904.29(b)(6) through 1904.29(b)(9)). [CD-ROM 15.8]

1904.11(a)

Basic requirement. If any of your employees has been occupationally exposed to anyone with a known case of active tuberculosis (TB), and that employee subsequently develops a tuberculosis infection, as evidenced by a positive skin test or diagnosis by a physician or other licensed health care professional, you must record the case on the OSHA 300 Log by checking the "respiratory condition" column. [CD-ROM 15.9]

Simply collecting this surveillance data is not enough. In order for it to be useful in preventing further injuries and illnesses, it must be available for analysis by OSHA and NIOSH. This rule is also important because of the safeguards against release of personal identifying information it incorporates. This rule allows OSHA and NIOSH to obtain employee medical records for the conduct of epidemiology studies to determine whether an employee's work experience has caused "impaired health or functional capacities" (Sec. 20(a)(3) of the Occupational Safety and Health Act).

> 29 CFR 1913.10 Rules of agency practice and procedure concerning OSHA access to employee medical records
>
> 1913.10(a) General policy. OSHA access to employee medical records will in certain circumstances be important to the agency's performance of its statutory functions. Medical records, however, contain personal details concerning the lives of employees. Due to the substantial personal privacy interests involved, OSHA authority to gain access to personally identifiable employee medical information will be exercised only after the agency has made a careful determination of its need for this information, and only with appropriate safeguards to protect individual privacy. Once this information is obtained, OSHA examination and use of it will be limited to only that information needed to accomplish the purpose for access, will be kept secure while being used, and will not be disclosed to other agencies or members of the public except in narrowly defined circumstances. This section establishes procedures to implement these policies. [CD-ROM 15.10]

Another of the critical surveillance standards is 29 CFR 1910.1020, Access to employee exposure and medical records. [CD-ROM 15.11] Simply collecting data and making it available to OSHA is not enough. This rule also requires that employees or their authorized representatives have access to exposure and medical records. The data must also be maintained for a period of time sufficient to allow for its analysis to determine whether an occupationally related chronic illness is or has occurred in the workplace. Because many serious diseases take decades to develop, OSHA established that such records must be kept for the duration of an employee's employment plus 30 years. Furthermore, should a health care facility close, it is required to send these records to NIOSH.

Some states have OSHA-approved state plans with their own standards and enforcement policies. For the most part, those states adopt standards that are identical to those of federal OSHA. However, some states have adopted different standards. Therefore, it is important to be familiar with the applicable regulations in the state where a facility is located.

Program Review

Regular evaluation of the medical surveillance program is important to ensure its effectiveness. Maintenance and review of medical records and test results aid health care providers, health and safety professionals, and facility leadership in assessing the effectiveness of the health and safety program. The Environmental Health and Safety Department should at least annually:

- ☐ Establish that each accident or illness was promptly investigated to determine the cause and make necessary changes in health and safety procedures.
- ☐ Evaluate the efficiency of specific medical surveillance in the context of potential site exposures.
- ☐ Revise medical surveillance as suggested by current industrial hygiene and environmental data.
- ☐ Review potential exposures and facility health and safety plans to determine if additional testing is required.
- ☐ Review emergency treatment procedures and update lists of emergency contacts.

Although medical surveillance focuses primarily on exposures to substances such as chemical and radiation, other important areas to consider are ergonomics, back safety, computer monitors, physical conditions (heat, cold, vibration, noise), and biological factors.

Specific OSHA Standards Requiring Medical Surveillance

Medical screening, medical monitoring, and exposure monitoring are the fundamental strategies for protecting workers.

Medical Screening

Medical screening is a method for detecting disease or body dysfunction before an individual would normally seek medical care. Screening tests are usually administered to individuals without symptoms, but who may be at high risk for certain adverse health outcomes. Medical screening is conducted on certain applicants and employees based on the health hazards of the job. The publication *Screening and Surveillance: A Guide to OSHA Standards* provides a quick reference to help an employer locate and implement the screening and surveillance requirements of the OSHA standards.[2] [CD-ROM 15.12]

Medical Monitoring

Whereas exposure monitoring is used to ensure that airborne concentrations of harmful chemicals (and also noise levels) are not exceeding their respective OSHA permissible exposure limits (PELs), medical monitoring is used to ensure that employees are not suffering adverse health effects even if exposures are well controlled. Examples of medical monitoring standards

Figure 15–2. Examples of Standards That Include Requirements for Medical Monitoring

---

- ☐ 1910.95, Occupational noise exposure
- ☐ 1910.120, Hazardous waste operations and emergency response
- ☐ 1910.134, Respiratory protection
- ☐ 1910.1001, Asbestos
- ☐ 1910.1020, Access to employee expsosure and medical records
- ☐ 1910.1025, Lead
- ☐ 1910.1028, Benzene
- ☐ 1910.1030, Bloodborne pathogens
- ☐ 1910.1047, Ethylene oxide
- ☐ 1910.1048, Formaldehyde
- ☐ 1910.1052, Methylene chloride
- ☐ 1910.1096, Ionizing radiation
- ☐ 1910.1200, Hazard communication
- ☐ 1910.1450, Occupational exposure to hazardous chemicals in laboratories

---

(found in 29 CFR 1910) having requirements that are of concern in health care facilities are listed in figure 15-2. These standards are included on the CD-ROM accompanying this book.

Though no longer used in construction in the United States, asbestos may be found in older health care facilities, where it was used as insulating material for piping and, in some cases, in floor tile.[3] Asbestos exposures in these health care facilities are most likely to occur during expansion, renovation, or maintenance activities.

Exposure Monitoring

The ability to precisely and accurately monitor the workplace air for contaminants is essential to understanding what chemicals workers may be exposed to, the concentrations of the chemicals in the air, and whether the controls that were put in place are effectively controlling exposures. Exposure monitoring is generally conducted by an industrial hygienist.

As is the case for medical monitoring, OSHA standards also provide requirements for exposure monitoring and the keeping of exposure records. Exposure records analyzed in concert with medical monitoring and injury and illness reports can be used to conduct a job hazard analysis (JHA) and are invaluable to the conduct of epidemiology studies. The standards listed in the previous section on medical monitoring should also be consulted to for exposure monitoring requirements.

BEST PRACTICES IN OCCUPATIONAL SURVEILLANCE AND PUBLIC HEALTH SURVEILLANCE

Public health surveillance is the ongoing systematic collection, analysis, and interpretation of health data for purposes of improving health and safety. Key to public health surveillance is the dissemination and use of data to improve health.

Occupational health surveillance can be defined as the tracking of occupational injuries, illnesses, hazards, and exposures. Occupational surveillance data are used to guide efforts to improve employee safety and health and to monitor trends and progress over time.

A commitment to effective surveillance represents a commitment to the individual dignity of every sick and injured worker. In the public health arena, certain injuries and diseases require careful surveillance so that the appropriate measures can be taken to either prevent them or minimize their impact.

Occupational Epidemiology

Epidemiology is the study of the distribution and determinants of health-related states or events in specific populations. In other words, it is the study of epidemics (widespread outbreaks). The well-conducted epidemiology study can provide important information on the causes of specific diseases. In the occupational environment it has been used to demonstrate the association between the magnitude and range of specific chemical exposures and the extent to which those exposures adversely affect a population. For example, depending on the magnitude of benzene exposure, some workers will exhibit neurological effects. However, other workers exposed under other conditions may develop leukemia. The determinant of which workers will suffer neurological effects and which ones will develop leukemia is based on the amount of benzene to which they were exposed and the duration of their exposure. The extent of the disease depends on the number of workers that were exposed. The ability to make such associations provides a basis for corrective action.

Federal, State, and Private Surveillance Activities

Numerous federal, state, and private organizations conduct injury and illness surveillance activities. Summaries of programs from four of these organizations follow.

Centers for Disease Control and Prevention (CDC)

Each year the Centers for Disease Control and Prevention (CDC) collects information from state health departments about cases of influenza. Using that information, the CDC can then provide information on steps that can be taken to reduce the likelihood of contracting the illness and can order the production of an appropriate vaccine.

National Institute for Occupational Safety and Health (NIOSH)

The National Institute for Occupational Safety and Health (NIOSH) has developed a list of 64 health "events" that each serve as an early warning to a more widespread occupational health problem. [CD-ROM 15.13] According to NIOSH:

> An Occupational Sentinel Health Event (SHE[O]) is a disease, disability, or untimely death, which is occupationally related and whose occurrence may:
>
> 1. Provide the impetus for epidemiologic or industrial hygiene studies; or
> 2. Serve as a warning signal that materials substitution, engineering control, personal protection, or medical care may be required.

The NIOSH SHE[O] list is no different from the cataloguing of occupational injuries and illnesses in the *Diseases of Tradesmen,* written by Bernardino Ramazzini in 1700. Knowing what to look for is half the battle. Whether it is "the sound of arms, and the tramp of feet, and the measured tread of the grenadiers" or malignant neoplasms of the trachea, bronchus, or lung, the warning cannot be ignored.

Chartbook The *Worker Health Chartbook,* prepared by NIOSH as a resource for agencies, organizations, employers, researchers, workers, and others who need to know about occupational injuries and illnesses, consolidates information from the network of tracking systems that forms the cornerstone of injury and illness surveillance in the United States.[4] [CD-ROM 15.14] The *Chartbook* is described by NIOSH as:

> a descriptive epidemiologic reference on occupational morbidity and mortality in the United States. A resource for agencies, organizations, employers, researchers, workers, and others who need to know about occupational injuries and illnesses, the *Chartbook* includes more than 400 figures and tables describing the magnitude, distribution, and trends of the Nation's occupational injuries, illnesses, and fatalities.

Figure 15-3 lists some of the occupational health priorities identified in the NIOSH *Worker Health Chartbook* (2004 ed.). Many of those NIOSH priorities are also current concerns in health care facilities.

Figure 15–3. Occupational Health Priorities Described in the NIOSH *Worker Health Chartbook,* **2004**

 ☐ Anxiety, stress, and neurotic disorders
 ☐ Bloodborne infections
 ☐ Fatal injuries
 ☐ Hearing loss
 ☐ Musculoskeletal disorders
 ☐ Nonfatal injuries
 ☐ Disorders due to physical agents
 ☐ Respiratory disease
 ☐ Skin diseases and disorders

While some of the data in the *Chartbook* is derived from the Bureau of Labor Statistics (BLS), a number of other sources are also used, including:

 ☐ U.S. Department of Agriculture, National Agricultural Statistics Service
 ☐ Mine Safety and Health Administration (MSHA)
 ☐ State health and labor departments
 ☐ Surveillance and prevention centers from the CDC, including the National Center for Health Statistics (NCHS); the National Center for Infectious Diseases (NCID); and the National Center for HIV, STD, and TB Prevention (NCHSTB)
 ☐ U.S. Bureau of the Census
 ☐ Consumer Product Safety Commission (CPSC)
 ☐ The Center to Protect Workers' Rights (CPWR)

Some of those sources are particularly useful in gauging the health status of the U.S. population as a whole and can be used in the development of a total health and safety program.

Health Hazard Evaluations   The NIOSH Health Hazard Evaluation (HHE) program may be able to help with the control of health hazards in health care facilities. This program allows employees and employers to request an investigation of a perceived health hazard. The evaluations are conducted at no cost to the health care facility. An HHE is a study of a workplace. It is done to determine whether workers are exposed to hazardous materials or harmful conditions. The NIOSH website provides information about the program and how to ask for help. It also has links to reports from thousands of HHEs conducted by NIOSH.[5]

Health Hazard Evaluations are conducted in health care facilities for situations that involve a variety of health hazards, such as indoor air quality, temperature extremes, chemicals, drugs, latex allergies, and ergonomics.

Sharps Injury Surveillance and Prevention Program

The Massachusetts Department of Public Health (MDPH) is working with the Massachusetts Hospital Association and the Massachusetts Nurses Association to provide tools and training to assist health care facilities in developing their own sharps injury surveillance and prevention programs. As part of this effort, MDPH, in collaboration with the CDC, is investigating the feasibility of a web-based sharps injury surveillance system that enables facilities to collect and analyze data regarding sharps injuries among their employees. The system will also provide MDPH and the CDC with anonymous data needed to track sharps injuries among health care workers statewide. The web-based application and data will be maintained centrally at CDC.[6] The initiative also addresses the role that state health agencies can play in helping health care facilities develop surveillance systems for work-related illnesses and injuries.

Bureau of Labor Statistics (BLS)

Data collected from OSHA Form 300 logs is summarized and presented in tabular form by the Bureau of Labor Statistics (BLS). [CD-ROM 15.15] Because it takes more than one year to collect, analyze, and prepare the data for publication, the most current data is from two years prior to publication. Thus, data published in 2005 reflects what occurred in 2003. The BLS data is a powerful tool for examining the recordable injury and illness data within a particular industry, which an individual facility can use as a basis of comparison.

JOB HAZARD ANALYSIS (JHA)

Bernardino Ramazzini observed workers and catalogued the potential hazards of their jobs and the illnesses and injuries that accompanied them.[7] Today, *Diseases of Tradesmen* remains a classic example of the job hazard analysis.

A job hazard analysis (JHA), sometimes called a job safety analysis or a hazard assessment, is the process of examining a job to identify any potential hazards associated with that job and redesigning the job, if necessary, to correct and prevent hazards. The potential hazards may be associated with exposures, equipment, the surroundings, or the way in which the worker performs the duties of the job. [CD-ROM 15.16]

A hazard, as defined by *The American Heritage Dictionary*, is a chance or accident; a danger; peril; risk.[8] Hazards fall into two major categories: physical hazards and health hazards. Physical hazards can include moving objects, temperature extremes, lighting, and sharp edges. Health hazards can be defined as exposures above the allowable limits to dusts, chemicals, and radiation. The circumstances that cause hazards can change from day to day.

Benefits of a Job Hazard Analysis

The general duty clause (5(a)(1)) of the OSH Act requires that:

> Each employer shall furnish to each of his employees employment and a place of employment which are free from recognized hazards that are causing or are likely to cause death or serious physical harm to his employees.

If a hazard is discovered, the JHA helps to determine the best way to protect an employee from injury or illness. Health care facilities can use JHAs as a tool to help identify the hazards associated with tasks performed by employees. They evaluate dangerous or potentially dangerous situations to determine if corrections can be made or in what ways employees can be protected from the situation or process. In addition, JHAs are useful training tools for new employees, and review of the JHA can serve as a refresher in terms of needed skills for the experienced employee. For a JHA to be effective, department managers must follow through to correct any uncontrolled hazards identified. Otherwise, the managers will lose credibility and employees may hesitate to go to them when they identify dangerous conditions.

Before Starting a Job Hazard Analysis

When conducting a JHA, be sure to consult appropriate OSHA standards or other guidelines that relate to the job. Compliance with these standards and guidelines is mandatory and will help the Environmental Health and Safety Department ensure that federal and other requirements are being met. Make an inventory of any chemicals that are routinely used by the employees and any tasks that require more than routine exertion.

Where to Begin

Under the direction of the Environmental Health and Safety Department, the department manager and department liaisons should conduct the JHA. The safety officer, department manager, and department liaison should meet to briefly discuss the job, any incidents that have resulted from tasks within the job, and the surroundings in which the job is performed. If any hazards exist that pose an immediate danger to an employee's life or health, immediate action should be taken to protect the employee. Any problems that can be corrected easily should be corrected as soon as possible. The department liaisons should remain involved because they are familiar with the jobs, tasks, and hazards found in their departments. In addition, the department liaisons and their colleagues will be instrumental in the implementation of any hazard elimination or control measures that may be necessary.

Employee Involvement

Employees should be involved in virtually every aspect of the Environmental Health and Safety program. For example, employees should participate in health and safety committees and in conducting training on a variety of safety and health topics if they are qualified. They should also be trained to identify and report health and safety hazards to their department liaisons and be actively involved in recommending safety and health–related improvements to management. Employees should also be asked to identify any aspect of their job that results in problems such as aches, pains, or rashes. Employees should be interviewed and asked to verify that what their position description says they are to do is what they are actually doing.

Reviewing the Accident History

Each department's injury and illness history should be reviewed with special attention paid to those injuries and illnesses that needed treatment, accidents that required repair or replacement of equipment, and any "near misses"— events in which an accident or loss did not occur, but could have. These events are indicators that the existing hazard controls (if any) may not be adequate and deserve more scrutiny, or that additional or refresher training is needed.

Selecting the Job for a JHA

The individual performing the safety function in the model program presented in this book is knowledgeable in safety standards and regulations and in the recognition of safety hazards. This individual should sit down with department managers and department liaisons and discuss concerns and situations in the department. It is the responsibility of the Environmental Health and Safety Department to work with each department's leadership to identify the jobs with the highest potential for injury or illness, such as chemical exposures, electrical hazards, or lifting hazards. The hazards of shift work in the facility should also be considered. [CD-ROM 15.17]

Other Selection Criteria

Other criteria that can be used to select jobs for hazard analysis include:

□ Jobs with the highest injury or illness rates. This information can be found by reviewing OSHA Form 300, Log of Work-Related Injuries and Illnesses, and selecting a place to start. In addition, workers' compensation records can be reviewed.

☐ Jobs with the potential to cause severe or disabling injuries or illness, even if there is no history of previous accidents.

☐ Jobs in which one simple human error could lead to a severe accident or injury.

☐ Jobs that are new to the facility or have undergone changes in processes and procedures.

☐ Jobs complex enough to require written instructions.

Identification of Tasks

To begin a JHA, watch the employee perform the job and list each task as the employee performs it. Be sure to record enough information to describe each job action without getting overly detailed. Avoid making the breakdown of steps so detailed that it becomes unnecessarily long or so broad that it does not include basic tasks. Later, review the job tasks with the employee to make sure nothing is omitted. Point out that the employee's job is being recorded, not the employee's job performance.

Sometimes, in conducting a JHA, it may be helpful to photograph or videotape the employee performing the job. These visual records can be handy references for a more detailed analysis of the work.

Performing a JHA is an exercise in detective work. The goal is to ask questions to learn about potential problems and hazards, as listed in figure 15-4.

To increase the usefulness of the job hazard analysis, document the answers to these questions in a consistent manner. Describing a hazard in this way helps to ensure that efforts to eliminate the hazard and implement hazard controls target the most important contributors to the hazard.

Redesigning Jobs to Correct and Prevent Hazards

After a review of the list of hazards with the department manager, department liaison, and employees assigned to the job, the next step is to develop a recommended safe job procedure that eliminates or controls hazardous conditions or operations. The principal solutions are finding a new way to do the job,

Figure 15–4. Questions to Ask during a JHA

☐ What can go wrong?

☐ What are the consequences?

☐ How could the hazard arise?

☐ What are other contributing factors?

☐ How likely is it that the hazard will occur?

changing the physical condition that creates the hazard, providing additional personal protective equipment (PPE) to the employee, and providing additional training to the employee. The order of precedence and effectiveness of hazard control is as follows:

1. **Substitution** of safer chemicals or other products to keep hazards from entering the workplace.
2. **Engineering controls** include using equipment that makes work safer.
3. **Administrative controls** (sometimes called work practice controls) include changing jobs to fit the needs of the workers.
4. **Personal protective equipment (PPE)** includes respirators, hard hats, face and eye protection, hearing protection, gloves, and protective clothing and footwear.

Substitution Keeps Hazards from Entering the Workplace

Employees do not have to worry about a hazard if it is not there. For example, the substitution of a hazardous chemical by a less hazardous chemical that is still effective in its intended use is always a goal of health and safety. Injuries from lifting heavy objects can be reduced by buying goods in smaller containers.

However, substitution is not always an option. If one chemical is being substituted for another, the new substance must be less toxic. For example, following the identification of the cold sterilant formaldehyde as a potential occupational carcinogen, there was a significant effort to substitute it with glutaraldehyde-containing sterilants. Unfortunately, that switch has proven to be a poor choice since after its introduction it was determined that glutaraldehyde caused both dermal and respiratory sensitization.

Engineering Controls to Make Work Safer

There are many types of devices that make work safer by eliminating or minimizing hazards:

- Patient-lifting devices reduce the strain on workers' backs and limbs.
- Enclosure of a hazard, such as closing off noisy equipment or locating it away from workers, reduces their exposure to loud noise, which can damage hearing. Glove boxes for handling hazardous materials (either chemical or biological) isolate the employee from the hazard.
- Needles that retract or are sheathed after use protect workers from needlestick injuries.

□ Guarding moving machine parts can prevent injury.

□ Removal or redirection of a hazard through ventilation is a good way to get rid of harmful substances in the air. "General ventilation" pertains to a large area, such as a building's air-handling system. "Local ventilation" pertains to small areas and includes hoods in laboratories or collection devices on power tools that generate dust.

Administrative Controls Change the Way Workers Do Their Jobs

Managing the way that jobs are done using administrative controls can reduce injuries and illnesses. For example:

□ Written operating procedures, work permits, and safe work practices

□ Exposure time limitations: Reducing exposure to hot or cold conditions by taking breaks in cool rest areas and drinking fluids for rehydration; reducing the frequency or length of exposure for tasks including computer work and tool vibration; rotating workers through various job assignments so they do not develop repetitive-motion injuries

□ Monitoring the use of hazardous materials and limiting the user's exposure time

□ Alarms, signs, and warning lights: Warning signs and lights for certain laser classes or laser systems to reduce exposure to eyes or skin; fire alarms, security alarms; caution signs

□ Buddy system: Reducing the weight that one worker must lift by having more than one person perform the lift

Personal Protective Equipment (PPE) Includes Safety Clothing and Equipment (29 CFR 1910.132)

If substitution, engineering, or administrative controls prove to be insufficient in protecting workers, then OSHA requires the use of personal protective equipment and clothing. However, PPE cannot be the first choice of the employer for mitigating a hazard and cannot be provided without first conducting a hazard assessment to help select the correct PPE. A hazard assessment is an important element of a PPE program because it produces the information needed to identify who will need to wear PPE and to select the appropriate PPE for any hazards present or likely to be present at the workplace. Standard 29 CFR 1910.132, Personal protective equipment general requirements, details hazard assessment requirements in paragraph (d), Hazard assessment and equipment selection. [CD-ROM 15.18] It is a performance-oriented provision that requires management to use their awareness of workplace hazards to enable them to select the appropriate PPE for the work being performed.

1910.132(d) Hazard assessment and equipment selection

1910.132(d)(1)
The employer shall assess the workplace to determine if hazards are present, or are likely to be present, which necessitate the use of personal protective equipment (PPE). If such hazards are present, or likely to be present, the employer shall:

1910.132(d)(1)(i)
Select, and have each affected employee use, the types of PPE that will protect the affected employee from the hazards identified in the hazard assessment;

1910.132(d)(1)(ii)
Communicate selection decisions to each affected employee; and,

1910.132(d)(1)(iii)
Select PPE that properly fits each affected employee. Note: Non-mandatory Appendix B contains an example of procedures that would comply with the requirement for a hazard assessment.

1910.132(d)(2)
The employer shall verify that the required workplace hazard assessment has been performed through a written certification that identifies the workplace evaluated; the person certifying that the evaluation has been performed; the date(s) of the hazard assessment; and, which identifies the document as a certification of hazard assessment.

Subpart I, Appendix B, of OSHA 1910 provides non-mandatory compliance guidelines for hazard assessment and personal protective equipment selection.[9] [CD-ROM 15.19]

Examples of PPE used in health care facilities include welding masks and goggles, cut-resistant gloves in kitchens, respirators in isolation areas, hard hats in construction zones, specialty glasses and goggles such as those used for laser and ultraviolet radiation protection, and disposable gloves in patient care and other areas.

PPE is the least effective way to protect workers because it does not eliminate or control the hazard. If the equipment fails, the worker is immediately exposed to the hazard.

Periodic Review of the JHA

Periodic review of the JHA ensures that it remains current and continues to be effective in reducing workplace accidents and injuries. Even if the job has not changed, it is possible that during the review process hazards will be identified that were not identified in the initial JHA.

The JHA should be reviewed if an illness or injury occurs on a specific job. Based on the circumstances, the job procedure may need to be changed to prevent similar injuries or illnesses. If an employee's failure to follow proper job procedures results in a "close call," discuss the situation with all employees who perform the job and remind them of proper procedures. Any time a JHA is revised, all employees affected by the changes must be trained in the new job methods, procedures, or protective measures adopted.

INCIDENT MANAGEMENT

The purpose of surveillance and job hazard analysis is to promote safe and healthful working conditions for all employees. Prevention systems provide managers, supervisors, and employees with a clear understanding of the facility's concern with protecting employees from job-related injuries and illnesses in compliance with federal, state, and local regulations. However, incidents and accidents do occur in health care facilities, and when they do, employees must be cared for. In addition, incidents and accidents must be reported and investigated and their causes must be determined to prevent them from recurring. The terms *incident* and *accident* are used interchangeably in this section.

Health care facilities have multiple systems for data collection encompassing a variety of parameters, such as employee injuries and illnesses, visitor injuries, patient injuries, vehicle/property damage, security incidents, and even near misses. In some health care facilities, there are no clear lines of authority for the safety and health function. When an incident occurs, it may not be reported; if it is, a report may be filed but the incident is not thoroughly investigated and facts are not used to find out why the incident happened and what can be done to prevent it in the future. In this case, managing incidents is difficult and ineffective. Providing statistics to the safety committee or senior administration may take weeks or even months, and the integrity of the data from these multiple systems can be questionable. To address these challenges, the Environmental Health and Safety Department must be an integral part of the incident management system. To result in an efficient and effective system, the process should:

- ☐ Ensure immediate, consistent, and accurate incident tracking.
- ☐ Track and sort all incident and accident data (employee, visitor, patient).
- ☐ Track all types of incidents, including investigation (i.e., type of incident unknown at this time), near miss, first aid only, no lost time, lost time, and fatality.
- ☐ Analyze and detect trends.
- ☐ Generate reports.
- ☐ Track all costs associated with incidents.

Computer-Based Reporting

Computer-based solutions can make incident reporting simple with little training. Computer-based reporting replaces forms and paperwork, may meet OSHA Form 300 log requirements, and can be customized to the facility's data needs. Other advantages of computer-based reporting include the ability to quickly examine possible hazards across the facility or in a specific department over the course of a shift, a week, a month, or a year. For multi-site health care facilities, users can compare incident reports among sites and determine the source and effectiveness of follow-up. Many computer-based incident tracking systems are designed to mimic the model that a user would follow in managing a claim in the paper world.

OSHA State Plan Resources

The Oregon OSHA office provides online training to inform Oregon employers of occupational safety and health requirements. This section presents portions of Oregon's course instruction and training in "Conducting an Accident Investigation." [CD-ROM 15.20] Any health care facilities can use any of OSHA's resources, whether federal or state.

An incident investigation should be started as soon as possible, not to establish blame but rather to accurately determine the surface and root causes for the incident. Two things disappear after an incident occurs:

☐ *Material evidence.* Tools, equipment, and sometimes people just seem to move or disappear from the scene. Material evidence should be protected so it does not get moved or disappear.

☐ *Memory.* As time passes after an incident, conversations with others and individual emotions distort what people believe they saw and heard. After a while, the memory of everyone affected by the incident will be altered in some way.

Effective Interviewing

When employees are interviewed following an incident, they may be uncomfortable. They may fear some form of reprisal, have personal problems, or may have had unpleasant interview experiences in the past. It is necessary to clarify that the investigation is not a blame or faultfinding mission, but rather a way to find out how the incident happened and how to avoid a recurrence that observation only might not otherwise detect.

Where an interview takes place can also have an influence on the outcome. If possible, conduct the interview at the employee's worksite. If an employee is having difficulty verbalizing what occurred, ask the employee to act it out. Showing what happened can often produce more effective results than statements alone.

Figure 15–5. "A MESS" Acronym That Spells Out the Steps to a Successful Interview

Acknowledge—Listen to people

Mirror—Rephrase what they say

Empathize—Understand their emotions

Solve—Determine correct action

Settle—Provide satisfactory solution

Reproduced with permission from *People Power*, published by Chaff & Co. Copyright © 1992 Chaff & Co.

A skilled interviewer listens for an employee's tone of voice, which may indicate emotional upset or concern. Body language is another helpful tool. An employee who is uncooperative—for any reason—might sit with arms folded across the chest. Any bodily signs of pulling back or shutting off can indicate the need to get through to the individual to enlist assistance. By showing appropriate sympathy, the interviewer can establish a stronger rapport. For example, the interviewer might say, "I realize this has to be very upsetting" or "Take your time, there is no rush."

At the end of the interview, thank employees for their time and assistance and end the interview on a positive note. If steps are in place to avoid a repeat incident, communicate this to the employee. The objective is to indicate that management is committed to a safe and healthy environment for its employees and patients, and is doing everything possible to ensure their well-being.

Effective interviewing skills are acquired through training and experience. Figure 15-5 provides steps, in acronym form, to help with a successful interview.

Analyzing the Accident Process

Event analysis is a very important process. This section discusses some theories of accident causation and the process of developing and analyzing the sequence of events occurring prior to, during, and immediately after an accident.

Developing the Sequence of Events   A challenge in the investigation process is to accurately determine the sequence of events to more effectively analyze the accident process. Once the steps in the process are developed, each event can be studied to determine related circumstances, as illustrated in figure 15-6.

In the multiple-cause approach to accident investigation, many events may occur, each contributing to the incident. For example, if supervisors ignore unsafe behaviors because following up on them is not thought to be

Figure 15-6. Steps to Determining the Sequence of Events

□ *Hazardous conditions:* Things and states that directly caused the accident.

□ *Unsafe behaviors:* Actions taken/not taken that contributed to the accident.

□ *System weaknesses*: Underlying inadequate or missing programs, plans, policies, processes, and procedures that contributed to the accident.

---

their responsibility, it can result in a cascade of events that may contribute to or increase the probability of another accident.

Each event in the accident process describes a unique individual or object and action. An individual or object directly influenced the flow of the sequence of events. Action is something that is done by an individual. Actions may or may not be observable. An action may describe something that is done or not done. Failure to act should be thought of as an act in itself.

When describing events, first indicate the individual, and then tell what the individual did—for example, "Jane placed the uncapped needle in her pocket." The statement is written in the active tense.

Paint a Word Picture   The sequence of events should clearly describe what occurred so that someone unfamiliar with the accident is able to "see it happen" as they read. If an event is hard to understand, it may be that the description is too vague or general. The solution to this problem is to increase the level of detail. Determine if anything else was said or done before or after the event being assessed.

Determining Surface and Root Causes

Most accidents in the workplace result from unsafe work behaviors. Oregon OSHA describes an unsafe behavior as one that is an action taken or not taken that increases the risk of injury or illness. An unsafe behavior can also be a process error and may occur at any level in the organization. According to the latest research, such behaviors represent the direct cause of about 95 percent of all workplace accidents. Hazardous conditions represent the direct cause of only about 3 percent of workplace accidents. "Acts of God" account for the remaining 2 percent. These statistics imply that management system weaknesses account for fully 98 percent of all workplace accidents. Effective fulfillment of accident investigation responsibilities requires that the investigation not be closed until the root causes have been identified.

It is a struggle to try to overcome long-held perceptions about safety and how accidents occur. Management, perceptions, and subsequent actions reflect both traditional and progressive approaches. Old and new ways of thinking come in to play.

The old theory: worker error. The old thinking about the causes of accidents assumes that the worker makes a choice to work in an unsafe manner. It implies that there are no outside forces acting on and influencing the actions of the worker and that there are simple reasons for an accident. The old thinking also considers accidents as resulting solely from worker error: a lack of "common sense." The employee is "the problem." To prevent accidents, the employee must work more safely. This thinking results in blame and short-term fixes, which are inefficient, ineffective, and in the long run more expensive to implement and maintain.

The new theory: systems approach. The systems approach takes into account the dynamics of systems that interact within the overall safety and health program. It concludes that accidents are defects in the system. People are only one part of a complex system composed of many complicated processes (more than we realize). Accidents are the result of multiple causes or defects in the system. It is the investigator's job to uncover the root causes (defects) in the system. Fixing the system, not the employee, is the goal of the investigation. To prevent accidents, the system must operate more safely. This thinking results in long-term fixes, which are less expensive to implement and maintain.

Analyze for Cause When information is gathered and used to develop an accurate sequence of events, the result is a good mental picture of what happened. The next step is to conduct an analysis of each event to determine causes.

As mentioned earlier, accidents are processes that may culminate in an injury or illness. An accident may be the result of many factors (simultaneous, interconnected, cross-linked events) that have interacted in some dynamic way. An effective accident investigation involves three levels of cause analysis:

Injury analysis. At this level of analysis, do not attempt to determine what caused the accident, but rather focus on trying to determine how the injury was caused. The outcome of the accident process is an injury.

Event analysis. Determine the surface cause(s) for the accident— those hazardous conditions and unsafe behaviors described throughout all events that dynamically interact to produce the injury. All hazardous conditions and unsafe behaviors are clues pointing to possible system weaknesses. This level of investigation is also called "special cause" analysis because the analyst can point to a specific thing or behavior.

Systems analysis. At this level, analyze the root causes contributing to the accident. Usually, surface causes can be traced to inadequate safety policies, programs, plans, processes, or procedures. Root causes always preexist surface causes and may function through poor component design to allow, promote, encourage, or even require systems that result in hazardous conditions and unsafe behaviors. This level of investigation is also called "common cause" analysis because a system component may contribute to common conditions and behaviors throughout the organization.

The Direct Cause of Injury   If a harsh acid splashes on an employee's face, the employee may suffer a chemical burn because the skin has been exposed to a chemical that destroys tissue. In this instance, the direct cause of the injury is a harmful chemical reaction. The related surface cause might be the acid (condition) or working without the proper face protection (unsafe behavior).

If an employee's workload is too strenuous, it may cause a muscle strain. The direct cause of injury is impact, causing injury to muscle tissue. A related surface cause of the accident might be fatigue (hazardous condition) or improper lifting techniques (unsafe behavior).

In these two cases, the direct cause of injury is not the same as the surface cause of the accident. The surface cause of the accident describes a condition or behavior. The result of the condition and/or behavior is the direct cause of injury. The surface causes of accidents are those specific hazardous conditions and unsafe employee/manager behaviors that have directly caused or contributed in some way to the accident.

Hazardous Conditions   Hazardous conditions:

- □ Are things or objects that cause injury or illness
- □ May also be viewed as defects in a process
- □ May exist at any level of the organization

Hazardous conditions may exist in any of the following categories:

- □ Materials
- □ Machinery
- □ Equipment
- □ Tools
- □ Chemicals
- □ Environment
- □ Facilities
- □ People
- □ Workload

Most hazardous conditions in the workplace are the result of specific unsafe behaviors. Unsafe behaviors are actions we take or don't take, resulting in increased risk of injury or illness. They may also be thought of as errors in a process, and they may occur at any level of the organization. Examples of unsafe employee and manager behaviors include the items listed in figure 15-7.

Incident Analysis   Each incident must be examined to determine the hazardous conditions and the unsafe or inappropriate behaviors representing the surface causes for the incident. Techniques that can be used to conduct the

Figure 15–7. Examples of Unsafe Behaviors

- ☐ Failing to comply with rules
- ☐ Using unsafe methods
- ☐ Taking shortcuts
- ☐ Horseplay
- ☐ Failing to report injuries
- ☐ Failing to report hazards
- ☐ Allowing unsafe behaviors
- ☐ Failing to train
- ☐ Failing to supervise
- ☐ Failing to correct
- ☐ Scheduling too much work
- ☐ Ignoring worker stress
- ☐ Failing to staff appropriately

incident analysis include the "fishbone diagram" used successfully by many as a general problem-solving tool in an incident analysis. Invented by Dr. Kaoru Ishikawa, a Japanese quality control statistician, the fishbone diagram is an analysis tool that provides a systematic way of looking at effects and the causes that create or contribute to those effects. For this reason the fishbone diagram may be referred to as a cause-and-effect diagram. The design of the diagram looks much like the skeleton of a fish.

The value of the fishbone diagram is to assist individuals or teams in categorizing the many potential causes of problems or issues in an orderly way and in identifying root causes. Identifying inadequate policies, programs, plans, processes, and procedures gets to the root causes. The root causes for accidents are the underlying safety system weaknesses that have somehow contributed to the existence of hazardous conditions and unsafe behaviors that represent surface causes of accidents. These weaknesses can take two forms:

Design root causes: Inadequate planning and design of the system. The development of formal (written) safety management system policies, plans, processes, and procedures is very important to make sure conditions, activities, behaviors, and practices are appropriate.

Implementation root causes: Inadequate implementation of the system. Care to effectively carry out the safety management system is critical to the success of the system. A wonderfully designed system that is not implemented correctly will not work.

Root causes always preexist surface causes. Inadequately designed and implemented system components have the potential to nurture hazardous conditions and unsafe behaviors. If root causes are left unchecked, surface causes will flourish.

Safety management systems are developed to:

☐ Promote commitment and leadership
☐ Increase employee involvement
☐ Establish accountability
☐ Identify and control hazards
☐ Investigate incidents/accidents
☐ Educate and train
☐ Evaluate the safety and health program

System components include:

☐ Policies
☐ Programs
☐ Plans
☐ Processes
☐ Procedures
☐ Budgets
☐ Reports
☐ Rules

Developing Effective Recommendations   An incident investigation is generally thought to be a reactive safety and health process because it is initiated only after an accident has occurred. However, when recommendations are proposed that include effective control strategies and systems improvements, the investigation is transformed into a valuable proactive process that ensures similar incidents do not occur. Effective recommendations will "sell" safety and health improvements.

To make sure recommendations are effective, control strategies must be addressed that will eliminate or reduce the specific surface causes of the incident. In addition, system improvements must be proposed to correct missing or inadequate safety system components that contributed to the incident.

System Improvements   Missing or inadequate safety system components represent root causes for workplace accidents. Surface causes represent symptoms indicating system weaknesses. Therefore, every effort should be made to improve system components to ensure long-term workplace safety. System improvements might include some of the following:

☐ Including employee health and safety in the organization's mission statement

- ☐ Improving safety and health policy so that it clearly establishes responsibility and accountability
- ☐ Changing a work process so that checklists are used that include safety checks
- ☐ Revising purchasing policy to include safety as well as cost considerations
- ☐ Changing the safety and health inspection process to include department liaisons, supervisors, and employees

Proactive Recommendations   The Environmental Health and Safety Department must learn to anticipate the concerns and questions that other departments face when deciding what actions to take. The more pertinent the information included in the recommendation, the greater the likelihood of approval. To make certain good information is provided, ask some important proactive questions. The following six questions will help develop and justify recommendations.

1. *Pinpoint the problem: What exactly is the problem?*

What are the specific hazardous conditions and unsafe work practices that caused the problem? What are the system components—the inadequate or missing policies, processes, or rules that allowed the conditions and practices to exist?

2. *What is the history of the problem?*

Have similar accidents occurred previously? If so, the probability of similar future accidents is highly likely to be certain. What were the previous direct and indirect costs for similar accidents? How have similar accidents affected production and morale?

3. *Pinpoint the solution: What are solutions that would correct the problem?*

What specific engineering, administrative, and PPE controls will eliminate or at least reduce exposure to the hazardous conditions? What are the specific system improvements needed to ensure a long-term fix?

4. *Who is the decision maker?*

Who can approve, authorize, and act on the corrective measures? What are the possible objections that the individual might have? What arguments will be most effective in overcoming objections?

5. *Why is that person supporting safety and health?*

It is important to know what is motivating the decision maker. For example:

- ☐ Fulfill the legal obligation? If so, emphasize possible penalties if corrections are not made.
- ☐ Fulfill the fiscal obligation? If so, emphasize the costs/benefits.
- ☐ Fulfill the moral obligation? If so, emphasize improved morale and public relations.

6. *What will be the cost/benefits if the recommendation is approved and the predictable cost/benefits if it is not?*

What are the estimated costs and benefits of taking corrective action, as contrasted with the possible costs and harm that might occur if the hazardous conditions and unsafe work practices remain? What are the employer obligations under administrative law? What is the "message" sent to the workforce as a result of action or inaction? Detail the costs associated with any training that might be required.

Cost-Benefit Analysis To be effective, recommendations should be supported by a bottom-line cost-benefit analysis that contrasts the relative high costs of accidents against the much lower costs associated with corrective actions. Doing a cost-benefit analysis is even more important for recommending corrective actions before an accident occurs. According to the National Safety Council, the estimated 2003 average direct and indirect costs of a lost-time injury are about $35,000.

The Environmental Health and Safety Department should work with heads of other departments to provide alternatives to make it more likely that corrective actions will be taken. Options include the following logic:

- ☐ *First option:* If the facility has all the money it needs, what can be done? Eliminate the hazard primarily using engineering controls, with additional administrative controls, if required.
- ☐ *Second option:* If the facility has limited funds, what can be done? Eliminate the hazard using work practice and/or administrative controls, along with engineering controls, if required.
- ☐ *Third option:* If the facility does not have money, what can be done? Reduce exposure to the hazard with administrative controls and/or PPE.

First, try to "engineer out" the hazard, if feasible, before using administrative controls or PPE. Some tasks, of course, require the use of PPE in accordance with OSHA requirements.

Writing the Report

Once the facts related to the incident have been accurately assessed and analyzed, the findings must be reported to those who have authority, account-ability, and the capacity to take action. The primary objective of incident investigation is to uncover the causal factors that contributed to the incident—not to place blame. The challenge is to be as objective and accurate as possible.

Findings

The findings and how they are presented will shape perceptions and subsequent corrective actions. If the report arrives at a conclusion such as "Bob should have used common sense" or "Bob forgot to use PPE," how effective will it be? If the report concludes with statements such as "It will be virtually impossible to take corrective actions that permanently eliminate the causes," it is likely that simi-lar accidents will repeatedly occur. If the incident investigation does not fix the system, the investigation has likely been a waste of time and effort.

Report the findings in a well-thought-out manner so that recommendations will be adopted for improving the facility's safety and health process, which can lead to the solution of problems in the long term. Some report forms force the investigator to list only surface causes for incidents. Consequently, the investigator may believe the job is done without searching for the root causes. Other forms offer very little space to report findings, and consequently the form may not list the root causes associated with each surface cause. It is not the objective of this section of the form to find fault or place blame. The facts and only the facts should be stated in complete, descriptive statements, not short, cryptic phrases.

Recommendations

If root causes are not addressed properly in the report, it is doubtful that recommendations will include improving system inadequacies. Effective recommendations describe ways to eliminate or reduce both surface and root causes. They also detail estimated investments connected with implementing corrective actions and system improvements.

Workers' Compensation

Workers' compensation protects employees who are injured or contract a disease on the job. Workers' compensation insurance in the United States originated roughly a century ago as a reform of the insurance system designed to maximize benefits to workers while minimizing administrative litiga-tion costs.

Workers' compensation is a state-based system. Statutes limit the com-pensation the worker receives, and the worker cannot sue in court for further damages. Medical benefits vary state to state. Key elements that are common to almost all states are:

1. All work-related injuries and illnesses must be compensated, regardless of fault.
2. There are varying types of benefits, such as temporary total, permanent total, temporary partial, permanent partial, and death.
3. The system does not allow payments for pain and suffering, nor may workers receive punitive damages from their employers.

Workers' compensation is required in most states. Even in states where it is not required, most employers provide it. (An employer that does not carry coverage runs the risk of being sued for major legal damages.)

Workers' Compensation Costs

The national annual average cost for an OSHA-recordable accident is $25,000 to $35,000. An injury resulting from repetitive motion can run up to $100,000. Total workers' compensation costs continue to rise as the average cost of a claim soars. The costs of workers' compensation have risen steadily through the years, with the rates for both the medical and disability components of workers' compensation far exceeding that of inflation.[10]

The following are some of the factors driving pricing in today's market:[11]

1. Higher claims frequency
2. Longer periods of disability
3. Rising medical costs
4. Double-digit increases in the prices of prescription drugs every year for the past five years
5. More preexisting risk factors—especially obesity, diabetes, and an aging workforce—contributing to the incidence and severity of injury and hampering recovery
6. More social complications, such as chemical dependency, mental health conditions, family problems, and violent history, impacting and complicating a greater proportion of claims
7. More benefits extending past the presumed retirement age

Figure 15-8 provides a formula for workers' compensation insurance premiums. The experience modification is a critical factor in the final cost of an employer's workers' compensation policy. Much like the experience rating system used by many states to develop auto insurance rates, a bad year can haunt an employer for years to come. Insurance premiums are based on three consecutive years of workers' compensation experience.

Figure 15–8. Formula for Workers' Compensation Insurance Premiums

---

\# of Accidents
<u>+ \$ Spent on Accidents</u>
Experience Modification

$\downarrow$

Which determines insurance premiums

If an employer can proactively avoid costly workers' compensation claims, money becomes available that would otherwise go toward compensation expenses. As accountants and business owners know, it is not what the health care facility earns, but what it saves that counts.

Workers' compensation fraud has become a high-profile issue, with media reports of "injured" workers painting houses, moving furniture, and conducting other activities that are contraindicated by their compensation claim, and exacting huge settlements for bogus claims. Those arrested for workers' compensation fraud are not just people who collect benefits they are not entitled to receive. Examples of fraud also include physicians who submit bills for patients who were never examined or for treatments that were not provided. Other examples involve employers regularly billing for more time than was actually spent with a patient, duplicate billing, and receiving payment from more than one insurance carrier for the same treatment—and not making restitution.

Workers' compensation reform legislation is spreading among states, and premium reduction strategies are working. These include joint employer-employee safety and health committees, managed care programs, aggressive antifraud initiatives, strict limits on claims litigation, and the use of medical fee schedules. Some states have enacted stiff penalties for compensation fraud, backed by media advertisements warning workers to "think twice" before filing false claims.

Incentives to Return to Work

Returning the employee to work as soon as medically possible is essential in properly managing workers' compensation claims, and it is better for the employee physically and psychologically.

Generally speaking, injured employees who cannot return to work are paid two-thirds of their salaries to recuperate at home. From a business standpoint, this expense translates to dollars that could have been spent on office equipment or employee benefits and raises and dollars not spent for replacement employees. Supervisors and managers benefit when they help employees return to work as soon as possible. Money is saved that would have been spent on hiring temporaries, costs for lost workdays are decreased, employee morale is promoted throughout the department, productivity is maintained, and the potential for adversarial relationships among employees is minimized.

Department managers can positively or negatively influence their net costs for workers' compensation coverage. This power is critical to health care facilities in both economic and human terms. When health and safety is a high priority, management, employees, and the public realize the direct benefits.

Risk Management Strategies

Effective workers' compensation management requires a risk management approach to minimize the risks and reduce costs associated with employee injuries and illnesses. Risk management, as it relates to workers' compensation, has a two-part focus: prevention and case management.

The prevention strategies discussed throughout this book should be the main thrust of the approach. Employees should be educated about the workers' compensation system, including what it covers, what it does not cover, the cost of workers' compensation, the facility's philosophy about workers' compensation, and the return-to-work policies.

Case management is effective follow-up after employee incidents. Department managers have a responsibility to injured workers and also to control workers' compensation dollars. Case management steps include a relationship with a designated medical provider for occupational health services and a return-to-work program that includes transitional jobs.

JOINT COMMISSION ACCREDITATION: A TOOL FOR ENSURING IMPROVED SURVEILLANCE AND DATA COLLECTION

The Joint Commission's procedures for responding to a sentinel event among patients are strikingly similar to the procedures used to identify the root causes of employee injuries and illnesses. Therefore, as each health care facility regularly assesses its compliance with Joint Commission standards (through the periodic performance review, on-site survey, and other mechanisms), it can use that opportunity to assess its OSHA compliance status as well. In addition to assessing the facility's compliance with OSHA regulations, the facility should look at the Joint Commission's Environment of Care standards, specifically:

    □ EC.1.10, The health care facility manages safety risks
    □ EC.1.20, The health care facility maintains a safe environment
    □ EC.9.10, The health care facility monitors conditions in the
      environment

☐ EC.9.20, The health care facility analyzes identified environment issues and develops recommendations for resolving them

☐ EC.9.30, The health care facility improves the environment

The elements of performance for EC.1.20 provide the health care facility with an ideal opportunity to review its record of performance concerning compliance with OSHA regulations. One way of doing this is by reviewing OSHA Form 300 logs.

THE ROLE OF THE ENVIRONMENTAL HEALTH AND SAFETY DEPARTMENT

Surveillance, data analysis, and incident management are among the most significant functions of the Environmental Health and Safety Department. The routine collection and analysis of the data will allow identification of controls that have failed or are inadequate, tasks for which additional or refresher training is needed, and emerging health and safety hazards.

The staff of the Environmental Health and Safety Department, in conjunction with the department liaisons and other appropriate staff, should conduct accident investigations. Investigations must be methodical and thorough and targeted at identifying causes rather than assessing blame.

The Environmental Health and Safety Department must work closely with the department liaisons to ensure that information is recorded promptly and accurately. The department liaisons will often be the first to observe or learn of health and safety problems that need immediate attention.

References

1. Portions of this section were adapted from the Michigan Hospital Association's medical surveillance program.
2. OSHA. *Screening and Surveillance: A Guide to OSHA Standards.* OSHA 3162 2000 (reprint). Available at http://www.osha.gov/Publications/osha3162.pdf (accessed 3/29/2006).
3. Newman, Mary A., and John B. Kachuba. *An Asbestos Abatement Program for Healthcare Institutions.* Cincinnati: Healthcare Environments, 1990.
4. NIOSH. *Worker Health Chartbook,* 2004 ed. HHS (NIOSH) Publication No. 2004-146. Available at http://www.cdc.gov/niosh/docs/chartbook/ (accessed 3/29/2006).
5. See NIOSH website, www.cdc.gov/niosh.
6. Laramie, Angela, and Letitia Davis. *The Link between Workplace and Public Health Surveillance: Example of a Web-Based Surveillance System for Sharps Injuries among Health Care Workers in Massachusetts.* Available at http://www.cdc.gov/niosh/sbw/public_health/pdfs/laramie.pdf (accessed 3/29/2006).
7. Ramazzini, Bernardino. *Diseases of Workers.* Translated from the Latin text *DeMorbis Articum* (1713) by Wilmer Cave Wright. OH&S Press, 1993.

8. Morris, William. *American Heritage Dictionary*. New College Edition. Boston: Houghton Mifflin, 1976.

9. OSHA Standard 29 CFR 1910 Subpart I, Appendix B. *Non-mandatory Compliance Guidelines for Hazard Assessment and Personal Protective Equipment Selection*. Available at http://www.osha.gov/pls/oshaweb/owadisp.show_document?p_table=STANDARDS&p_id=10120 (accessed 3/29/2006).

10. Menard, R.A. II. *Talking Dollars & Sense: Occupational Health & Safety*. Dallas: Stevens Publishing Corporation, 2001, pp. 62–65.

11. Farmers Insurance Pool. Available at http://www.farmersinsurancepool.com/report.html (accessed 3/29/2006).

CHAPTER 16

TRAINING AND DEVELOPMENT

He arrived in late August. Eager and filled with the anticipation of his first biochemistry course, he couldn't wait for the first class to begin. Oddly, there was no text; but then this was graduate school, and he knew that it would be different. The expectation of a higher level of thought and discussion was seductive. He entered the classroom early. He was never late for anything, not even a dentist's appointment. He took a seat and waited. The professor entered, wrote his name on the board, and with no introductory discussion began drawing molecular chemical structures the young man had never seen before. They were odd mixtures of rings and straight chains with lots of "functional groups" hanging on. The names were strange and didn't conform to any of the terminology he had learned during several years of advanced organic chemistry. Every now and then the professor would draw an arrow from one molecule to another, slightly different one. The arrow was the symbol typically used to show that two or more substances had reacted to produce something different. But in this case the diagram began with only one chemical, and over the arrow the professor wrote strange words that all ended with "-ase." The young man assumed that at some point the professor would provide an explanation of what he was doing, particularly since long strings of such reactions were connected one to the other, ending in a compound that bore no resemblance to the original substance. Days became weeks, but the explanation that the young man had hoped would be forthcoming never came. And then it was time for the first examination.

He reviewed his notes but had no idea what it was he was to be tested on. Though he had learned that words ending with "ase" were things called "enzymes," he had no idea what an enzyme did, how it did it, or what its composition was. The first test was brutal. He thought that he would be required to provide explanations of chemical reactions, but the professor expected only one simple thing: the complete regurgitation of everything he had written on the board. In some cases, the professor had provided the name of one of the odd chemicals and asked for its structure to be given as the answer. Those "questions" had a value of 3 points. Although the chemical may have been composed of 15 or more atoms, if just one hydrogen atom was omitted or misplaced, 1 point out of the 3 was deducted.

After failing the first two examinations, the discouraged young man finally understood that all he had to do to be successful was to memorize each and every thing the professor wrote on the board. By the end of the course, his ability to memorize had dramatically increased (though at the expense of his personal life and psyche) and he achieved the desired B, which was the best he could expect after such a shaky beginning. He also learned that the long chain of reactions represented what was called a metabolic pathway, and that his previous education, which had taught him how to think, analyze, and apply the principles of chemistry, was useless in this course.

Education is the acquisition of the art of the utilization of knowledge. This is an art very difficult to impart. Whenever a textbook is written of real educational worth, you may be quite certain that some reviewer will say that it will be difficult to teach from it. Of course it will be difficult to teach from it. If it were easy, the book ought to be burned; for it cannot be educational. In education, as elsewhere, the broad primrose path leads to a nasty place. This evil path is represented by a book or a set of lectures which will practically enable the student to learn by heart all the questions likely to be asked at the next external examination.

Alfred North Whitehead, *The Aims of Education*

There are many theories of education and training, but Whitehead articulated a core value:

> The point of education is to learn but not for the sake of simply passing an examination or obtaining a certificate.

In the arena of Environmental Health and Safety, the requirement to learn is bolstered by the fact that the lives and well-being of others are dependent on proper training and the daily application of that training.

To simply comply with the worker training requirements imposed by a variety of public and private organizations is not enough. The material must be understood, practiced, and relearned. While the Occupational Safety and Health Administration (OSHA), the Food and Drug Administration (FDA), the Environmental Protection Agency (EPA), the Department of Health and Human Services (HHS), and a variety of state and local health and safety agencies and accreditation organizations each have requirements and guidelines that impact the health care facility, there is not only overlap among them but an interconnection as well. It is the discovery and application of the underlying principles that is the key to grasping why those standards and regulations exist and why they are written as they are. Harbored within that understanding is the ability to see the interconnections and realize the fruits of proper training.

Some insight regarding the value that organizations place on training can be gained from the American Society for Training and Development (ASTD). In its annual report published in 2005, *State of the Industry: ASTD's Annual Review of Trends in Workplace Learning*, ASTD provided data showing how various industry sectors allocate funds for training and development.[1] The trade and wholesale sector, government, and health care spent less per full-time employee on training and development than any other industry sector. While the overall average spent per employee in 2004 was about $955.00, the health care industry spent just $658.00 per employee. Furthermore, the average amount of instruction across all industries was more than 32 hours per full-time employee, while in health care fewer than 28 hours per employee were devoted to training and development. However, only the agriculture, mining, and construction sector spent a larger percent of its profit on training and development (13.90 percent) compared with health care (10.34 percent).

According to the ASTD survey, the majority of the health care training (18.2 percent) was devoted to topics specific to the health care industry, but a disproportionate amount of training time compared with all other industry sectors was spent on new-employee orientation (12.37 percent for health care vs. 6.06 percent for all industries). It is noteworthy that the health care industry devoted about 16.5 percent of its training and development time to issues concerning compliance.

Training should not be viewed as a requisite burden imposed by agencies and organizations, but rather as an opportunity to build corporate competency and morale. A secondary outcome is that training requirements help protect patients and the general public. Many federal health and safety standards require that training and information be provided to employees and that the employees' training be documented. Facilities should also contact the appropriate state agency to determine which, if any, state requirements may apply.

TRAINING AND TRAINING GUIDELINES

There a number of circumstances that require training:

- Training new employees about the facility's health and safety policy as well as the requirements of the standards and regulations that directly affect them
- Retraining in the event that surveillance data indicates a lapse in compliance
- The introduction of new chemicals, equipment, or procedures
- Annual refresher training
- Professional development or enhancing an employee's competencies

The intent behind every health and safety standard is that certain employees be trained. Requirements on the nature and extent of the training vary. It is the responsibility of the department manager in consultation with the Environmental Health and Safety Department to determine what training is needed, who needs the training, and how often training is to be provided, and to develop training guidelines around those requirements.

Every health care facility employee does not need to be trained on every standard. Training programs should be tailored to the needs and responsibilities of both supervisors and employees as well as to specific job and departmental responsibilities. Supervisors must also receive training so that they can understand the hazards associated with a job and their potential effects on employees, and the supervisor's role in ensuring that employees follow the rules, procedures, and work practices for controlling hazards. Employees must understand the hazards to which they may be exposed, how to prevent harm to themselves and others, and the importance of following the employer's safety and health rules.

Some OSHA state plan agencies publish training materials that health care facilities can use to train employees. [CD-ROM 16.1] Many of these agencies also promote health and safety through community outreach efforts, Spanish-language courses, and youth initiatives. The training provided aids employers in the recognition, avoidance, and prevention of unsafe and unhealthful working conditions.

The OSHA Training Institute provides training and education in occupational safety and health for federal and state compliance officers, state consultants, other federal agency personnel, and the private sector.[2] The length and complexity of OSHA standards may make it difficult to find all the references to training. Therefore, to help employers, safety and health professionals, training directors, and others with a need to know, OSHA's training-related requirements have been excerpted and collected in its publication *Training Requirements in OSHA Standards and Training Guidelines* in the form of a model.[3] [CD-ROM 16.2] Requirements for posting information, warning signs, labels, and the like are excluded, as are most references to the qualifications of people assigned to test workplace conditions or equipment.

This model is designed to help employers develop instructional programs as part of their total education and training effort. The model addresses the questions of who should be trained, on what topics, and for what purposes. It also helps employers determine how effective the program has been and enables them to identify employees who are in greatest need of education and training. The model is general enough to be used in any area of occupational safety and health training, and it allows employers to determine for themselves the content and format of training. Use of this model in training activities is just one of many ways that employers can comply with the OSHA standards on training and enhance the safety and health of their employees. The training guideline model is organized as follows:

a) Determining if training is needed
b) Identifying training needs

    c) Identifying goals and objectives

    d) Developing learning activities

    e) Conducting the training

    f) Evaluating program effectiveness

    g) Improving the program

The model is designed to be one that even facilities with very few employees can use. With this model, employers or supervisors can develop and administer safety and health training programs that address problems specific to their own facility, fulfill the learning needs of their own employees, and strengthen the overall safety and health program of the workplace.

Determining If Training Is Needed

The first step in the training process is a basic one: to determine whether training can solve a problem. When employees are not performing their jobs properly, it is often assumed that training will bring them up to standards. However, it is possible that other actions (such as hazard abatement or the implementation of engineering controls) would better enable employees to perform their jobs properly.

Ideally, safety and health training should be provided before problems or accidents occur. This training would cover both general safety and health rules and work procedures, and would be repeated if an accident or near-miss incident occurred.

Problems that can be addressed effectively by training include those that arise from lack of knowledge of a work process, unfamiliarity with equipment, or incorrect execution of a task. Training is less effective (but still can be used) for problems arising from an employee's lack of motivation or lack of attention to the job. Whatever its purpose, training is most effective when designed in concert with the goals of the facility's total safety and health program.

Identifying Training Needs

If the problem is one that can be solved, in whole or in part, by training, then the next step is to determine what training is needed. For this, it is necessary to identify (1) what the employee is expected to do and (2) in what ways, if any, the employee's performance is deficient. This information can be obtained by conducting a job analysis that pinpoints what an employee needs to know in order to perform the job.

In designing a new training program or preparing to instruct an employee in an unfamiliar procedure or system, a job analysis can be developed by examining engineering data on new equipment or the safety data sheets on unfamiliar substances. The content of the specific federal or state standards applicable to a facility can also provide direction in developing training content. Another option is to conduct a job hazard analysis (JHA). This is a procedure for studying and recording each step of a job, identifying existing or potential hazards, and determining the best way to reduce or eliminate the risks to ensure acceptable performance of the job. Information obtained from a JHA can be used as the content for the training activity.[4] [CD-ROM 16.3]

If an employer's learning needs can be met by the revision of an existing training program rather than the development of a new one, or if the employer already has some knowledge of the process or system to be used, appropriate training content can be developed through such means as:

- □ Using the health care facility's accident and injury records to identify how accidents occur and what can be done to prevent them from recurring.
- □ Requesting employees to provide, in writing and in their own words, descriptions of their jobs. These should include the tasks performed and the tools, materials, and equipment used.
- □ Observing employees at the worksite as they perform tasks, asking about the work, and recording their answers.
- □ Examining similar training programs offered by other health care facilities or obtaining suggestions from such organizations as the Bureau of Labor Statistics (BLS), OSHA-approved services and programs, other regulatory agencies and associations, or private companies.

The employees themselves can provide valuable information on the training they need. Safety and health hazards can be identified through the employees' responses to such questions as whether anything about their jobs concerns them, if they have had any near-miss incidents, if they feel they are taking risks, or if they believe that their jobs involve hazardous operations or substances.

Identifying Goals and Objectives

Once the kind of training that is needed has been determined, it is equally important to determine what kind of training is not needed. Employees should be made aware of all the steps involved in a task or procedure, but training should focus on those steps for which skills or improved performance is needed. This approach tailors the training to the needs of the employees.

Once the employees' training needs have been identified, employers can prepare objectives for the training. Instructional objectives, if clearly stated, provide employers with an idea of what they want their employees to do, to do better, or to stop doing.

Learning objectives do not necessarily have to be written, but in order for the training to be as successful as possible, clear and measurable objectives should be thought out before the training begins. For an objective to be effective, it should identify as precisely as possible what the individuals will do to demonstrate that they have learned, or that the objective has been reached. Learning objectives should also describe the important conditions under which the individual will demonstrate competence and should define what constitutes acceptable performance.

Using specific, action-oriented language, the instructional objectives should describe the preferred practice or skill and its observable behavior. For example, rather than using the statement "The employee will understand how to use a respirator" as an instructional objective, it would be better to say, "The employee will be able to describe how a respirator works, when it should be used, and when it is being used properly." Objectives are most effective when worded in sufficient detail that other qualified persons can recognize when the desired behavior is exhibited.

Developing Learning Activities

Once employers have precisely stated the objectives for the training program, learning activities can be identified and described. Learning activities enable employees to demonstrate that they have acquired the desired skills and knowledge. To ensure that employees transfer the skills or knowledge from the learning activity to the job, the learning situation should simulate the objectives and activities in a sequence that corresponds to the order in which the tasks are to be performed on the job, if a specific process is to be learned. For example, if an employee must learn the beginning processes of using a machine, the sequence might be:

1. Check that the power source is connected.
2. Ensure that the safety devices are in place and are operative.
3. Know when and how to throw the switch.
4. Other required procedures.

A few factors will help to determine the type of learning activity to be incorporated into the training. One is the training resources available to the health care facility. Can a group training program that uses an outside trainer be organized, or should the facility personally train the employees on a one-to-one basis? Should a train-the-trainer program be initiated? Another factor is the kind of skills or knowledge to be learned. Is the learning oriented toward physical skills (such as the use of special tools) or toward mental processes and attitudes? The training activity can be group oriented, with lectures, role play, and demonstrations, or designed for the individual (e.g., self-paced instruction).

The methods and materials chosen for the learning activity can be as varied as the employer's imagination and available resources will allow. The employer may want to use charts, diagrams, manuals, slides, skits, games, music, eLearning, videos, or simply a blackboard and chalk—or any combination of these and other instructional aids. Whatever the method of instruction, the learning activities should be developed in such a way that the employees can clearly demonstrate acquisition of the desired skills or knowledge.

Figure 16–1. Examples of Training Techniques

- ☐ Provide overviews of the material to be learned.
- ☐ Relate, wherever possible, the new information or skills to the employee's goals, interests, or experience.
- ☐ Reinforce what the employees have learned by summarizing the program's objectives and the key points of information covered. These steps will assist employers in presenting the training in a clear, unambiguous manner.

Conducting the Training

With the completion of the steps outlined above, the facility is ready to begin conducting the training. To the extent possible, the training should be presented so that its organization and meaning are clear to the employees. Toward this end, employers or supervisors should conduct the training using the techniques listed in figure 16-1.

In addition to organizing the content, employers must develop the structure and format of the training. The content developed for the program, the nature of the workplace or other training site, and the resources available for training will help facilities determine for themselves the frequency of training activities, the length of the sessions, the instructional techniques, and the individual(s) best qualified to present the information.

For employees to be motivated to pay attention and learn the material that the employer or supervisor is presenting, they must be convinced of the importance and relevance of the material. Among the ways of developing motivation are:

- ☐ Explaining the objectives of instruction
- ☐ Relating the training to the interests, skills, and experiences of the employees
- ☐ Outlining the main points to be presented during the training session(s)
- ☐ Pointing out the benefits of training (i.e., the employee will be better informed, more skilled, and thus more valuable on the job, or the employee will be able to work at reduced risk if the skills and knowledge learned are applied)

An effective training program allows employees to participate in the training process and to practice their skills or knowledge. This will help to ensure that they are learning the required knowledge or skills and will permit correction, if necessary. Employees can become involved in the training process by participating in discussions, asking questions, contributing their knowledge and expertise, learning through hands-on experiences, and engaging in role-playing exercises.

Evaluating Program Effectiveness

To make sure that the training program is accomplishing its goals, an evaluation of the training can be undertaken. Training should have, as one of its critical components, a method of measuring its effectiveness. A plan for evaluating the training session(s), either written or decided by the employer, should be developed in conjunction with the course objectives and content; it should not be delayed until the training has been completed. Evaluation will help employers or supervisors determine the amount of learning that has been achieved and whether an employee's performance has improved on the job. Among the methods of evaluating training are:

☐ *Employee opinion:* Questionnaires or informal discussions with employees can help the employer determine the relevance and appropriateness of the training program.

☐ *Supervisors' observations:* Supervisors are in a good position to observe an employee's performance both before and after the training and to note improvements or other changes.

☐ *Workplace improvements:* The ultimate measure of success of a training program may be changes throughout the workplace that result in reduced injury or accident rates.

An evaluation of training can give employers the information necessary to decide whether or not the employees have achieved the desired results and whether the training session should be offered again at some future date.

Improving the Program

If, after evaluation, it is clear that the training did not provide employees with the level of knowledge and skill that was expected, it may be necessary to revise the training program or provide periodic retraining. At this point, asking questions of employees and of those who conducted the training may be of some help. Examples of questions that could be asked are listed in figure 16-2.

Figure 16–2. Examples of Questions to Ask in the Event of Retraining

---

☐ Were parts of the content already known and, therefore, unnecessary?

☐ What material was confusing or distracting?

☐ Was anything missing from the program?

☐ What did the employees learn, and what did they fail to learn?

It may be necessary to repeat steps in the training process, that is, to return to the first steps and retrace one's way through the training process. As the program is evaluated, the employer should ask:

- ☐ If a job analysis was conducted, was it accurate?
- ☐ Was any critical feature of the job overlooked?
- ☐ Were the important gaps in knowledge and skill included?
- ☐ Was material that was already known by the employees intentionally omitted?
- ☐ Were the instructional objectives presented clearly and concretely?
- ☐ Did the objectives state the level of acceptable performance that was expected of employees?
- ☐ Did the learning activity simulate the actual job?
- ☐ Was the learning activity appropriate for the kinds of knowledge and skills required on the job?
- ☐ When the training was presented, were the organization of the material and its meaning made clear?
- ☐ Were the employees motivated to learn?
- ☐ Were the employees allowed to participate actively in the training process?
- ☐ Was the employer's evaluation of the program thorough?

A critical examination of the steps in the training process will help the facility to determine where course revision is necessary.

FUNDAMENTALS OF TRAINING AND EDUCATION

Malcolm Knowles is one of the most frequently cited theorists in adult education. In *The Modern Practice of Adult Education* (1970), Knowles articulated four assumptions concerning adult learning. According to Knowles, adults in learning situations:

1. Move from dependency to self-directedness
2. Draw upon their reservoir of experience for learning
3. Are ready to learn when they assume new roles
4. Want to solve problems and apply new knowledge immediately

Accordingly, Knowles suggested that adult educators should:

- ☐ Set a cooperative learning climate.
- ☐ Create mechanisms for mutual planning.
- ☐ Arrange for a diagnosis of learner needs and interests.

- Enable the formulation of learning objectives based on the diagnosed needs and interests.
- Design sequential activities for achieving the objectives.
- Execute the design by selecting methods, materials, and resources.
- Evaluate the quality of the learning experience while assessing the need for further learning.

In 1995 Marcia Conner wrote a white paper for Wave Technologies titled "Learning: The Critical Technology," in which she described learning as "the act, process, or experience of gaining knowledge or skills." Conner assumed that learning is (1) any increase in knowledge, (2) memorizing information, (3) acquiring knowledge for practical use, (4) abstracting meaning from what we do, and (5) a process that allows us to understand.[5] Conner continued:

> Western society once believed adults didn't learn. Even today, if you ask a group why adults cannot learn, it may surprise you how many begin answering the question without challenging the premise. Unfortunately, many adults deny themselves what should be one of the most enriching parts of life because they assume they can't learn.
>
> We can learn from everything the mind perceives (at any age). Our brains build and strengthen neural pathways no matter where we are, no matter what the subject or the context.
>
> In today's business environment, finding better ways to learn will propel organizations forward. Strong minds fuel strong organizations. We must capitalize on our natural styles and then build systems to satisfy needs. Only through an individual learning process can we re-create our environments and ourselves.

The views of Whitehead, Knowles, and Conner lead to the following fundamental precepts of adult learning:

- Learning is the acquisition and the application of knowledge.
- Rote memorization is not necessarily learning.
- Adults often base their acquisition of new knowledge on their past experiences.
- Individuals learn in different ways.
- Training and education of employees enhance the corporate bottom line.

The success of training depends on the establishment of a climate conducive to learning. A positive climate is one that stimulates discussion and the sharing of information. A group that has the freedom to express thoughts clearly and freely and feels secure in doing so is far ahead in the growth experience of the education process.

Technology-Based Learning

Effective safety training activities include techniques such as discussion, group brainstorming, demonstrations, and hands-on experiences. Traditional self-study permits trainees to progress at the pace that best suits them, and this approach should be combined with activities that involve instructor participation, opportunity for questions, and learning by doing.

As health care facilities continue to merge or partner with other facilities, additional safety training options become available. Many facilities are making dramatic changes in the way they develop the safety knowledge and skills of their workforce with technology-based learning. Self-directed learning, using such resources as interactive CDs, and distance learning via the Internet are examples of technology-based learning.

In OSHA's view, self-paced, interactive computer-based training can serve as a valuable training tool in the context of an overall training program. However, the use of computer-based training by itself is not sufficient to meet the intent of most OSHA training requirements.[6] On this type of training, OSHA's policy is essentially the same as its policy on the use of training videos, since the two approaches have similar shortcomings. Employers are urged to avoid relying solely on generic, packaged training programs to meet their training requirements. For example, training under the Bloodborne pathogens standard includes site-specific elements and should also be tailored to workers' assigned duties. In an effective training program, it is critical that trainees have an opportunity to ask questions if material is unfamiliar to them. In a computer-based program, this requirement may be met by providing a telephone hotline so that trainees have direct access to a qualified trainer.

Hands-on training and exercises provide trainees with an opportunity to become familiar with equipment, personal protective equipment, and safe work practices in a nonhazardous setting. Sole reliance on computer-based training programs will not provide the same level of understanding and competency as those programs that require direct interaction.

The reason for OSHA's warning about packaged programs is that health and safety training involves the presentation of technical material to audiences who typically have not had formal education in technical or scientific disciplines, such as in areas of chemistry or physiology. In an effective training program, it is critical that trainees have the opportunity to ask questions when material is unfamiliar to them. Traditional, hands-on training is OSHA's preferred method of preparing workers to safely perform job tasks.

Safety Training Requirements in OSHA Standards and Training Guidelines

Many standards promulgated by OSHA explicitly require the employer to train employees in the safety and health aspects of their jobs. Other OSHA standards make it the employer's responsibility to limit certain job assignments to employees who are "competent" or "qualified"—meaning that they have had special prior training in or outside the workplace or are experienced in the job.

Certain OSHA standards require a "competent person" to perform specific functions under the standard. In 18 subparts of the 1926 construction standards and 6 of the 1910 general industry standards, OSHA refers to requirements for a "competent person," meaning someone who has had special previous training in or out of the workplace. One of OSHA's top 10 citations among construction industry employers relates to the failure to provide a "competent person." A "competent person" is defined in 29 CFR 1926.32(f)[7] [CD-ROM 16.4] as:

> one who is capable of identifying existing and predictable hazards in the surroundings or working conditions which are unsanitary, hazardous, or dangerous to employees, and who has authorization to take prompt corrective measures to eliminate them.

The definition has two distinct parts:

> "Capable of identifying existing and predictable hazards in the surroundings or working conditions which are unsanitary, hazardous, or dangerous to employees"
>
> "Who has authorization to take prompt corrective measures to eliminate them"

Although training courses exist that are intended to build specific competencies, there are no courses that will by themselves make someone a "competent person." These OSHA standards simply require the employer to place competent persons in those positions in which they are required. Although there are no specific criteria for formal training, in assessing the facility's choice OSHA may review the "competent person's" safety training background; it may, of course, also review the training records of any and all workers in the facility during an inspection. A person is not required by OSHA to be "certified" using a rigid set of criteria or by any organization or agency; the person must simply meet the requirements of competency defined in 1926.32(f).

Identifying Employees at Risk

One method of identifying employee populations at high risk (and thus in greater need of safety and health training) is to pinpoint hazardous occupations. Even within industries that are hazardous in general, some employees operate at greater risk than others. In other cases, the hazardousness of an occupation is influenced by the conditions under which it is performed, such as noise, heat or cold, or safety/health hazards in the surrounding area. In these situations, employees should be trained not only on how to perform their jobs safely, but also on how to operate within a hazardous environment.

A second method of identifying employee populations at high levels of risk is to examine the incidence of accidents and injuries, both within the health care facility and within the industry. If employees in certain occupational categories are experiencing higher accident and injury rates than other employees, training may be one way to reduce these rates. In addition, thorough accident investigation procedures cannot only identify specific employees who could benefit from training, but also identify company-wide training needs.

Research has indicated the following variables as being related to a disproportionate share of employee injuries and illnesses at the worksite:

□ The age of the employee (younger employees have higher incidence rates)

□ The length of time on the job (new employees have higher incidence rates)

□ The size of the firm (in general, medium-size firms have higher incidence rates than small or large firms)

□ The type of work performed (incidence and severity rate vary significantly by NAICS/SIC code)

□ The use of hazardous substances (by NAICS/SIC code)

These variables should be considered in the process of identifying employee groups for training in occupational safety and health. Information is readily available to help employers identify which employees should receive safety and health information, education, and training, and which employees should receive it before others.

Training Employees at Risk

Determining the content of training for employee populations at higher levels of risk is similar to determining what any employee needs to know, but more emphasis is placed on the requirements of the job and the possibility of injury. One useful tool for determining training content from job requirements is the job hazard analysis. This procedure examines each step of a job, identifies existing or potential hazards, and determines the best way to perform the job in order to reduce or eliminate the hazards. Its key elements are:

□ Job description

□ Job location

□ Key steps (preferably in the order performed)

□ Tools, machines, and materials used

     ☐ Actual and potential safety and health hazards associated with
these key job steps

     ☐ Safe and healthful practices, apparel, and equipment required for
each job step

Material safety data sheets (MSDSs) can also provide information for training employees in the safe use of chemicals. These data sheets, developed by chemical manufacturers and importers, are supplied with manufacturing or construction materials and describe the ingredients of a product, its hazards, protective equipment to be used, safe handling procedures, and emergency first-aid responses. The information contained in these sheets can help employers identify employees in need of training (i.e., workers handling substances described in the sheets) and train these employees in the safe use of the substances. Material safety data sheets are generally available from suppliers or manufacturers of the substance. They are particularly useful for employers who are developing training on chemical use as required by OSHA's Hazard communication standard.

AUDITING TRAINING

Occupational safety and health training remains a fundamental element in workplace hazard control programs. Training objectives, recognition of job hazards, learning safe work practices, and appreciating other preventive measures contribute to the goal of reducing occupational risk of injury and disease. The publication *Assessing Occupational Safety and Health Training: A Literature Review* [CD-ROM 16.5], available from NIOSH, reviews data found in the literature reflecting the significance of training in meeting these objectives and outcomes. In addition to presenting an analysis to identify factors underlying a successful training experience, the document offers an agenda for addressing outstanding needs and ways to strengthen the role of training in improving workplace safety and health.

The review sought data from the literature bearing on two questions: Are occupational safety and health training requirements, as cited in many federal standards governing workplace conditions and operations, effective in reducing work-related injury and illness? Does the available evidence show certain training factors or practices to be more important than others in positively influencing these outcome measures?

SAFETY TRAINING FOR MULTICULTURAL EMPLOYEES

During the last 20 years there has been an increase in the number of people in the American workforce for whom English is a second language. To ensure that training is uniform and consistent, careful consideration should be given to providing training in the native languages of employees—particularly those of Hispanic origin, since the number of Spanish-speaking workers has increased significantly. Federal agencies such as OSHA and NIOSH and many organizations have translated their publications into Spanish, and many websites offer their material in a variety of languages. Non–English-speaking employees' cultural backgrounds may influence their approach to learning. Many websites present resources for multicultural workers.[8,9,10,11]

THE JOINT COMMISSION AS A RESOURCE FOR TRAINING AND DEVELOPMENT

The Joint Commission wants to ensure that health care facility staff receive the information they need to do their jobs properly and to provide high-quality, safe care for patients. Joint Commission Management of Human Resources standard HR.1.20 specifically addresses this issue. Standard HR.1.20 requires that the organization have a process to ensure that employees' qualifications are consistent with their job responsibilities. Another Joint Commission standard requires initial job training and information for employees during orientation (standard HR.2.10). Standard HR.2.20 requires health care facilities to ensure that all employees, licensed independent practitioners, students, and volunteers can describe or demonstrate their roles and responsibilities based on specific job duties or responsibilities relative to safety.

An employee's ongoing education needs required by HR.2.20 are based on the information obtained during the risk assessment steps described in the "Management of the Environment of Care" standards, and thus will vary based on the employee's potential risk. Standard HR.2.30, Element of Performance (EP) 8, requires that employees' ongoing education be documented. To ensure that an employee's ongoing education has been effective, standard HR.3.10 calls for an assessment of each employee's continuing ability to perform the responsibilities of the job. While these standards are essential to ensuring that employees understand the duties and potential hazards of their jobs, they are not a substitute for complying with the specific training requirements provided in OSHA standards.

THE ROLE OF THE ENVIRONMENTAL HEALTH AND SAFETY DEPARTMENT

As a first step in providing a strong and dynamic training program, the Environmental Health and Safety Department must work closely with the Human Resources Department to develop materials for new employees that explain the organizational structure and function of the department. At a minimum, those materials should include the facility's health and safety policy and the employees' rights and responsibilities articulated in the Occupational Safety and Health Act (OSH Act).

The Environmental Health and Safety Department has two significant functions to ensure that the facility's employees are properly trained.

☐ Determining training needs, course contents, schedules, and the method by which employees are trained

☐ Ensuring that its own staff and the department liaisons are able to provide training under the direction of the Environmental Health and Safety training director

Training should begin with an explanation of the OSH Act and the roles of federal, state, and local governments and independent accrediting organizations in relation to employee safety and health.

Training the Environmental Health and Safety Department

It is expected that the staff of the Environmental Health and Safety Department will have already acquired a significant understanding of Environmental Health and Safety as a result of either formal education or significant experience. Nevertheless, they should be encouraged to continue building their competencies through interaction with other Environmental Health and Safety professionals in other venues and formal training courses taught outside the facility either by well-qualified private organizations or through the Occupational Safety and Health Administration, which operates training institutes in several cities throughout the United States. Among the courses offered by OSHA are those that are required in OSHA's 10- and 30-hour programs, as well as on those that address the most hazardous occupations, as determined by OSHA. Other OSHA courses cover occupational safety and health standards for construction, permit-required confined-space entry, electrical standards, introduction to safety and health management, introduction to accident investigation, recordkeeping rule seminar, industrial hygiene, health hazard awareness, and bloodborne pathogens exposure control for health care facilities. The goal of such training is not simply to pass an accreditation survey or an OSHA inspection, but rather to build a first-tier Environmental Health and Safety program.

Training Department Liaisons

The department liaisons can provide department-specific training to their colleagues. Thus, one function of the training provided by the Environmental Health and Safety Department is to "train the trainer." Such training should be directed at building standard-specific competency as well as problem solving in the event that the department liaison detects a breakdown in compliance with a standard. The Small Business Outreach Training Program by OSHA is one source for teaching department liaisons. [CD-ROM 16.6] Course

501, Trainer Course in OSHA Standards for General Industry, is designed for individuals, such as Environmental Health and Safety staff, who are interested in teaching OSHA's 10- and 30-hour programs to department liaisons or other health care facility employees. There are prerequisites and continuing-education requirements, which are outlined in OSHA's Training Institute Education Center course descriptions. [CD-ROM 16.7]

References

1. Sugrue, Brenda, and Ray J. Rivera. *State of the Industry. ASTD's Annual Review of Trends in Workplace Learning and Performance*. Alexandria, VA: American Society for Training and Development, 2005.

2. Information available at http://www.osha.gov/fso/ote/training/edcenters/index.html (accessed 3/29/2006).

3. OSHA 2254 1998 (revised), *Training Requirements in OSHA Standards and Training Guidelines*. Available at http://www.osha.gov/Publications/osha2254.pdf (accessed 3/29/2006).

4. OSHA 3071, *Job Hazard Analysis*. Available at http://www.osha.gov/Publications/osha3071.pdf (accessed 3/29/2006).

5. Conner, Marcia L. "Learning: The Critical Technology (An Industry Whitepaper). St. Louis: Wave Technologies International, February 1995. Available at http://www.learnativity.com/download/Learning_Whitepaper96.pdf (accessed 3/29/2006).

6. OSHA Standard Interpretations. *Appropriateness of Computer-Based Interactive Training Programs to Satisfy Required OSHA Training*. June 11, 1997. Available at http://www.osha.gov/pls/oshaweb/owadisp.show_document?p_table=INTERPRETATIONS&p_id=22425 (accessed 3/29/2006).

7. OSHA 1926.32. *Safety and Health Regulations for Construction: Definitions*. Available at http://www.osha.gov/pls/oshaweb/owadisp.show_document?p_table=STANDARDS&p_id=10618 (accessed 3/29/2006).

8. Hayes, Casey. "Emergency Response for the Multicultural Work Force," *Occupational Hazards* (March 20, 2006). Available at http://www.occupational-hazards.com/articles/14895 (accessed 3/27/2006).

9. Cable, Josh. "The Multicultural Work Force: The Melting Pot Heats Up," *Occupational Hazards* (March 13, 2006). Available at http://www.occupational-hazards.com/articles/14866 (accessed 3/27/2006).

10. "Keeping the Multicultural Workforce Safe," *Workers' Comp Insider* (March 14, 2006). Available at http://www.workerscompinsider.com/archives/000456.html (accessed 3/30/2006).

11. New Jersey Department of Health & Senior Services. Office of Minority and Multicultural Health. *Cultural Competency Information and Resources*. Available at http://www.nj.gov/health/commiss/omh/competency.shtml (accessed 3/29/2006).

CHAPTER 17

FACILITIES RESPONSIBILITIES AND ENVIRONMENTAL ISSUES

Once upon a time, there was a great famine in which people hoarded their food, hiding it even from their friends and neighbors. One day a wandering soldier came into a village and began asking questions as if he planned to stay for the night.

"There's not a bite to eat in the whole province," he was told. "Better keep moving on." "Oh, I have everything I need," he said. "In fact, I was thinking of making some stone soup." He pulled an iron cauldron from his wagon, filled it with water, and built a fire under it. Then, with great ceremony, he drew an ordinary-looking stone from a velvet bag and dropped it into the water.

Hearing the rumor of this most curious recipe, many villagers came to the square to see for themselves how the foolish soldier was going to make soup from a stone. You can imagine the snickering and jokes that surrounded the soldier as he sniffed the "broth" and licked his lips in anticipation.

"Ahh," the soldier said to himself rather loudly. "I do like a tasty stone soup." He dipped his spoon in once more, blowing on it to cool the broth; "Of course, stone soup with cabbage—that's hard to beat."

Soon a villager approached hesitantly, holding a cabbage he'd retrieved from its hiding place, which he offered to the soldier. "Capital!" cried the soldier. "You know, I once had stone soup with cabbage and a bit of salt beef as well, and it was fit for a king."

The village butcher scurried away and returned with a nice slab of salt beef . . . And so it went—potatoes, onions, carrots, mushrooms, and so on, until there was indeed a delicious meal for all. The villagers offered the soldier a great deal of money for the magic stone, but he refused to sell and traveled on the next day.

French folk tale

In the health care facility, the wandering soldier is the head of the Environmental Health and Safety Department and the magic stone is the Occupational Safety and Health Act (OSH Act). [CD-ROM 17.1] But just as a single stone was only the basis for the magical concoction, the OSH Act by itself is insufficient to protect workers. Worker protection and the ancillary patient protection begin with the addition of various intense ingredients, much like the cabbage and salt beef in the stone soup.

Regulations concerning such matters as hazard communication, record-keeping, personal protective equipment and clothing, fire safety, and electrical safety are the coarse-cut "vegetables" of the soup of Environmental Health and Safety. The itinerant soldier most certainly realized that coarse-cut vegetables are not enough; salt and pepper and a handful of herbs and spices are needed to make stone soup a fine meal. And so it is with the Environmental Health and Safety program.

The successful Environmental Health and Safety program must be based on a solid understanding by staff in each department of the specific hazards, regulations, and standards that apply to their work area. This chapter discusses many of the specific regulations that are the herbs and spices of the stone soup called Environmental Health and Safety. However, unlike the town folk who volunteered the ingredients for the soup, compliance with these standards is not optional. They are intended to make the workplace free from "recognized hazards" and to ensure the safety of all workers. It is incumbent on each department head in the facility to be aware of which standards apply to their respective departments. [Selected OSHA standards for this chapter are included on the CD-ROM.]

CONSTRUCTION STANDARDS (29 CFR 1926)

A health care facility often is undergoing remodeling or new construction. There are a myriad of standards that address virtually every aspect of such work. As with the other standards discussed in this book, compliance with the worker health and safety requirements for construction will help protect all of the building's occupants as well. The facility is responsible for ensuring that any contractors on the facility's property comply with these standards and regulations. [Selected OSHA construction standards are provided on the CD-ROM.]

HAND AND PORTABLE POWER TOOLS (29 CFR 1910.242–244 AND 1926.300)

Tools are such a common part of our lives that we sometimes forget that they may pose hazards. Most tools are manufactured to comply with a variety of requirements developed by nongovernmental organizations to help ensure that they are used safely. Employees who use hand and power tools must be protected from falling, flying, abrasive, and splashing objects, or from harmful dusts, fumes, mists, vapors, or gases that may result from the use of power tools. Therefore, they must be provided with the personal protective equipment (PPE) necessary to protect them from those hazards. Figure 17-1 provides some basic safety rules that can help prevent hazards associated with the use of hand and power tools. [CD-ROM 17.2–17.5]

Figure 17–1. Basic Safety Rules for Hand and Power Tools

☐ Perform regular maintenance on tools to keep them in good condition.

☐ Use the right tool for the job.

☐ Examine each tool for damage before each use.

☐ Operate the tool according to the manufacturer's instructions.

☐ Use the right PPE when working with the tool.

☐ Never carry a tool by the cord or hose.

☐ Never yank the cord or the hose to disconnect it from a receptacle.

☐ Keep cords and hoses away from heat, oil, and sharp edges.

☐ Disconnect tools when not in use, before servicing, and when changing accessories, such as blades, bits, and cutters.

☐ Keep all observers at a safe distance from the power tool work area.

☐ Secure work with clamps or a vise, keeping both hands free to operate the tool.

☐ Avoid the accidental starting of a tool by keeping fingers away from the switch button while carrying a plugged-in tool.

☐ Maintain tools with care; for best performance, keep them sharp and clean. Be sure to follow the instructions in the user's manual.

☐ When working with power tools, be sure to maintain good footing and balance.

☐ Wear the proper apparel for the task. Loose clothing, ties, or jewelry can become caught in moving parts.

☐ Remove damaged portable electric tools from use, and tag them DO NOT USE.

☐ Safeguard all moving parts of power tools, such as belts, gears, sprockets, and chains, so that workers cannot come into contact with them.

☐ Ensure that employees are aware of the dangers associated with the use of power tools, such as electric shock and burns. Never use a power tool in wet or damp locations.

☐ Do not allow cords to present a tripping hazard.

☐ Keep work areas well lit.

☐ Store tools in a dry place when not in use.

SIGNS AND TAGS (29 CFR 1910.145)

Signage is a significant factor in protecting workers, patients, and visitors from harm. Just as signs are posted outside a patient's room to warn of communicable disease risk or to indicate that the patient has limited mobility, signs with specific language, color, and size are required to warn workers, patients, and visitors of specific hazards. In addition to these general requirements for signs, many OSHA standards for specific chemicals have their own signage requirements.

A tag is a temporary way to warn of an equipment malfunction or to alert workers and others that a piece of equipment has been "deenergized" while undergoing repair or maintenance. Sometimes a piece of equipment is disabled or "locked out" to prevent its inadvertent operation. This is often referred to as lockout/tagout or LOTO.

Standard 29 CFR 1910.145, Specification for accident prevention signs and tags, contains specific information concerning proper sign and tag requirements. [CD-ROM 17.6] Other OSHA standards also have requirements for signs, such as 1910.37, Maintenance, safeguards, and operational features for exit routes. [CD-ROM 17.7] Examples of signage requirements for specific chemicals that may be used or found in a health care facility are provided in figure 17-2. [Selected OSHA standards for these items are on the CD-ROM.]

TEMPERATURE EXTREMES: HEAT AND COLD EXPOSURE

In health care facilities, several jobs require outdoor work, which means that workers may be subject to extreme seasonal weather and temperatures. These include loading dock employees, security officers making their rounds, groundskeeping staff, and maintenance workers. However, other workers may also be exposed to temperature extremes, such as kitchen workers.

Figure 17–2. Examples of Signage Requirements for Specific Chemicals

---

□ Asbestos (29 CFR 1910.1001)

□ Carcinogens (29 CFR 1910.1003)

□ Vinyl chloride (29 CFR 1910.1017)

□ Lead (29 CFR 1910.1025)

□ Cadmium (29 CFR 1910.1027)

□ Benzene (29 CFR 1910.1028)

□ Ethylene oxide (29 CFR 1910.1047)

□ Formaldehyde (29 CFR 1910.1048)

□ Methylene chloride (29 CFR 1910.1052)

□ Labels complying with the Hazard communication standard (29 CFR 1910.1200)

There are several approaches that can be used to protect workers from the effects of extreme temperatures, including:

☐ Performing outside work during either the cooler or warmer times of the day

☐ Using the "buddy" system (working in pairs)

☐ Drinking plenty of cool water in warm or hot weather and warm beverages in cold weather

☐ Wearing appropriate clothing (hat and light, loose-fitting, breathable clothing in warm or hot weather; and warm, layered clothing in cold weather, including hat and gloves)

☐ In cold weather, paying special attention to protecting feet, hands, face, and head; up to 40 percent of body heat can be lost when the head is exposed

☐ Applying sunscreen on sunny days

☐ Taking frequent, short breaks indoors to cool off or warm up

☐ Educating employees to recognize symptoms of cold- or heat-related stress and to seek medical help for workers that have such symptoms

☐ Wearing PPE when unpacking and sorting meat and other food products in freezers (such as hats, gloves, and rubber-soled non-slip shoes)

Hot Environments

There are several heat-related illnesses attendant to working in a hot environment, particularly for the unacclimatized worker. These illnesses include heat exhaustion and heat stroke. Workers in hot environments should be trained to recognize the signs and symptoms of these illnesses:

☐ Headaches, dizziness, light-headedness, weakness, mood changes, feeling sick to the stomach, pale and clammy skin, vomiting, and fainting characterize heat exhaustion.

☐ Heat stroke is caused by an increase in the body's core temperature and is characterized by dry, pale skin; mood changes; seizure; collapse; and possibly death.

Numerous resources for protecting workers in hot environments are available from OSHA. These include Fact Sheet 95-16, *Protecting Workers in Hot Environments* [CD-ROM 17.8]; Quick Card 3154, *Protect Yourself: Heat Stress* [CD-ROM 17.9]; and *The Heat Equation* [CD-ROM 17.10].

Cold Environments

Cold environments can cause frostbite on unprotected skin and hypothermia. Frostbite is the freezing of deep skin tissue layers and leads to hardening and numbing of the skin. It usually affects the fingers, hands, toes, feet, ears, and nose. Hypothermia occurs when the body's temperature falls below 95°F. The person becomes tired and drowsy, begins to shiver uncontrollably, moves clumsily, and is irritable and confused. As the hypothermia progresses, the victim's speech becomes slurred, behavior may become irrational, and unconsciousness and full heart failure can occur.

Resources for protecting workers in cold environments are also available from OSHA. Publications include OSHA 3156, *The Cold Stress Equation* [CD-ROM 17.11]; and OSHA 98-55, *Protecting Workers in Cold Environments* [CD-ROM 17.12].

Slips, Trips, and Falls (29 CFR 1910.22)

Slips, trips, and falls are a leading cause of injuries in health care facilities. Employees are at risk of slips, trips, and falls from foods or liquids that have fallen to the floor, power cords that run across pathways, bulging or bunched carpets, or uneven walking surfaces and cracked pavement. Falls can occur from elevated walkways or as a result of tripping or slipping. Some OSHA standards require employers to mark hazards or safety zones in the workplace (e.g., changes in elevation or walking aisles). Other standards require an area of clear space for access (e.g., around fire extinguishers). In some cases, the regulation specifies a particular distance. Other standards use more general language, such as "sufficient safe clearances shall be allowed for aisles." Examples of OSHA standards that are intended to prevent slips, trips, and falls include:

- □ Walking-working surfaces, guarding floor and wall openings and holes (29 CFR 1910.23) [CD-ROM 17.13]
- □ Maintenance, safeguards, and operational features for exit routes (29 CFR 1910.37) [CD-ROM 17.14]

Preventing slips, trips, and falls requires a team effort to identify potential hazards and take corrective action before an injury occurs. Although slips and trips often result in falls, it is not necessary to fall to sustain an injury. The following precautions are important to help prevent slips, trips, and falls in health care facilities.

Slips

To prevent slips in the workplace or on the outside grounds, it is important to:

- □ Promptly clean up spills.
- □ Post signs to warn of wet areas.
- □ Keep walking surfaces free of ice and snow. Have ice and snow cleared as quickly as possible.

☐ Shelter doorways from ice, snow, sleet, and rain.

☐ Have slip-resistant coatings or non-slip surfaces installed in areas likely to become slippery and on stair treads, or use non-slip mats.

☐ Be careful when wearing wet shoes on a dry floor. They can be just as slippery as dry shoes on a wet floor. Wear appropriate non-slip footwear.

☐ Use proper lifting techniques.

☐ Keep walk-in freezer and refrigerator floors free from slip hazards such as spills or clutter, and use non-slip matting for potentially slippery surfaces.

☐ Promote a program that provides for appropriate work shoes for employees. Shoe policy programs require workers or employers to purchase non-slip footwear for work use.

Trips

In an effort to prevent trips in the workplace or on the outside grounds, employees should:

☐ Turn on lights before entering an area and have light bulbs replaced when burned out.

☐ Use footstools with rubber feet.

☐ Use step stools for reaching high places.

☐ See that damaged sidewalks, parking areas, and other walking surfaces are repaired as quickly as possible.

☐ Have loose or broken grab bars and handrails repaired.

☐ Have loose carpeting tacked or taped down. Stretch carpets that bulge or have become bunched to prevent tripping hazards.

☐ Use throw rugs with a skid-resistant backing.

☐ Cover cables that cross walkways to prevent trips.

☐ Keep walkways and hallways free of objects and clutter.

☐ Put trash in the trashcans.

☐ Close file cabinet drawers.

☐ When carrying items, limit their height to one over which the upcoming area can be safely seen.

☐ Lighten loads or get help carrying a load.

☐ Monitor hallways to be certain they are not blocked by delivery items.

Falls

With observance of the following safety precautions, most falls can be avoided.

☐ Keep chairs, tables, and other equipment in good repair.

☐ Use ladders properly.

□ Take steps one at a time and use the handrail. Never skip or jump from one level to another.

□ Never use the stairs as a storage area.

□ Slow down when approaching steps or a staircase.

An effective prevention program focuses on the potential for these hazards and should include:

□ Training in the identification of potential slip, trip, and fall hazards

□ Immediate reporting of any potential physical hazards due to slips, trips, and falls, including those identified by patients and visitors

□ Records of incidents and information regarding slips, trips, and falls

□ Routine inspection of the facility for possible hazards

□ Provisions for the Environmental Health and Safety Department to work with the contractor and architect in remodeling or building new facilities

NOISE EXPOSURE AND HEARING CONSERVATION (29 CFR 1910.95)

Noise is defined as any unwanted sound and is one of the most common health problems in American workplaces. Sound is the result of air being moved in a wave, much like water, and striking the hearing mechanisms of the ear. The magnitude of the noise depends on the force with which the air is moved and the pressure with which it strikes the human eardrum. If the pressure of the sound wave is great enough, it can damage one's hearing. The OSHA Hearing conservation standard is intended to prevent noise-induced hearing loss. The unit of measurement used for noise is the decibel. Noise levels that reach or exceed 90 decibels are considered potentially damaging to the human ear. OSHA requires employers to determine if workers are exposed to excessive noise in the workplace. If so, the employers must implement feasible engineering or administrative controls to eliminate or reduce hazardous levels of noise. Where controls are not sufficient, employers must implement an effective hearing conservation program.

Noise exposure standards have been established by OSHA to protect the hearing of employees. Other federal agencies and organizations have established similar criteria.

> **General industry.** Standard 29 CFR 1910.95, Occupational noise exposure, is designed to protect general industry employees, such as those working in health care facilities [CD-ROM 17.15]; it does not cover the construction industry. The standard establishes permissible noise exposures and outlines requirements according to two primary cate-

gories: (1) engineering and administrative controls and (2) hearing conservation program.

Construction industry. Standard 29 CFR 1926.52, Occupational noise exposure, covers permissible noise exposures and engineering and administrative controls. [CD-ROM 17.16] Requirements for permissible noise exposures and controls under the standard for construction are the same as those in the standard for general industry (1910.95).

Standard 29 CFR 1926.101, Hearing protection, covers a hearing conservation program. [CD-ROM 17.17] In all cases where sound levels exceed the values shown in 1926.52(d)(1), Table D-2, a continuing effective hearing conservation program must be administered. There are no specific provisions for the hearing conservation program in construction.

Effects of Excessive Exposure

Although noise-induced hearing loss is one of the most common occupational illnesses, it is often ignored because there are no visible effects, it usually develops over a long period of time, and, except in very rare cases, there is no pain. What does occur is a progressive loss of communication, socialization, and responsiveness to the environment. In its early stages, when hearing loss occurs above 2,000 hertz (Hz), it affects the ability to understand or discriminate speech patterns. As it progresses to the lower frequencies, it begins to affect the ability to hear sounds in general.

The three main types of hearing loss are conductive, sensorineural, and a combination of the two.

The effects of noise can be broken down into three general categories:

1. *Primary effects*, which include noise-induced temporary threshold shift, noise-induced permanent threshold shift, acoustic trauma, and tinnitus
2. *Effects on communication and performance*, which may include isolation, annoyance, difficulty concentrating, absenteeism, and accidents
3. *Other effects*, which may include stress, muscle tension, ulcers, increased blood pressure, and hypertension

In some cases, the effects of hearing loss may be classified by cause. Additional information about the effects of excessive noise exposure can be found in OSHA Standard 29 CFR 1910.95, Occupational noise exposure, Appendix C, Audiometric measuring instruments. [CD-ROM 17.18]

Ultrasonics

Ultrasound is high-frequency sound that is unaudible, or cannot be heard by the human ear. However, it can still affect hearing and produce other health effects. There are some factors to consider regarding ultrasonics:

The upper frequency of human audibility is approximately 15–20 kilohertz (kHz). This is not a set limit, and some individuals have higher or (usually) lower limits. The frequency limit normally declines with age.

Most of the audible noise associated with ultrasonic sources, such as ultrasonic welders or ultrasonic cleaners, consists of subharmonics of the machine's major ultrasonic frequencies. For example, many ultrasonic welders have a fundamental operating frequency of 20 kHz, which is at the upper frequency of human audibility. However, a good deal of noise may be present at 10 kHz, the first subharmonic frequency of the 20 kHz operating frequency, and will therefore be audible to most people.

Additional information on ultrasonics and the applicability of OSHA's Occupational noise exposure standard can be found in OSHA Standard 29 CFR 1910.95 Appendix D, Audiometric test rooms. [CD-ROM 17.19]

GUARDING FLOOR AND WALL OPENINGS AND HOLES (29 CFR 1910.23)

Floor openings and holes, wall openings and holes, and the open sides of platforms may create hazards. People may fall through the openings or over the sides to the level below. Objects, such as tools or parts, may fall through the holes and strike people or damage machinery on lower levels. Violations of 1910.23 are among the 10 standards most frequently cited by OSHA in health care facilities. Regulations for preventing injuries of this type are contained in OSHA Standard 29 CFR 1910.23, Guarding floor and wall openings and holes. [CD-ROM 17.20]

COMPRESSED GASES (29 CFR 1910.101)

Hazards associated with compressed gases include oxygen displacement, fires, explosions, and toxic gas exposures, as well as the physical hazards associated with high-pressure systems. Special storage, use, and handling precautions are necessary to control these hazards.

To prevent accidents involving compressed-gas cylinders, OSHA enforces Standard 29 CFR 1910.101, Compressed gases (general requirements) [CD-ROM 17.21], and incorporates by reference many standards developed by the Compressed Gas Association [CD-ROM 17.22]. Compressed gas and equipment are also addressed in other OSHA standards, including those listed in figure 17-3. [Selected OSHA standards are provided on the CD-ROM.]

Compressed gases are prevalent in many areas of the health care facility. Depending on the particular gas, there is a potential for simultaneous exposure to both mechanical and chemical hazards. Gases may be flammable or combustible, explosive, corrosive, poisonous, inert, or a combination thereof.

Careful procedures are necessary for handling the various compressed gases, the cylinders containing the compressed gases, the regulators or valves used to control gas flow, and the piping used to confine gases during flow.

Figure 17–3. Examples of Specific OSHA Standards Governing the Use of Compressed Gas and Equipment

---

29 CFR 1910 Subpart H, Hazardous Materials
- 1910.102, Acetylene
- 1910.103, Hydrogen
- 1910.104, Oxygen
- 1910.105, Nitrous oxide

29 CFR 1910 Subpart M, Compressed Gas and Compressed Air Equipment
- 1910.169, Air receivers

29 CFR 1910 Subpart Q, Welding, Cutting, and Brazing
- 1910.253, Oxygen–fuel gas welding and cutting
- 1910.254, Arc welding and cutting

29 CFR 1926 Subpart D, Occupational Health and Environmental Controls
- 1926.65, Hazardous waste operations and emergency response

29 CFR 1926 Subpart J, Welding and Cutting
- 1926.350, Gas welding and cutting

Additional regulations applicable to compressed-gas containers and examples of precautions for compressed gas are detailed in the Montana Department of Labor & Industry's *Compressed Gas Safety General Safety Guidelines* (2000). [CD-ROM 17.23]

EMERGENCY EYEWASH AND SHOWER EQUIPMENT (29 CFR 1910.151(2)(c))

The first 10 to 15 seconds after exposure to a hazardous substance, especially a corrosive substance, are critical. Delaying treatment, even for a few seconds, may cause serious injury. Emergency showers and eyewash stations provide on-the-spot decontamination. They allow workers to flush away hazardous substances that can cause injury.

Accidental chemical exposures can occur even with good engineering controls and safety precautions. As a result, it is essential to look beyond the use of goggles, face shields, and procedures for using personal protective equipment. Emergency showers and eyewash stations are a necessary backup to minimize the effects of accidental exposure to chemicals.

The ANSI-Z358.1 standard is commonly accepted for use in the selection, installation, and maintenance of emergency fixtures. It is understood that OSHA uses the requirements from the ANSI standard for compliance with its 29 CFR 1910.151(c), even though this is not specified in its Code of Federal

Regulations. [CD-ROM 17.24] Therefore, it is important to understand the standard to ensure compliance in selecting and installing emergency equipment. In addition to the ANSI Z358.1 standard, all local codes should be reviewed before any emergency fixture installation.

Electrical Equipment (29 CFR Subpart S, Electrical, 1910.301–399)

Electrical current exposes workers to a serious, widespread occupational hazard. Practically all members of the workforce are exposed to electrical energy during the performance of their daily duties, and electrocutions occur to workers in various job categories. Many workers are unaware of the potential electrical hazards present in their work environment, which makes them more vulnerable to the danger of electrocution.

Electrical injuries consist of four main types: electrocution (fatal), electric shock, burns, and falls resulting from contact with electrical energy.

The OSHA electrical standards are designed to protect employees exposed to dangers such as electric shock, electrocution, fires, and explosions. Electrical hazards are addressed in specific standards for health care facilities. The electrical standards for general industry, 29 CFR Subpart S, Electrical, 1910.301–399, are performance-oriented regulations that include requirements for protecting employees from electrical hazards, training, safety-related work practices to prevent shock or other injuries, use of equipment, and safeguards for personnel protection.

The National Fire Protection Association's *NFPA 70E: Standard for Electrical Safety in the Workplace* can be helpful in understanding and complying with the requirements in OSHA's Subpart S. This standard includes the following chapters and annexes that can be of particular assistance to health care facilities:

☐ Chapter 1, Safety-Related Work Practices
☐ Chapter 2, Safety-Related Maintenance Requirements
☐ Chapter 3, Safety Requirements for Special Equipment
☐ Chapter 4, Installation Safety Requirements
☐ Annex E, Electrical Safety Program
☐ Annex F, Hazard Risk Evaluation Procedure
☐ Annex G, Sample Lockout/Tagout Procedure
☐ Annex I, Job Briefing and Planning Checklist
☐ Annex J, Energized Electrical Work Permit
☐ Annex K, General Categories of Electrical Hazards
☐ Annex M, Cross-Reference Tables

The booklet *Controlling Electrical Hazards* (OSHA 3075) provides an overview of basic electrical safety on the job. [CD-ROM 17.25]

THE CONTROL OF HAZARDOUS ENERGY (LOCKOUT/TAGOUT) (29 CFR 1910.147)

"Lockout/tagout" (LOTO) refers to specific practices and procedures to safeguard employees from the unexpected energization or start-up of machinery and equipment, or the release of hazardous energy during service or maintenance activities. This requires that a designated individual turn off and disconnect the machinery or equipment from its energy source(s) before performing service or maintenance, and that the authorized employee(s) either lock or tag the energy-isolating device(s) to prevent the release of hazardous energy and take steps to verify that the energy has been isolated effectively. If the potential exists for the release of hazardous stored energy or for the re-accumulation of stored energy to a hazardous level, the employer must ensure that the employee(s) take steps to prevent injury that may result from the release of the stored energy.

Lockout devices hold energy-isolating devices in a safe or "off" position. They provide protection by preventing machines or equipment from becoming energized. They are positive restraints that no one can remove without a key or other unlocking mechanism, or through extraordinary means, such as bolt cutters. Tagout devices, by contrast, are prominent warning devices that an authorized employee fastens to energy-isolating devices to warn employees not to reenergize the machine while he or she is servicing or maintaining it. Tagout devices are easier to remove and, by themselves, provide employees with less protection than do lockout devices.

Employees can be seriously or fatally injured if the machinery they service or maintain unexpectedly energizes, starts up, or releases stored energy. Standard 29 CFR 1910.147, The control of hazardous energy (lockout/tagout), spells out the steps employers must take to prevent accidents associated with hazardous energy. The standard addresses practices and procedures necessary to disable machinery and equipment and to prevent the release of potentially hazardous energy while maintenance or servicing activities are being performed. [CD-ROM 17.26]

Some standards relating to specific types of machinery or equipment contain de-energization requirements. The provisions of 1910.147 apply in conjunction with these machine-specific standards to ensure that employees will be adequately protected against hazardous energy. The booklet *Control of Hazardous Energy Lockout/Tagout* (OSHA 3120) presents the agency's general requirements for controlling hazardous energy during service or maintenance of machines or equipment. [CD-ROM 17.27]

MEDICAL DEVICES AND EQUIPMENT

Certain organizations and government bodies have developed guidelines and standards that address the maintenance of medical equipment. Many of these guidelines and standards are also referred to as "industry standards" and may be used in a court of law during a case that involves injury or death caused by malfunctioning medical equipment.

The Safe Medical Device Act (SMDA) of 1990 requires health care facilities to report all medical device–related serious injuries and deaths to the manufacturer. The Food and Drug Administration (FDA) must be notified if the incident results in the death of a staff member and/or the hospitalization of three or more staff members. The SMDA gives FDA investigators access to the facility and to organization equipment records. [CD-ROM 17.28]

Effective procurement planning enables health care facilities to select devices that, in addition to being safe and productive, offer the best combination of ease of use, effortlessness of servicing, and performance reliability with the least amount of preventive maintenance.

All patient care equipment should be included in an organized program. A comprehensive program also addresses preventive maintenance. The first step in planning the medical equipment safety program is an analysis of the risks presented by such equipment in both the patient care and staff safety processes. An effective risk analysis should address engineering and the medical equipment.

There is no OSHA standard that specifically addresses medical equipment hazards. The enforcement of the medical equipment safety program falls under the OSHA general duty clause (5a1) and OSHA Standard 29 CFR Subpart S 1910.301–399, Electrical.

Health care facilities are required to develop and implement plans for the management of medical equipment under standards issued by accreditation organizations. Individual states may have requirements for medical equipment safety management programs and reporting requirements under the state department of health, local fire department, or other entities. Health care facilities should check with the state and local governing bodies before preparing programs, policies, and procedures.

Lasers

LASER is an acronym that stands for "light amplification by stimulated emission of radiation." The laser produces an intense, highly directional beam of light. The most common cause of laser-induced tissue damage is thermal in nature; the tissue proteins are denatured due to the temperature rise following absorption of laser energy.

The American National Standards Institute (ANSI) has developed standards Z136.1, Safe Use of Lasers, and specifically Z136.3, Safe Use of Lasers in Health Care Facilities. These standards provide guidance for the safe operation and use of lasers and laser systems by defining control measures for each of four laser classifications. The basis of the laser classification scheme is the ability of the primary or reflected beam to cause biological damage to the eye or skin during its intended use. Most medical laser systems are designated Class 4 and may by definition present a skin, ocular, or fire hazard by direct or reflected laser radiation. The ANSI standards provide guidelines for developing appropriate control measures to minimize these potential hazards.

The OSHA Technical Manual [CD-ROM 17.29, 17.30] also provides guidance in recognizing laser hazards:

□ Section III: Chapter 6, *Laser Hazards.* Provides information to assist industrial hygienists in the assessment of worksites for potential laser hazards. The document provides information on biological effects, hazard classifications, investigation guidelines, control measures, and safety programs.

□ Section III: Chapter 6, Appendix III: 6-2, *FDA/CDRH Federal Product Performance Standard Evaluation Outline.* Provides a checklist for evaluating lasers. Regulatory references are included for each checklist item.

□ Section VI: Chapter 1, *Hospital Investigations: Health Hazards.* Contains information that will assist in the recognition and evaluation of laser hazards within health care facilities. Describes lasers as a potential hazard in the hospital environment and identifies areas to investigate.

□ Section VI: Chapter 1, Appendix VI: 1-3, *Physical Agents.* Identifies the acute effects of laser exposure. It also states that chronic effects are unknown.

The National Fire Protection Association and the Food and Drug Administration's Center for Devices and Radiological Health are also sources for laser safety standards.

Other OSHA Standards

Examples of other OSHA standards that apply to health care facilities, but are not discussed in detail in this book, are listed in figure 17-4. [Each of the standards is included on the CD-ROM.]

Indoor Air Quality (IAQ)

In many situations, the term *indoor air quality* (IAQ) is used to refer to the source of health problems among workers in non-industrial buildings, such as health care facilities. However, some scientists believe that *indoor environmental quality* (IEQ) is a more appropriate term because it covers a wider range of problems and their sources. This lack of agreement in terminology reflects the lack of consensus concerning the scientific evidence for the association between poor IAQ and reported illnesses. Terms such as *sick-building syndrome* and *environmental illness* have been used to describe certain health conditions reported by occupants of non-industrial buildings. However, these terms are no longer widely used by the scientific community. There are no federal regulations that specifically address indoor air quality.

Figure 17–4. Examples of Other OSHA Standards That Apply to Health Care Facilities

- □ 29 CFR 1910.25, Portable wood ladders
- □ 29 CFR 1910.27, Fixed ladders
- □ 29 CFR 1910.28, Safety requirements for scaffolding
- □ 29 CFR 1910.94, Ventilation
- □ 29 CFR 1910.141, Sanitation
- □ 29 CFR 1910.144, Safety color code for marking physical hazards
- □ 29 CFR 1910.146, Permit-required confined space
- □ 29 CFR 1910.178, Powered industrial trucks
- □ 29 CFR 1910.183, Helicopters
- □ 29 CFR 1910.212, General requirements for all machines
- □ 29 CFR 1910.215, Abrasive wheel machinery
- □ 29 CFR 1910.251–255, Welding, cutting, and brazing
- □ 29 CFR 1910.264, Laundry machinery and operations
- □ 29 CFR 1910.1096, Ionizing radiation

The typical spectrum of reported symptoms includes headache, unusual fatigue, varying degrees of itching or burning of the eyes, skin irritation, nasal congestion, dry or irritated throat, and other respiratory irritation. These symptoms do not suggest any particular medical diagnosis, nor can they be readily associated with any particular causative agent. Usually, the workplace environment is implicated because workers reported that their symptoms lessened or resolved when they left the building.

Although employees may attribute their health problems to poor IAQ, implying air contamination as the cause, many scientists investigating these issues believe that multiple factors may contribute to reports of such health problems. These factors include ventilation system problems, exposures to chemicals, increased concentrations of airborne dusts, microbiological contamination, and factors that affect comfort, such as odors, temperature, humidity, lighting, and noise. In some studies, occupant perceptions of the indoor environment were more closely related to the occurrence of symptoms than any measured indoor contaminant or condition. Other studies have shown relationships between psychological, social, and organizational factors in the workplace and the occurrence of symptoms and discomfort.

That poor indoor air quality is detrimental to both the integrity of the building and the health of its occupants is illustrated in documents published by NIOSH. [CD-ROM 17.31] Many IAQ problems can be solved with in-house expertise. In conjunction with the Environmental Protection Agency (EPA), NIOSH has published a guide to provide help in solving these problems. This publication, *Building Air Quality: A Guide for Building Owners and Managers*, provides practical advice for evaluating IAQ problems. [CD-ROM 17.32]

Sources of Indoor Air Pollutants

Indoor air pollutants can originate within the building or be drawn in from outdoors, as described in figure 17-5.

In addition to the number of potential pollutants, a complicating factor is that indoor air pollutant concentrations can vary by time and location within the building. For example, floor stripping and waxing is typically performed during the night shift, and the odors from that process may have been

Figure 17–5. Typical Sources of Indoor Air Pollutants

External Sources	Internal Sources
□ Pollen, dust, fungal spores	□ Microbiological growth in drip pans, ductwork, coils, and humidifiers
□ Industrial emissions	□ Microbiological growth on or in soiled or water-damaged materials and furnishings
□ Vehicle emissions	□ Improper venting of combustion products
□ Loading docks	□ Dust or debris in ductwork
□ Odors from dumpsters	□ Emissions from office equipment such as copy and print machines
□ Unsanitary debris or building exhausts near outdoor air intakes	□ Emissions from shops, labs, cleaning processes, food prep areas
□ Radon	□ Materials containing volatile organic compounds, inorganic compounds, or damaged asbestos
□ Pesticides	□ Materials that produce particles (dust)
□ Leakage from underground storage tanks	□ Emissions from new furnishings and floorings
	□ Cleaning materials
	□ Emissions from trash
	□ Odors from paint, caulk, or adhesives
	□ Occupants with communicable diseases
	□ Insects and other pests
	□ Personal care products
	□ Mold from moisture accumulating from sources such as pipe leaks, roof leaks, or condensation

Adapted from Indoor Air: IAQ Tools for Schools Program. *IAQ Coordinator's Guide*, Publication EPA 402-K-95-001.

removed by the HVAC system before the beginning of the next shift. On the other hand, fungal growth in the HVAC system is a continuous process.

Pollutants can also be emitted from point sources, such as an open solvent container in a laboratory, or from an area such as a freshly painted hallway.

The Joint Commission as a Guardian of the Facility's Infrastructure

Apart from health care employees, the most important component of health care delivery is a facility's infrastructure. There are a number of Joint Commission standards that are intended to help ensure the integrity of the facility's infrastructure, including the following:

- □ EC.1.10, The health care facility manages safety risks
- □ EC.5.20, Newly constructed and existing environments are designed and maintained to comply with the *Life Safety Code*®
- □ EC.5.40, The health care facility maintains fire-safety equipment and building features
- □ EC.5.50, The health care facility develops and implements activities to protect occupants during periods when a building does not meet the applicable provisions of the *Life Safety Code*®
- □ EC.6.10, The health care facility manages medical equipment risks
- □ EC.6.20, Medical equipment is maintained, tested, and inspected
- □ EC.7.10, The health care facility manages its utility risks
- □ EC.7.20, The health care facility provides an emergency electrical power source
- □ EC.7.30, The health care facility maintains, tests, and inspects its utility systems
- □ EC.7.40, The health care facility maintains, tests, and inspects its emergency power systems
- □ EC.8.10, The health care facility establishes and maintains an appropriate environment
- □ EC.8.30, The health care facility manages the design and building of the environment when it is renovated, altered, or newly created
- □ EC.9.10, The health care facility monitors conditions in the environment
- □ HR.2.10, Orientation provides initial job training and information
- □ HR.2.20, Staff members, licensed independent practitioners, students, and volunteers, as appropriate, can describe or demonstrate their roles and responsibilities, based on specific job duties or responsibilities, relative to safety
- □ HR.2.30, Ongoing education, including in-services, training, and other activities, maintains and improves competence
- □ HR.3.10, Competence to perform job responsibilities is assessed, demonstrated, and maintained

There are additional requirements for the maintenance of equipment used in home care.

Achieving Joint Commission accreditation is not equivalent to OSHA compliance. By the same token, compliance with OSHA regulations alone does not ensure that the requirements of the Joint Commission have been met.

THE ROLE OF THE ENVIRONMENTAL HEALTH AND SAFETY DEPARTMENT

The Environmental Health and Safety Department serves much the same function as the soldier with the stone. The Environmental Health and Safety Department must ensure that the staff of each department in the facility are aware of the federal, state, and local regulations and accreditation standards that apply to their area. But compliance with those regulations and standards is not the sole responsibility of the Environmental Health and Safety Department. Department heads must understand which regulations and standards apply to their respective departments and ensure that their staff are in compliance. Because of the nature of the bulk of the regulations and standards described in this chapter, the majority of the responsibility for compliance resides with the Engineering Department.

The department liaisons are a vital part of the internal compliance process, and it is incumbent on them to assist their department heads in ensuring compliance and noting any areas in which compliance may be questionable.

During semi-annual and annual surveys, the Environmental Health and Safety Department needs to identify any areas in which there are issues of noncompliance and assist the particular department(s) in correcting the deficiency. The Environmental Health and Safety Department should also work with the other departments to correct any areas of noncompliance that have resulted in a work-related injury or illness.

CHAPTER 18

PROGRAM EVALUATION AND BENCHMARKING

Liza and Henry ran their home like a well-oiled machine. Each had routine responsibilities that they had agreed on and they performed them without complaint, most of the time. Some couples have detailed lists of who is to do what, and when and how they are to do things. Some very well-organized partners even detail a course of action to ensure that their routine continues smoothly and can be modified, if needed. Liza and Henry didn't seem to need such a cumbersome document. But one day Liza encountered a minor problem: she needed some water, so she turned to her devoted mate and asked him to fetch some water for her. We can only imagine Henry gladly finding the bucket and walking to the well, whistling and humming along the way. Suddenly, however, Henry encountered a dilemma, and he rushed back to the house to tell Liza:

There's a hole in the bucket,
Dear Liza, dear Liza
There's a hole in the bucket,
Dear Liza, a hole.

Liza, being a natural-born leader, had the solution:

Then fix it, dear Henry,
Dear Henry, dear Henry
Then fix it, dear Henry,
Dear Henry, fix it.

Henry believed this to be a reasonable approach: the bucket has a hole in it, so he would simply fix it; but he needed a plan. Henry needed to know what he was going to fix it with, what tools he might need, and how he would test the bucket to see if his "fix" worked. Furthermore, Henry would need to closely monitor his work to make certain that his "fix" would last. And so began his quest:

With what shall I fix it,
Dear Liza?

With a straw, dear Henry.

That took care of Henry's first question, but he soon encountered another problem. Liza was ready with a solution:

But the straw is too long,
Dear Liza.

Then cut it, dear Henry.

Liza's exasperation began to mount, as she was confronted with one seemingly annoying question or problem after another.

With what shall I cut it?
With an axe.

The axe is too dull,
Dear Liza.
Then sharpen it, dear Henry.

With what shall I sharpen it?
With a stone, dear Henry.

The stone is too dry,
Dear Liza.
Then wet it.

With what shall I wet it, dear Liza?
With water, dear Henry.

The exchange had become rapid. Henry cited one impediment after another, but Liza just as quickly posed a solution. Nevertheless, the outcome was inevitable.

How shall I get it
Dear Liza, dear Liza,
How shall I get it,
Dear Liza, how?

In the bucket, dear Henry,
Dear Henry, dear Henry
In the bucket, dear Henry,
Dear Henry, in the bucket.

There's a hole in the bucket, dear Liza, dear Liza.

There's a Hole in the Bucket (traditional American folk song)

If Henry and Liza had developed a plan for drawing water from the well, they surely would have included bucket maintenance and routine testing to make sure the bucket didn't leak. And if a hole did develop, all of the necessary materials and tools would have been readily available and in good working order. Had they been truly fortunate, Liza would have socked away a little extra in the bucket fund so that they could have purchased a spare bucket in case the repairs couldn't be made as quickly as planned. While Liza was in charge of overseeing the collection of water and providing the resources for bucket repair, maintenance, and replacement, Henry was responsible for water collection, bucket and tool maintenance, and reporting any potential problems to Liza. Furthermore, every now and then Liza and Henry would have sat down and discussed water collection to ensure that the plan they had put in place was working and that Henry would not lose any fingers or toes to a dull axe. But Liza and Henry apparently had no such plan. One can only imagine that by now they are both very thirsty.

For the Environmental Health and Safety program to continue operating effectively, it needs periodic review and modification. While senior leadership is obligated to provide the resources for program implementation and maintenance—including a sufficient budget, technical information, assigned responsibility, adequate expertise and authority, line accountability, and program evaluation procedures—employees are obligated to follow the program faithfully. Those resources are the core program elements outlined in OSHA's *Safety and Health Program Management Guidelines*: management leadership and employee participation, hazard identification and assessment, hazard prevention and control, information and training, and evaluation of program effectiveness.[1] [CD-ROM 18.1] An evaluation looks at the systems that have been created to carry out the program to determine if they are working effectively. All systems that contribute to the safety and health program should be reviewed. Document review, employee interviews, and review of site conditions are useful evaluation tools and are the basis for an effective evaluation report.

The key to a successful and efficient evaluation is to combine elements when using each technique. First review the available documentation that relates to each element. Then walk through the worksite to observe how effectively what is on paper is apparently being implemented. While walking around, interview employees to verify that what is read and what is seen reflects the state of the facility's health and safety program.

Effective health and safety program evaluation is a dynamic process. If evaluators see or hear about aspects of the program not covered in the document review, they should ask to receive any documents relating to these aspects. If the documents include program elements not visible during the walk-around or not known to employees, probe further. Utilizing this cross-checking technique will help result in an effective, comprehensive evaluation of the facility's health and safety program.

METHODS FOR EVALUATING PROGRAM EFFECTIVENESS

Sometimes the ability to lead and the willingness to perform are simply not enough to prevent problems. Liza had the ability to lead, and Henry was more than willing to perform the task that Liza had given him. Unfortunately, they had no contingency plan for what to do if there was a hole in the bucket. Once they recognized the flaw in their system, it is quite possible that Liza and Henry sat down and chatted about how to prevent a recurrence of their untimely problem. Although they had the will to solve the problem, they simply did not have the capacity to solve all aspects of the problem at once. So they may have decided to lay out a series of incremental goals that they could use to chart their progress toward ensuring that they would never run out of water because of a hole in the bucket. Liza and Henry were now functioning in a partnership based on mutual respect and trust and a common goal.

The evaluation process that Liza and Henry undertook was no different from the process of evaluating the effectiveness of the health and safety program. The foremost goal is to prevent work-related injuries and illnesses. When that is done, several tangible benefits will accrue. Most notably, there will be fewer days away from work because of lost-time accidents, the costs of workers' compensation will decrease, productivity and morale will be enhanced, and the quality of patient care will improve. Better management through critical evaluation of the health and safety program can also prevent standards violations that can lead to citations and fines.

For example, over the past several years, OSHA has added more and more safety and health management provisions to its promulgated standards. These provisions include self-inspections for specific conditions, employee training, and specific types of hazard analysis. It has also focused more on the management of workplace safety and health when enforcing the "general duty clause" (OSH Act, Sec. 5(a)(1), 29 U.S.C. 654), which requires that each employer "furnish to each of his employees employment and a place of employment that are free from recognized hazards that are causing or likely to cause death or serious physical harm to his employees." Like industrial facilities, health care facilities have a responsibility to take reasonable steps to maintain a workplace that is "free of recognized hazards." This responsibility places the burden on senior leadership to establish and maintain the management practices that are necessary for establishing safe and healthful work practices and ensuring that they are followed.

Like Liza and Henry, senior management must work with all levels of the organization to identify problems, arrive at solutions, and develop reasonable milestones that can be used to track progress and monitor the effectiveness of the existing program. For example, if a facility is concerned about a high rate of needlestick injuries, it is unreasonable to establish as a goal the immediate elimination of needlestick injuries. However, if the reasons for those injuries are identified and intermediate goals for reducing their number are established, significant progress can be made toward reducing their incidence.

This chapter describes the three basic methods for assessing health and safety program effectiveness and provides information on how to use these tools to evaluate each element and subsidiary component of the program. The three basic methods for assessing health and safety program effectiveness are:

1. Checking documentation of activity
2. Interviewing employees at all levels for knowledge, awareness, and perceptions
3. Reviewing site conditions and, where hazards are found, finding the weaknesses in management systems that allowed the hazards to occur or to be "uncontrolled"

Some elements of the health and safety program are best assessed using one of these methods. Others lend themselves to assessment using two or all three methods.

Documentation

Checking documentation is a standard audit technique. It is particularly useful for understanding whether identified hazards have been effectively corrected. It can also be used to determine the quality of certain activities, such as self-inspections or routine hazard analysis.

Inspection records can reveal whether new hazards are being identified or whether the same hazards are being found repeatedly. If no new hazards are being found but accidents keep occurring, there may be a need to retrain evaluators or employees.

If certain hazards recur repeatedly, even after corrective action has been taken, it is possible that someone is not taking responsibility for keeping the hazards under control or that the lines of responsibility are not clear.

Employee Interviews

Talking to randomly selected employees at all levels can provide an indication of the quality of employee training and of employee perceptions of the program. If health and safety training is effective, employees will be able to discuss the hazards they work with and how they protect themselves and others by keeping those hazards controlled. Employees should also be able to precisely describe what they are expected to do as part of the program. And all employees should know what to do during an emergency.

Employee perceptions can provide other useful information. An employee's opinion of how easy it is to report a hazard and get a response will tell evaluators a lot about how well the hazard reporting system is working. If employees indicate that the system for enforcing health and safety rules and safe work practices is inconsistent or confusing, evaluators will know that the system needs improvement.

Interviews should not be limited to hourly employees. Much can be learned from talking with first-line supervisors. It is also helpful to query managers and department heads about their understanding of their safety and health responsibilities.

Site Conditions and Root Causes of Hazards

Examining workplace conditions can reveal existing hazards and provide information about the breakdown of the management systems meant to prevent or control these hazards.

Carefully examining conditions and practices is a well-established technique for assessing the effectiveness of health and safety programs. For example, in areas where personal protective equipment (PPE) is required, it should be obvious that the equipment is being properly maintained and stored. There should also be documented evidence that employees who must wear PPE have received the required training. In some areas, there should be signs notifying all employees that PPE is required for them to work in the area.

Another way to obtain information about health and safety program management is through root analysis of observed hazards. This approach to hazards is much like sophisticated accident investigation techniques, in which many contributing factors are located and then corrected or controlled.

ASSESSING THE COMPONENTS OF A QUALITY HEALTH AND SAFETY PROGRAM

Throughout this book, the four core program elements of OSHA's *Safety and Health Program Management Guidelines* are presented (see figure 18-1).

The following discussion focuses on evaluation of the four elements and describes useful ways to assess these components, as detailed in OSHA's

Figure 18–1. Major Elements of an Effective Safety and Health Program

☐ Management commitment and employee involvement
☐ Worksite analysis
☐ Hazard prevention and control
☐ Safety and health training

Tools for a Safety and Health Program Assessment.[2] [CD-ROM 18.2] Many of the evaluation items are appropriate for inclusion in the facility's hazard surveillance program required by OSHA and accreditation organizations.

1. Assessing the Key Components of Leadership, Participation, and Line Accountability

Worksite Policy on Safe and Healthful Working Conditions

- ☐ *Documentation*
  - The first step is to develop a clear and concise written Environmental Health and Safety policy that clearly establishes worker health and safety as a significant priority item, on the same level as organizational values such as patient safety. Questions can be used to assess the facility's success in doing this.
- ☐ *Interviews*
  - When asked, can employees at all levels express the facility's policy on worker safety and health?
  - If the policy is written, can hourly employees say where they have seen it?
  - Can employees at all levels explain the priority of worker safety and health as it relates to other organizational values, as the policy intends?
- ☐ *Site conditions and root causes of hazards*
  - Have injuries occurred because employees at any level did not understand the importance of safety precautions in relation to other organizational values?

Goal and Objectives for Worker Safety and Health

- ☐ *Documentation*
  - If there is a written goal for the health and safety program, is it updated annually?
  - If there are written objectives, such as an annual plan to reach the goal, are they clearly stated?
  - If managers and supervisors have written objectives, do these documents include objectives for the health and safety program?
- ☐ *Interviews*
  - Do managers and supervisors have a clear idea of their objectives for employee health and safety?
  - Do hourly employees understand the current objectives of the health and safety program?
- ☐ *Site conditions and root causes of hazards (only helpful in a general sense)*

Visible Top Management Leadership

☐ *Documentation*

- Are there one or more written programs that involve top-level management in health and safety activities? For example, top management receives and signs off on inspection reports either after each inspection or in a quarterly summary. These reports are then posted for employees to see. Top management rewards the best safety suggestions each month or at other specified intervals.

☐ *Interviews*

- Can hourly employees describe how management officials are involved in health and safety activities?
- Do hourly employees perceive that managers and supervisors follow health and safety rules and work practices, such as wearing appropriate PPE?

☐ *Site conditions and root causes of hazards*

- When employees are found not wearing required PPE or not following safe work practices, have any of them said that managers or supervisors also did not follow these rules?

Employee Participation

☐ *Documentation*

- Are there one or more written programs that provide for employee participation in decisions affecting their health and safety?
- Is there documentation of these activities (e.g., employee inspection reports, or minutes of joint employee–management or employee health and safety committee meetings)?
- Is there written documentation of any management response to employee health and safety program activities?
- Does the documentation indicate that employee health and safety activities are meaningful and substantive?
- Are there written guarantees of employee protection from harassment resulting from health and safety program involvement?

☐ *Interviews*

- Are employees aware of ways they can participate in decisions affecting their health and safety?
- Do employees appear to take pride in the achievements of the worksite health and safety program?
- Are employees comfortable answering questions about health and safety programs and conditions at the facility?
- Do employees feel they have the support of management for their health and safety activities?

☐ *Site conditions and root causes of hazards* (not applicable)

Assignment of Responsibility

- ☐ *Documentation*
  - Are responsibilities written out so they can be clearly understood?
- ☐ *Interviews*
  - Do employees understand their own responsibilities and those of others?
- ☐ *Site conditions and root causes of hazards*
  - Are hazards caused in part because no one was assigned the responsibility to control or prevent them?
  - Are hazards allowed to exist in part because someone in management did not have the clear responsibility to hold a lower-level manager or supervisor accountable for carrying out assigned responsibilities?

Adequate Authority and Resources

- ☐ *Documentation* (only generally applicable)
- ☐ *Interviews*
  - Does the Environmental Health and Safety Department and the department liaisons, or any other personnel with responsibilities for ensuring safe operations, have the authority to shut down equipment or to suggest maintenance or parts?
  - Do employees talk about not being able to get health and safety improvements because of cost?
  - Do employees mention the need for more health and safety personnel or expert consultants?
- ☐ *Site conditions and root causes of hazards*
  - Do recognized hazards go uncorrected because of lack of authority or resources?
  - Do hazards go unrecognized because greater expertise is needed to diagnose them?

Accountability of Managers, Supervisors, and Hourly Employees

- ☐ *Documentation*
  - Do performance evaluations for managers, department heads, and supervisors include specific criteria relating to health and safety protection?
  - Is there documented evidence of employees at all levels being held accountable for health and safety responsibilities, including safe work practices? Is accountability accomplished through either performance evaluations affecting pay and/or promotions or disciplinary actions?

□ *Interviews*

- When evaluators ask employees what happens to people who violate health and safety rules or safe work practices, do they indicate that rule breakers are clearly and consistently held accountable?
- Do hourly employees indicate that supervisors and managers genuinely care about meeting health and safety responsibilities?
- When asked what happens when rules are broken, do hourly employees complain that supervisors and managers do not follow rules and are never disciplined for infractions?

□ *Site conditions and root causes of hazards*

- Are hazards occurring because employees, supervisors, and/or managers are not being held accountable for their health and safety responsibilities?
- Are identified hazards not being corrected because those persons assigned the responsibility are not being held accountable?

Evaluation of Contractor Programs

□ *Documentation*

- Are there written policies for on-site contractors?
- Are contractor health and safety programs reviewed before selection?
- Do contracts require the contractor to follow facility health and safety rules?
- Do contractors receive requisite training to comply with health and safety rules unique to the facility?
- Are there means for removing a contractor that violates the rules?

□ *Interviews*

- Do employees describe hazardous conditions created by contract employees?
- Are employees comfortable reporting hazards created by contractors?
- Do contract employees feel they are covered by the same, or the same-quality, health and safety program as regular facility employees?

□ *Site conditions and root causes of hazards*

- Do areas where contractors are working appear to be in the same condition as areas where regular facility employees are working? Better? Worse?
- Does the working relationship between facility and contract employees appear cordial?

2. Assessing the Key Components of a Worksite Analysis

Comprehensive Surveys, Change Analysis, Routine Hazard Analysis

☐ *Documentation*
- Are there documents that provide comprehensive analysis of all potential safety and health hazards of the facility?
- Are there documents that provide both the analysis of potential health and safety hazards for each facility, equipment, material, or process and the means for eliminating or controlling such hazards?
- Does documentation exist of the step-by-step analysis of the hazards in each part of each job, so that evaluators can clearly discern the evolution of decisions on safe work procedures?
- If complicated processes exist, with a potential for catastrophic impact from an accident but a low probability of such accident, are there documents analyzing the potential hazards in each part of the processes and the means to prevent or control them?
- If there are processes with a potential for catastrophic impact from an accident but a low probability of an accident, have risk assessment techniques (such as fault tree analysis (FTA); failure modes and effects analysis (FMEA); or failure modes, effects, and criticality analysis (FMECA)) been documented to ensure the presence of enough backup systems for worker protection in the event of multiple control failure? (The nuclear, aerospace, automobile, and airline industries routinely use these techniques to mitigate and prevent potential problems that can affect human life, and these tools can easily be applied to health care.)

☐ *Interviews*
- Do employees complain that new equipment, materials, or processes are hazardous?
- Do any employees say they have been involved in a job hazard analysis (JHA) (also known as a job safety analysis) or process review and are satisfied with the results?
- Does the health and safety staff indicate unfamiliarity with existing or potential hazards at the facility?
- Does the occupational health physician and/or employee health professional understand the potential occupational diseases and health effects in the facility?

☐ *Site conditions and root causes of hazards*
- Have hazards appeared where no one in management realized there was potential for their development?
- Where workers have faithfully followed job procedures, have accidents or near misses occurred because of hidden hazards?

- Have hazards been discovered in the design of new facilities, equipment, materials, and processes after their use has begun?
- Have accidents or near misses occurred when two or more failures in the hazard control system occurred at the same time, surprising everyone?

Regular Site Safety and Health Inspections

☐ *Documentation*
  - If inspection reports are written, do they show that inspections are done on a regular basis?
  - Do the hazards found indicate good ability to recognize those hazards typical of the health care industry?
  - Are hazards found during inspections tracked to complete correction?
  - What is the relationship between hazards uncovered during inspections and those implicated in injuries or illnesses?
☐ *Interviews*
  - Do employees indicate that they see inspections being conducted and that these inspections appear thorough?
☐ *Site conditions and root causes of hazards*
  - Are the hazards discovered during accident investigations ones that should have been recognized and corrected by the regular inspection process?

Employee Reports of Hazards

☐ *Documentation*
  - Is the system for written reports being used frequently?
  - Are valid hazards that have been reported by employees tracked to complete correction?
  - Are the responses timely and adequate?
☐ *Interviews*
  - Do employees know whom to contact and what to do if they see something they believe to be hazardous to themselves or co-workers?
  - Do employees think that responses to their reports of hazards are timely and adequate?
  - Do employees say that sometimes when they report a hazard, they hear nothing further about it?
  - Do any employees say that they or other workers are being harassed, officially or otherwise, for reporting hazards?
☐ *Site conditions and root causes of hazards*
  - Are hazards ever found where employees could reasonably be expected to have previously recognized and reported them?

- When hazards are found, is there evidence that employees had complained repeatedly but to no avail?

Accident and Near-Miss Investigations

☐ *Documentation*
- Do accident investigation reports show a thorough analysis of causes, rather than a tendency to automatically blame the injured employee?
- Are near misses (property damage or close calls) investigated using the same techniques as for accident investigations?
- Are hazards that are identified as contributing to accidents or near misses tracked to correction?

☐ *Interviews*
- Do employees understand and accept the results of accident and near-miss investigations?
- Do employees mention a tendency on management's part to blame the injured employee?
- Do employees believe that all hazards contributing to accidents are corrected or controlled?

☐ *Site conditions and root causes of hazards*
- Are accidents sometimes caused at least partly by factors that might also have contributed to previous near misses that were not investigated or accidents that were too superficially investigated?

Injury and Illness Pattern Analysis

☐ *Documentation*
- In addition to the required OSHA Form 300 log, are careful records kept of first-aid injuries and/or illnesses that might not immediately appear to be work related?
- Is there any periodic, written analysis of the patterns of near misses, injuries, and/or illnesses over time, seeking previously unrecognized connections between them that indicate unrecognized hazards needing correction or control?
- Looking at the OSHA Form 300 log and, where applicable, first-aid logs, are there patterns of illness or injury that should have been analyzed for previously undetected hazards?
- If employees suffering from ordinary illness are encouraged to see a health care provider, are the lists of those visits analyzed for clusters of illness that might be work related?

☐ *Interviews*
- Do employees mention illnesses or injuries that seem work related to them but that have not been analyzed for previously undetected hazards?

☐ *Site conditions and root causes of hazards* (not generally applicable)

3. Assessing the Key Components of Hazard Prevention and Control

Appropriate Use of Engineering Controls, Administrative Controls, and Personal Protective Equipment

☐ *Documentation*
- If there are documented comprehensive surveys, are they accompanied by a plan for the systematic prevention or control of hazards found?
- If there is a written plan, does it show that the best method of hazard protection was chosen?
- Are there written safe-work procedures?
- If respirators are used, is there a written respirator program?
- Is there a qualified program administrator?

☐ *Interviews*
- Do employees say they have been trained in, and have ready access to, reliable and safe work procedures?
- Do employees say they have difficulty accomplishing their work because of unwieldy controls meant to protect them?
- Do employees ever mention PPE, work procedures, or engineering controls as interfering with their ability to work safely?
- Do employees who use PPE understand why they use it and how to maintain it?
- Do employees who use PPE indicate that the rules for PPE use are consistently and fairly enforced?
- Do employees indicate that safe work procedures are fairly and consistently enforced?

☐ *Site conditions and root causes of hazards*
- Are controls meant to protect workers actually putting them at risk or not providing enough protection?
- Are employees engaging in unsafe practices or creating unsafe conditions because rules and work practices are not fairly and consistently enforced?
- Are employees in areas designated for PPE wearing it properly, with no exceptions?
- Are hazards that could feasibly be controlled through improved design being inadequately controlled by other means?

Facility and Equipment Preventive Maintenance

☐ *Documentation*
- Is there a preventive maintenance schedule that provides for timely maintenance of the facilities and equipment?
- Is there a written or computerized record of performed maintenance that shows the schedule has been followed?

- Do maintenance request records show a pattern of certain facilities or equipment needing repair or breaking down before maintenance was scheduled or actually performed?
- Do any accident/incident investigations list facility or equipment breakdown as a major cause?

☐ *Interviews*

- Do employees mention difficulty with improperly functioning equipment or facilities in poor repair?
- Do maintenance employees believe that the preventive maintenance system is working well?
- Do employees believe that hazard controls needing maintenance are properly cared for?

☐ *Site conditions and root causes of hazards*

- Is poor maintenance a frequent source of hazards?
- Are hazard controls in good working order?
- Does equipment appear to be in good working order?

Establishing a Medical Screening and Surveillance Program

☐ *Documentation*

- Are good, clear records kept of medical screening and exposure monitoring?

☐ *Interviews*

- Do employees say that test results were explained to them?
- Does the employee health professional understand the potential hazards of the worksite, so that occupational illness symptoms can be recognized?

☐ *Site conditions and root causes of hazards*

- Have occupational illnesses possibly gone undetected because no one with occupational health specialty training reviewed employee symptoms as part of the medical screening and surveillance program?

Emergency Planning and Preparation

☐ *Documentation*

- Are there clearly written procedures for every likely emergency, with clear evacuation routes, assembly points, and emergency telephone numbers?

☐ *Interviews*

- When asked about any kind of likely emergency, can employees tell exactly what they are supposed to do and where they are supposed to go?

☐ *Site conditions and root causes of hazards*

- Have hazards occurred during actual or simulated emergencies due to confusion about what to do?

- Are emergency evacuation routes clearly marked?
- Are emergency telephone numbers and fire alarms in prominent, easy-to-find locations?

4. Assessing the Key Components of Health and Safety Training

Ensuring That All Employees Understand Hazards

☐ *Documentation*
  - Does the written training program include complete training for every employee in emergency procedures and in all potential hazards to which employees may be exposed?
  - Do training records show that every employee received the planned training?
  - Do the written evaluations of training indicate that the training was successful and that the employees learned what was intended?

☐ *Interviews*
  - Can employees tell the evaluator what hazards they are exposed to, why those hazards are a threat, and how they can help protect themselves and others?
  - When PPE is used, can employees explain why they use it and how to use and maintain it properly?
  - Do employees feel that health and safety training is adequate?

☐ *Site conditions and root causes of hazards*
  - Have employees been hurt or made ill by hazards of which they were completely unaware, or whose dangers they did not understand, or from which they did not know how to protect themselves?
  - Have employees or emergency response staff ever been endangered by employees not knowing what to do or where to go in a given emergency situation?
  - Are there hazards in the workplace that exist, at least in part, because one or more employees have not received adequate hazard control training?
  - Are there any instances of employees not wearing required PPE properly because they have not received proper training? Because they simply do not want to and the requirement is not enforced?

Ensuring That Supervisors Understand Their Responsibilities

☐ *Documentation*
  - Do training records indicate that all supervisors have been trained in their responsibilities to analyze work under their supervision for unrecognized hazards, to maintain physical protections, and to

reinforce employee training through performance feedback and, where necessary, enforcement of safe work procedures and health and safety rules?

☐ *Interviews*
  ▪ Are supervisors aware of their responsibilities?
  ▪ Do employees confirm that supervisors are carrying out these duties?

☐ *Site conditions and root causes*
  ▪ Has a supervisor's lack of understanding of health and safety responsibilities played a part in creating hazardous activities or conditions?

Ensuring That Managers Understand Their Health and Safety Responsibilities

☐ *Documentation*
  ▪ Do training plans for managers and department heads include training in health and safety responsibilities?
  ▪ Do records indicate that all managers and department heads have received this training?

☐ *Interviews*
  ▪ Do employees indicate that managers and department heads know and carry out their safety and health responsibilities?

☐ *Site conditions and root causes of hazards*
  ▪ Has an incomplete or inaccurate understanding by management of its health and safety responsibilities played a part in the creation of hazardous activities or conditions?

STRENGTHS, WEAKNESSES, OPPORTUNITIES, AND THREATS (SWOT) ANALYSIS

A key problem facing Environmental Health and Safety departments is how to focus limited business resources of time and money. "SWOT" analysis provides an efficient way to evaluate the range of factors that influence the department and can give valuable guidance in making decisions about what to do next. It also provides a highly productive way to get key personnel involved in the management decision-making process.[3,4]

Some industry Environmental Health and Safety departments routinely use the SWOT analysis tool for annual and longer-term planning. A functional area, such as safety or occupational health, or a geographical region, such as North America, will apply the tool to look at the strengths, weaknesses, opportunities, and threats to their programs. This process also takes into consideration the key stakeholders involved and potential obstacles.[5]

The SWOT analysis process consists of carefully inspecting the department and its environment through the various dimensions of "strengths, weaknesses, opportunities, and threats." "Strengths" are the department's core competencies and include technology, skills, resources, market position, and other features. "Weaknesses" are conditions within the department that can lead to poor performance and can include poor health and safety performance, obsolete equipment, no clear strategy, poor product or market image, and weak management. "Opportunities" are outside conditions or circumstances that the department could turn to its advantages, and may include a specialty niche skill or technology that suddenly realizes growth in broad market interest. "Threats" are current or future conditions in the outside environment that may harm the department, and might include population shifts, changes in purchasing preferences, new technologies, changes in governmental or environmental regulations, or an increase in competition.

Like most management analysis tools, SWOT in of itself will not give specific answers. Rather, it is a way to organize information and assign probabilities to potential events—both good and bad—as the basis for developing business strategy and operational plans.

Using SWOT analysis is a straightforward process. The key is to limit the number of issues under each category. This forces evaluation of the relative importance of each issue, with only the most critical being selected. To achieve this, a reduction process is used.

Each function of the model program presented in chapter 1 of this book should go through the same process, and a master list of the ideas should be gathered. This list now becomes the basis for further strategic planning. Each of the "strengths, weaknesses, opportunities, and threats" should be inspected and a determination made as to what each of them implies for the department. Feedback and support from senior administration is critical, as many of the goals will rise to the formal, facility-wide level and often be integrated into the performance management objectives of the administration. In some companies, achieving or missing performance management objectives is linked to certain elements of one's compensation for that year. Goals may include environmental goals, environmental incident goals, occupational health and safety goals, occupational health and safety incident goals, and industrial hygiene goals.

The "proposed goals," once finalized and approved by senior administration, should become part of the Environmental Health and Safety Department's annual scorecard and strategic plan. These proposed goals provide a glimpse of the department's program priorities. Once the goals are established, the Environmental Health and Safety Department will work with other departments and senior administration to help achieve the facility's goals and the expected financial savings, business advantages, and employee and patient satisfaction associated with them.

BENCHMARKING

Benchmarking is the search for best practices that lead to superior performance. Through looking outward, the Environmental Health and Safety Department can learn from others and achieve quantum leaps in performance that could take years to achieve through internal incremental improvements. Benchmarking is the process of continuously comparing and measuring the department against health and safety leaders everywhere in the world in order to gain information that will help the department take action to improve its performance. However, it is imperative that the Environmental Health and Safety Department first understand its own processes and practices. Only then can the department be quantified to show its effects, compared to the best, and then changed to achieve greater overall effectiveness.

Because health and safety is integral to all key business processes, benchmarking health and safety can contribute to improvements in all management systems. It is a powerful strategy for promoting the attitude that health and safety is everyone's responsibility in the health care facility.

In any health care facility or company, all areas of management interact. Sometimes health and safety is seen just as accidents and incidents, inspections and audits, hazard management, and policies and procedures. But in fact, Environmental Health and Safety is an integral part of general management and plays a role in all key areas, including maintenance, training, purchasing, work system design, and patient care. Health care facilities that deal successfully with Environmental Health and Safety integrate it into the systems used to manage the facility.

Levels of Benchmarking

In its guide *Benchmarking Occupational Health and Safety: Team Leader's Manual,*[6] the National Occupational Health & Safety Commission of Australia reports that companies undertake benchmarking at a range of different levels.

Some examine the products of competitors and call this benchmarking. This is a simplistic form of benchmarking and is relatively easy to do, but it tends to yield little useful information.

Others seek to quantify the differences between themselves and their competitors. Statistics, while comforting to some as tangible proof of performance or change, can be very misleading.

Other companies say that the most useful form of benchmarking involves self-analysis of processes and procedures, the analysis of other companies, and the adaptation of the findings to guide improvements. This approach gives valuable information about the changes that are necessary in the facility. It is generally a better use of the resources applied to benchmarking.

Using Statistics with Caution

Benchmarking health and safety can involve comparisons of outcome measures such as lost-time injury frequency rates. However, using statistics of accidents and injuries as performance indicators for benchmarking has its problems. For example, accident data measures failure and not success, is subject to random fluctuations, and measures injury severity and not necessarily the potential seriousness of the accident.

Selecting Benchmarking Partners

Companies that have benchmarked health and safety successfully emphasize the importance of choosing the right benchmarking partners. The best benchmarking partners are willing to participate in benchmarking and have good performance in the management systems in which the department is interested. As well as being ready to share information, partners should be undertaking work that is of interest to the department. They should be able to teach the partner something about how to do it better.

Benchmarking partners should not be selected by comparing numerical data or "metrics." This method alone tends to give unreliable results. It is much more important to have information on the management processes that are used by the potential partner.

Programs and Studies to Help Benchmark the Environmental Health and Safety Program

There are many ways to benchmark the facility's Environmental Health and Safety Department. Information can be learned from data reported in studies, from health care facilities and companies that are leaders in health and safety, and from associations and agencies that provide leadership in health and safety.

In addition, the concepts involved in quality measurement–based strategies that focus on process improvement are tools that the Environmental Health and Safety Department can utilize.

Example 1

Participation in the OSHA Voluntary Protection Program (VPP) is an excellent way for senior management to demonstrate and benchmark their commitment to employee health and safety.

Since the start of the VPP in 1982, OSHA has verified that participating worksites have experienced a lost-workday case rate that is 60 to 80 percent lower than their industry averages. Program requirements consist of management systems consistent with OSHA's *Safety and Health Program Management Guidelines*.

Figure 18–2. Grading the Performance of the Health Care Facility

---

    ☐ "A"—World-class performance

    ☐ "B"—Minor gaps or shortcomings

    ☐ "C"—Major pieces are in place

    ☐ "D"—Significant holes or lapses; a more serious focus needed

    ☐ "F"—Major shortcomings, and a long way to go

The OSHA *Guidelines* and this book can be used to benchmark the successes of the facility's safety and health program. Consideration can be given to grading the performance of each department or compliance with specific standards (see figure 18-2).

Example 2

The National Institute of Occupational Safety and Health (NIOSH) recommends that health care facilities use safer medical devices to protect workers from needlestick and other sharps injuries. Since the passage of the Needlestick Safety and Prevention Act in 2000 (P.L. 106-430, 106th Congress) [CD-ROM 18.3] and the subsequent 2000 revision of OSHA Standard 29 CFR 1910.1030, Bloodborne pathogens [CD-ROM 18.4, 18.5, 18.6], all health care facilities are required to use safer medical devices.

Upon request by NIOSH, a small number of health care facilities shared reports on how they implemented safer medical devices in their settings. They described how each step was accomplished, and also discussed the barriers they encountered and how they were resolved, and most important, lessons learned. The resulting document, *Safer Medical Device Implementation in Health Care Facilities: Sharing Lessons Learned*, provides a report of this project, including the estimated staff hours involved in the priority-setting phase. [CD-ROM 18.7]

Example 3

The American National Standards Institute (ANSI) is a consensus standards-setting organization that has no regulatory authority. However, many ANSI standards have been adopted as enforceable OSHA standards. In 2005 ANSI and the American Industrial Hygiene Association (AIHA) published ANSI/AIHA Z10, American National Standard for Occupational Health and Safety Management Systems.[7] This voluntary consensus standard provides management systems with requirements and guidelines for improvement of occupational health and safety. It provides a blueprint for widespread benefits in health and safety, as well as in productivity, financial, performance, quality, and other organizational and business objectives. The voluntary standard is based on the following:

- ☐ Management system principles that are compatible with quality and environmental management system standards ISO 9000 and ISO 14000
- ☐ International Labor Organization (ILO) Guidelines on Occupational Health and Safety Management Systems
- ☐ Systems in use in U.S. organizations

Adherence to ANSI's standard will help provide an organized structure to existing or new programs.

Example 4

The Health Care Health & Safety Association of Ontario (HCHSA)[8] benchmarked ergonomics approaches to patient handling through its Award of Merit to the Tillsonburg District Memorial Hospital Safe Moves Committee. [CD-ROM 18.8] The Award of Merit criteria highlight the accomplishments of health care–sector individuals or organizations. The Safe Moves Committee has demonstrated leadership in the following ways:

- ☐ By sharing lessons learned from lift and transfer practices with other health care sector partners
- ☐ By showing initiative through partnering with relevant community experts to create a video to address organization-specific issues
- ☐ By raising its community profile as an excellent resource for health and safety
- ☐ By engaging workers within the organization and from the broader community to strive for the prevention or reduction of workplace injuries

In May 2005 HCHSA was recognized with the Health Care Public Relations Association of Canada Hygeia Award for its educational approach to personal protective equipment to help health care workers avoid infectious disease. The training video, *Don of a New Day*, placed second in the Multi-Media Production category. The Hygeia Award recognizes excellence in health care communications. It is awarded to public relations professionals in the health care industry to honor outstanding media pieces and accomplishments across Canada. The annual awards program encourages Canadian health care public relations professionals to strive to meet the highest standards in their communications work, regardless of the size, resources, or location of their place of employment.

Example 5

Organizations and associations such as the Bureau of National Affairs (BNA), the National Electrical Manufacturers Association (NEMA), and the National Occupational Health and Safety Commission in Australia benchmark data on Environmental Health and Safety staffing, budgeting, responsibility, and program effectiveness.

Many companies have health and safety programs designed to improve the health and safety stewardship of their employees and their industry, and they need to determine whether they are investing the right amount of money in their programs. During periods of change, this information can prove extremely important to organizations as they strive to remain competitive while ensuring an appropriate level of staffing and program leadership.

Example 6

In a study conducted in 2004,[9] health and safety data was collected from 53 organizations across several industries in the following areas:

- □ Resources and responsibilities for safety
- □ Trust and buy-in for the safety function
- □ Measuring the performance of health and safety programs
- □ Performance of the safety function
- □ Leading and lagging indicators for workplace safety

Key findings of the study include:

- □ Across the benchmark class, health and safety organizations empower their front-line staff to proactively prevent safety incidents. One company features an online close-call program where employees can submit health and safety best practices and ultimately are entered for a prize drawing. Another identifies informal "walk-arounds" and discussions as effective in encouraging health and safety–conscious behavior in workers.
- □ For 47 percent of the benchmark class, the implementation and promotion of health and wellness programs led to a reduction in minor physical injuries at the workplace. Some companies achieved more than a 50 percent reduction rate in one year or less.

The Environmental Health and Safety Department can use this type of data to learn about the health and safety tools and programs of other health care facilities and companies, and can ultimately streamline its health and safety programs to reduce injury rates and maintain workplace productivity.

Benchmarking Questions

Peers in the Environmental Health and Safety profession follow up on certain key issues and trends. Is the Environmental Health and Safety Department running with the pack or marching to the beat of a different drummer?

☐ Do Environmental Health and Safety staff value communication skills? For years Environmental Health and Safety professionals have been told to supplement technical knowledge with communication skills. The ability to communicate is considered more important than technical knowledge. If technical and regulatory information cannot be articulated to managers and employees, Environmental Health and Safety professionals are left stranded in health care facilities. It is clear professionals do not want to be in that position.

☐ Does the Environmental Health and Safety Department "sell" Environmental Health and Safety? Selling senior management to gain their commitment to health and safety is a very important issue.

☐ Does the Environmental Health and Safety Department pay attention to the bottom line? It will be hard for the department to join the business mainstream without a demonstration that they are as concerned about profit and loss as other departments.

☐ How centered on compliance is the facility's health and safety program? Understanding OSHA regulations is the most important issue on the job. These regulations continue to dominate the day-to-day plans and activities of proactive Environmental Health and Safety professionals.

☐ Will OSHA shape the facility's Environmental Health and Safety professional's job in the future?

☐ Who are the customers of the facility's health and safety program?

☐ Is the department confronting ergonomic issues?

☐ How important are health and safety media issues to the department?

Health and Safety Performance Monitoring by Senior Management and Boards of Directors

Health and safety management success requires identification of the key elements of an effective health and safety management system. By measuring the performance of the health and safety program, senior management will also be able to benchmark aspects of the patient safety program relating to the interaction between employees and patients. Effective program management and benchmarking will enable senior management to provide accurate information to members of the board of directors and will identify areas that need additional attention. If the data and information show that an effective program that has helped reduce injuries and illnesses is in place, this success can be used to negotiate insurance premiums and services and serve as an excellent marketing tool that demonstrates the facility's quality of care.

No matter what system is adopted, it should include both active and reactive monitoring. Active monitoring provides feedback on performance before risks result in injury, ill health, or other damage. It includes procedures to monitor progress toward specific health and safety program objectives. The effectiveness of controls can be assessed through systematic inspections of the facility and equipment and compliance with safe work practices. Program effectiveness can also be tracked by analyzing the results of environmental monitoring and health surveillance to confirm the effectiveness of health control measures and detect any early signs of harm to the health of employees.

Reactive monitoring includes gathering data about injuries and illnesses. Senior management and the board of directors should ensure that the management systems are adequate to provide the factual basis for regular reports on health and safety performance, which they will need to make reasoned decisions concerning allocation of resources.

THE ROLE OF THE JOINT COMMISSION IN ASSESSING AND BENCHMARKING PROGRAM PROGRESS

The Joint Commission recognizes the value of analyzing collected data as a way to assess program effectiveness and identify areas for improvement. Joint Commission standards that address recordkeeping include the following:

- ☐ EC.9.10, Monitoring environmental conditions
- ☐ EC.9.20, Analyzing environmental issues
- ☐ EC.9.30, Improving the environment

Under standard EC.9.10, health care facilities are required to annually evaluate their management plans in each area of the environment of care.

THE ROLE OF THE ENVIRONMENTAL HEALTH AND SAFETY DEPARTMENT

The Environmental Health and Safety Department is the principal organizational component for the collection of data and the preparation of reports showing progress toward the goal of reducing injuries and illnesses. Through the network of department liaisons, the Environmental Health and Safety Department is uniquely suited to that task. More important, because of its close organizational relationship with senior management, the Environmental

Health and Safety Department can help establish short-term and long-range goals for improving employee health and safety. Once those goals have been established, the Environmental Health and Safety Department can work with the department liaisons to benchmark progress toward those goals. The surveillance activities of the department are essential to that effort.

References

1. *Safety and Health Program Management Guidelines: Issuance of Voluntary Guidelines.* OSHA Federal Register Notice 54 (18) (January 26, 1989), pp. 3908–3916. Available at http://www.osha.gov/pls/oshaweb/owadisp.show_document?p_table=FEDERAL_REGISTER&p_id=12909 (accessed 3/28/2006).
2. OSHA Office of Training and Education. *Tools for a Safety and Health Program Assessment.* (1997) Available at http://www.osha.gov/doc/outreachtraining/htmlfiles/evaltool.html (accessed 3/29/2006).
3. Osgood, William R. *Where Is My Business Headed and Why?* (Adapted.) Available at http://www.buzgate.org/nh/bft_swot.html?redirectedFrom=/dc/bft_swot.html (accessed 3/29/2006).
4. *Common Sense Strategic Analysis.* Strategic Management Learning System (SMLS), U.S. Small Business Administration. Available at http://www.bdki.com/smls.php (accessed 3/29/2006).
5. *Next-Generation Environment, Health and Safety Goals.* Baxter Worldwide. Available at http://www.baxter.com/about_baxter/sustainability/our_environment/programs/sub/goals.html (accessed 3/29/2006).
6. Worksafe Australia. *Benchmarking Occupational Health and Safety: Team Leader's Manual.* Commonwealth of Australia, 1996. Available at http://www.nohsc.gov.au/PDF/Standards/BenchmarkingOHS.pdf (accessed 3/29/2006).
7. *American National Standard for Occupational Health and Safety Management Systems.* ANSI/AIHA Z10-2005. Available at http://webstore.ansi.org/ansidocstore/product.asp?sku=ANSI%2FAIHA+Z10-2005 (accessed 4/28/2006).
8. Health Care Health & Safety Association (HCHSA), www.hchsa.on.ca.
9. Best Practices, LLC. *Benchmarks for Establishing and Measuring Successful Health & Safety Functions.* August 31, 2004. Available at http://www3.best-in-class.com/bestp/domrep.nsf/Content/2D893575FC556EF785256F01005B0DDF!OpenDocument (accessed 3/29/2006).

[AuQ1] Please confirm this is set correctly.

Appendix: Additional Resources

The CD-ROM on the inside back cover contains additional resources to supplement the electronic documents identified in the preface and chapters. (See "About the CD-ROM" in the front matter for a full description of the CD-ROM.) The following tables serve as an index to these additional resources.

Table A-1. Additional Resources Organized by Book Chapter

CD File Number	Document Title
Preface	
P-AR.1	OSH Act of 1970
Chapter 1: The Current State of Health Care Employee Safety Programs and a Model for the Future	
1-AR.1	CCOHS, Bringing Health to Work
1-AR.2	CCOHS, Bringing Health to Work: Employees
1-AR.3	CCOHS, Bringing Health to Work: Employers
1-AR.4	The OSHA Alliance Program
1-AR.5	The Alliance Program: A Cooperative and Collaborative Approach to Workplace Safety and Health
1-AR.6	An Overview of OSHA's Compliance Assistance Resources: 2005 National Equal Opportunity Conference
1-AR.7	Leadership—*The* Driver for Safety and Health
1-AR.8	Module 4—Safety and Health Program Management: Fact Sheets—Management Leadership
1-AR.9	Safety and Health Management Systems eTool—Management Leadership
1-AR.10	OSHA Strategic Partnership Program (OSPP)
1-AR.11	Safety and Health Add Value
Chapter 2: Getting the Environmental Health and Safety Program Started	
2-AR.1	CA OSHA, Guide to Developing Your Workplace Injury and Illness Prevention Program with Checklists for Self-Inspection
2-AR.2	Updated U.S. Public Health Service Guidelines for the Management of Occupational Exposures to HBV, HCV, and HIV and Recommendations for Postexposure Prophylaxis

(Continued on next page)

Table A-1. *(Continued)*

CD File Number	Document Title
2-AR.3	Getting in the Door: Language Barriers to Health Services at New York City's Hospitals
2-AR.4	Health and Safety Guidelines for Home-Based Health Care Services
2-AR.5	Put It in Writing: The Complete Guide to OR-OSHA's Written Requirements for the Workplace
2-AR.6	Safety Committees for the Real World: OR-OSHA's Guide to Starting an Effective Workplace Safety Committee
2-AR.7	You Have a Right to a Safe and Healthful Workplace. It's the Law!
2-AR.8	OSHA Medical Surveillance Requirements
2-AR.9	OSHA Self-Inspection Checklists
2-AR.10	Overcoming Language Barriers Part II: For Administrators. A Volunteers in Health Care Guide
2-AR.11	NIOSH Alert: Preventing Deaths, Injuries, and Illnesses of Young Workers
2-AR.12	OSHA Federal Agency Programs
2-AR.13	Section 5: Overview of Occupational Safety and Occupational Health/Industrial Hygiene
2-AR.14	Occupational Health and Safety Program: Client Self-Assessment Checklist

Chapter 3: Positioning and Marketing the Environmental Health and Safety Program and Achieving National Recognition

3-AR.1	"Change—It's Up to You!" (Poem by Charles Sexton)
3-AR.2	"Valuing You" (Poem by Charles Sexton)

Chapter 4: Occupational Safety and Health Agencies and Organizations

4-AR.1	Centers for Medicare & Medicaid Services (CMS)
4-AR.2	CMS Life Safety Code Requirements
4-AR.3	United States Government Accountability Office: CMS Needs Additional Authority to Adequately Oversee Patient Safety in Hospitals
4-AR.4	CMS Certification & Compliance: Overview

Chapter 5: Integrating Workplace and Family Safety and Health: The Holistic Approach

5-AR.1	A Workplace Toolkit: Model Family Violence Policy, Safety Plans and Messages
5-AR.2	Building Safe Communities: A Publication of the National Highway Traffic Safety Administration
5-AR.3	Handling Chemotherapy Drugs Safely at Home
5-AR.4	NIOSH, Plain Language about Shiftwork

(Continued on next page)

Table A-1. *(Continued)*

CD File Number	Document Title
5-AR.5	Washington Traffic Safety Commission Harborview Injury Prevention and Research Center: Training Programs for Bicycle Safety
5-AR.6	CCOHS, Active Living at Work
5-AR.7	CCOHS, Bringing Health to Work: Employees—Why Should I Bring Health to Work?
5-AR.8	CCOHS, Bringing Health to Work: Employees—Healthy Living Choices
5-AR.9	CCOSH, Rotational Shiftwork

Chapter 6: Infection Control

CD File Number	Document Title
6-AR.1	CDC, Key Facts about Avian Influenza (Bird Flu) and Avian Influenza A (H5N1) Virus
6-AR.2	Public Health Foundation, Exposure to Blood: What Healthcare Personnel Need to Know
6-AR.3	CDC, Guidelines for Environmental Infection Control in Health-Care Facilities
6-AR.4	CDC: Hand Hygiene Guidelines Fact Sheet
6-AR.5	Updated U.S. Public Health Service Guidelines for the Management of Occupational Exposures to HBV, HCV, and HIV and Recommendations for Postexposure Prophylaxis
6-AR.6	Guidelines for Preventing the Transmission of *Mycobacterium tuberculosis* in Health-Care Settings, 2005
6-AR.7	Needlestick Safety and Prevention Act
6-AR.8	NIOSH Alert: Preventing Needlestick Injuries in Health Care Settings
6-AR.9	NIOSH, How to Protect Yourself from Needlestick Injuries
6-AR.10	NIOSH, Eye Protection for Infection Control
6-AR.11	NIOSH, Safer Medical Device Implementation in Health Care Facilities
6-AR.12	OSHA Fact Sheet for Bloodborne Pathogens
6-AR.13	OSHA, 29 CFR Part 1910: Occupational Exposure to Bloodborne Pathogens; Needlesticks and Other Sharps Injuries; Final Rule
6-AR.14	OSHA, Most Frequently Asked Questions Concerning the Bloodborne Pathogens Standard
6-AR.15	OSHA Frequently Asked Questions: Needlestick Safety and Prevention Act
6-AR.16	How (and Why) to Make a Display Board of Sharps Devices
6-AR.17	How to Calculate Sharps Injury Rates
6-AR.18	How to Develop a Sharps Policy for Your Facility

(Continued on next page)

Table A-1. *(Continued)*

CD File Number	Document Title
Chapter 7: Chemicals	
7-AR.1	HHS, "If I'm Pregnant, Can the Chemicals I Work with Harm My Baby?"
7-AR.2	Understanding Toxic Substances
7-AR.3	NIOSH, Contact Lens Use in a Chemical Environment
7-AR.4	OSHA Safety and Health Topics: Chemical Reactivity Hazards
7-AR.5	OSHA Draft Model Training Program for Hazard Communication
7-AR.6	OSHA Hazard Communication: Foundation of Workplace Chemical Safety Programs
7-AR.7	OSHA Compliance Assistance: Hazard Communication in the 21st Century Workplace
7-AR.8	NIOSH Alert: Preventing Occupational Exposures to Antineoplastic and Other Hazardous Drugs in Health Care Settings
7-AR.9	Changing Materials and Practices in Anatomical Pathology Laboratories: An Overview for Managers and Administrators
7-AR.10	Interpreting Analytical Results for Mercury and Other Substances
7-AR.11	Pilot Study of Alternatives to the Use of Xylene in a Hospital Histology Laboratory
Chapter 8: Waste Management	
8-AR.1	Hazardous Waste & Toxics Reduction Program: Best Management Practices
8-AR.2	Healthy Hospitals: Environmental Improvements through Environmental Accounting
8-AR.3	EPA, Preventing and Managing Mixed Waste
8-AR.4	National Safety Council, A Guide to the U.S. Department of Energy's Low-Level Radioactive Waste
8-AR.5	Handbook for Hazardous Waste Generators
8-AR.6	Healthcare Pollution Prevention
8-AR.7	10 CFR Part 62—Criteria and Procedures for Emergency Access to Non-Federal and Regional Low-Level Waste Disposal Facilities
8-AR.8	NRC, Who Regulates Radioactive Materials and Radioactive Exposure?
8-AR.9	National Safety Council, Radioactive Waste
8-AR.10	OSHA, Industrial Hygiene
8-AR.11	OSHA, 03/28/2005—Containment and Disposal Requirements for Disposable Razors Used in Long-Term Health Care Facilities for Personal Grooming
8-AR.12	Radiation Safety Manual for Laboratory Users, Section 7: Radioactive Waste Disposal

(Continued on next page)

Table A-1. *(Continued)*

CD File Number	Document Title
8-AR.13	Radioactive Waste
8-AR.14	What Is Dangerous Waste?
8-AR.15	H2E Tools/Resources: Waste Reduction Guide
8-AR.16	Removing Mercury from Hospital Labs
8-AR.17	Mercury Spills—How Much Do They Cost?

Chapter 9: Personal Protective Equipment

9-AR.1	CCOHS, Designing an Effective PPE Program
9-AR.2	Biosafety in Microbiological and Biomedical Laboratories
9-AR.3	Personal Protective Equipment Program
9-AR.4	Personal Protective Equipment
9-AR.5	NIOSH, Protective Clothing
9-AR.6	NYCOSH, Personal Protective Equipment
9-AR.7	OR OSHA Module Three: Eye and Face Protection
9-AR.8	Respiratory Protection
9-AR.9	OSHA 01/01/1993—Eye Protection in the Workplace
9-AR.10	OSHA Safety and Health Topics: Noise and Hearing Conservation
9-AR.11	OSHA Safety and Health Topics: Personal Protective Equipment (PPE)
9-AR.12	OSHA Personal Protective Equipment Fact Sheet
9-AR.13	Small Entity Compliance Guide for the Revised Respiratory Protection Standard
9-AR.14	OSHA Technical Manual—Section VIII, Chapter 1: Chemical Protective Clothing
9-AR.15	Questions to Ask When Selecting Medical Gloves for Handling Chemotherapy Drugs
9-AR.16	Selecting Medical Gloves
9-AR.17	Vinyl Medical Gloves: What Are the Concerns?

Chapter 10: Ergonomics

10-AR.1	Incidents of Jeopardy/Harm to Patient/Resident Health and Safety
10-AR.2	NIOSH/ERGO Conference: Healthcare (Presentation by Bernice Owen)
10-AR.3	OSHA, Healthcare Facilities: Back Facts—Activity 6
10-AR.4	OSHA, Ergonomics: Guidelines for Nursing Homes

Chapter 11: Workplace Violence

11-AR.1	Stalking in America: Findings from the National Violence Against Women Survey
11-AR.2	NIOSH, Violence: Occupational Hazards in Hospitals
11-AR.3	A Guide to the Development of a Workplace Violence Prevention Program

(Continued on next page)

Table A-1. *(Continued)*

CD File Number	Document Title
Chapter 12: Emergency Management	
12-AR.1	California Hospital Bioterrorism Response Planning Guide
12-AR.2	CCOSH, Emergency Planning
12-AR.3	CDC, Maintaining a Healthy State of Mind
12-AR.4	CDC, Fact Sheet: Anthrax Information for Health Care Providers
12-AR.5	CDC, Botulism Case Definition
12-AR.6	CDC, Burns
12-AR.7	CDC, Shelter-in-Place during a Chemical or Radiation Emergency
12-AR.8	CDC, Clean Up Safely after a Natural Disaster
12-AR.9	CDC, Controlling the Spread of Contagious Diseases: Quarantine and Isolation
12-AR.10	CDC, Coping with a Traumatic Event
12-AR.11	CDC, Emergency Water and Food Supplies
12-AR.12	CDC, Frequently Asked Questions about a Nuclear Blast
12-AR.13	CDC, Hand Hygiene in Emergency Situations
12-AR.14	CDC, Helping Patients Cope with a Traumatic Event
12-AR.15	CDC, Interim Health Recommendations for Workers Who Handle Human Remains
12-AR.16	CDC, After a Hurricane: Key Facts about Infectious Disease
12-AR.17	CDC, Key Facts about Hurricane Readiness
12-AR.18	CDC, Infection Control Prevention Guidance for Community Shelters Following Disasters
12-AR.19	CDC, Facts about Lewisite
12-AR.20	CDC, Disaster Mental Health for *Responders:* Key Principles, Issues and Questions
12-AR.21	CDC, Case Definition: Plague
12-AR.22	CDC, Frequently Asked Questions about Plague
12-AR.23	CDC, Prevent Illness after a Natural Disaster
12-AR.24	CDC, Prevent Injury after a Natural Disaster
12-AR.25	CDC, Facts about Ricin
12-AR.26	Self-Care Tips for Emergency and Disaster Response Workers
12-AR.27	CDC, The Threat of Biological Attack: Why Concern Now?
12-AR.28	CDC, Tularemia Case Definition
12-AR.29	CDC, Abstract: "Consensus Statement: Tularemia as a Biological Weapon: Medical and Public Health Management"
12-AR.30	CDC, Facts about VX
12-AR.31	Chemical Facility Security
12-AR.32	Guidelines for Mass Casualty Decontamination during a Terrorist Chemical Agent Incident
12-AR.33	CDC, Facts about Pneumonic Plague

(Continued on next page)

Table A-1. *(Continued)*

CD File Number	Document Title
12-AR.34	FEMA, Emergency Response to Terrorism
12-AR.35	FEMA Public Service Announcements
12-AR.36	FEMA, Backgrounder: Thunderstorms and Lightning
12-AR.37	FEMA, Tornado Safety Tips Brochure
12-AR.38	FEMA, Factsheet: Winter Storms
12-AR.39	FEMA, Emergency Management Guide for Business and Industry: A Step-by-Step Approach to Emergency Planning, Response and Recovery for Companies of All Sizes
12-AR.40	Guidelines for Responding to a Chemical Weapons Incident
12-AR.41	National Strategy for Homeland Security
12-AR.42	National Incident Management System National Standard Curriculum Training Development Guidance
12-AR.43	Emergency Responder Guidelines
12-AR.44	Hospital-Based First Receivers of Victims from Mass Casualty Incidents Involving the Release of Hazardous Substances
12-AR.45	OSHA, Section 10: Emergency Preparedness and Response
12-AR.46	NRC, Fact Sheet: Dirty Bombs
12-AR.47	NRC, Fact Sheet on Emergency Planning and Preparedness

Chapter 13: Fire Prevention and Control

13-AR.1	All Structure Fires in 2000
13-AR.2	CCOSH, Emergency Planning
13-AR.3	Fire Safety
13-AR.4	Am I Ready for My CMS Survey?
13-AR.5	FDA Public Health Notification: Safety Tips for Preventing Hospital Bed Fires
13-AR.6	NIOSH Alert: Preventing Electrocutions Due to Damaged Receptacles and Connectors
13-AR.7	Surges Happen! How to Protect the Appliances in Your Home
13-AR.8	AUBE '01: 12th International Conference on Automatic Fire Detection
13-AR.9	Fire Hazards
13-AR.10	Flammable and Combustible Materials
13-AR.11	Sacramento City Fire Department, Fire Links
13-AR.12	Is Your Fire Brigade Up to Snuff?

Chapter 14: Improving Patient Safety through Improved Employee Health and Safety

14-AR.1	Measures of Patient Safety Based on Hospital Administrative Data: The Patient Safety Indicators
14-AR.2	Fact Sheet: Tools for Hospitals and Health Care Systems
14-AR.3	Home Study Program: Advanced Practice Nurse Entrepreneurs in a Multidisciplinary Surgical-Assisting Partnership

(Continued on next page)

Table A-1. *(Continued)*

CD File Number	Document Title
14-AR.4	CDC, For Healthcare Providers: Guidelines for the Management of Acute Diarrhea
14-AR.5	Medicaid Program; Use of Restraint and Seclusion in Psychiatric Residential Treatment Facilities Providing Psychiatric Services to Individuals Under Age 21; Final Rule
14-AR.6	NIOSH, Safer Medical Device Implementation in Health Care Facilities
14-AR.7	The Operating Room Charge Nurse: Coordinator and Communicator
14-AR.8	OSACH Handle with Care: A Comprehensive Approach to Developing and Implementing a Client Handling Program

Chapter 15: Surveillance, Data Analysis, and Incident Management

CD File Number	Document Title
15-AR.1	Hazard Analysis and Critical Control Point Principles and Application Guidelines
15-AR.2	Tracking Occupational Injuries, Illnesses, and Hazards: The NIOSH Surveillance Strategic Plan
15-AR.3	NIOSH, Occupational Sentinel Health Events SHE(O)
15-AR.4	NIOSH, Occupational Sentinel Health Events SHE(O)—Abstracts
15-AR.5	Accident Investigation Report
15-AR.6	OSHA, Asbestos—1910.1001
15-AR.7	Job Hazard Analysis
15-AR.8	Screening and Surveillance: A Guide to OSHA Standards
15-AR.9	OSHA, Section 6: Accident Investigation
15-AR.10	OSHA, Injury and Illness—Recordkeeping
15-AR.11	Job Safety Analysis
15-AR.12	Appendix A: Hazard Assessment and Personal Protective Equipment Selection

Chapter 16: Training and Development

CD File Number	Document Title
16-AR.1	CA Safety and Health Training and Instruction Requirements
16-AR.2	Occupational Health and Safety Issues for the Older Worker
16-AR.3	How to Implement Safer Workplace Practices
16-AR.4	Policies, Practices, & Procedures for Health Care Facilities
16-AR.5	Be Trained: A Guide to OR-OSHA's Safety & Health Training Requirements
16-AR.6	Competent Persons: OSHA Standards
16-AR.7	OSHA, Draft Model Training Program for Hazard Communication
16-AR.8	OSHA Outreach Training Program Guidelines: General Industry Safety and Health
16-AR.9	OSH Basics—OSHA Training Guidelines
16-AR.10	OSHA Outreach Training Program

(Continued on next page)

Table A-1. *(Continued)*

CD File Number	Document Title
Chapter 17: Facilities Responsibilities and Environmental Issues	
17-AR.1	CCOSH, How Do I Work Safely with Compressed Gases?
17-AR.2	Standpipe and Hose Fire Protection Systems: Self-Inspection Checklist
17-AR.3	Hazards of Compressed Gas Cylinders in the Magnetic Resonance Imaging (MRI) Environment
17-AR.4	Acetylene Safety Alert
17-AR.5	Department of Energy (DOE) OSH Technical Reference, Chapter 3, Appendix A: Lockout/Tagout Safety Checklist
17-AR.6	Control of Hazardous Energy Sources: Self-Inspection Checklist
17-AR.7	Working Safely in the Cold
17-AR.8	OR OSHA Fact Sheet: Compressed Gas Safety
17-AR.9	OSHA, Self-Inspection Checklists
17-AR.10	OSHA, Hospital Hazards
17-AR.11	OSHA, Indoor Air Quality—59:15968–16039
17-AR.12	OSHA, STD 01-12-002, PUB 8-1.3: Guidelines for Robotics Safety
17-AR.13	Machines and Machine Guarding Self-Audit Checklist
17-AR.14	Compressed Gas Cylinders
17-AR.15	Design + Safety Handbook for Specialty Gas Delivery Systems
17-AR.16	CCOSH, Prevention of Slips, Trips and Falls
Chapter 18: Program Evaluation and Benchmarking	
18-AR.1	Workplace Safety Evaluation Programme

Table A-2. Text of Selected Portions of Federal OSHA Standards from Parts 1904, 1910, 1913, 1926, and 1960

CD File Number	Source Publication No.	Document Title
Part 1910: Occupational Safety and Health Standards		
O-AR.1	1910	Table of Contents
O-AR.2	1910 Subpart A	Authority for 1910 Subpart A
O-AR.3	1910.1	Purpose and scope
O-AR.4	1910.2	Definitions
O-AR.5	1910.3	Petitions for the Issuance, Amendment, or Repeal of a Standard
O-AR.6	1910.4	Amendments to This Part
O-AR.7	1910.5	Applicability of Standards
O-AR.8	1910.6	Incorporation by Reference
O-AR.9	1910 Subpart B	Adoption and Extension of Established Federal Standards
O-AR.10	1910.11	Scope and Purpose
O-AR.11	1910.18	Changes in Established Federal Standards
O-AR.12	1910.19	Special Provisions for Air Contaminants
O-AR.13	1910 Subpart C	Adoption and Extension of Established Federal Standards
O-AR.14	1910 Subpart D	Walking-Working Surfaces: Authority for 1910 Subpart D
O-AR.15	1910.21	Definitions
O-AR.16	1910.22	General Requirements
O-AR.17	1910.23	Guarding Floor and Wall Openings and Holes
O-AR.18	1910.24	Fixed Industrial Stairs
O-AR.19	1910.25	Portable Wood Ladders
O-AR.20	1910.26	Portable Metal Ladders
O-AR.21	1910.27	Fixed Ladders
O-AR.22	1910.28	Safety Requirements for Scaffolding
O-AR.23	1910.30	Other Working Surfaces
O-AR.24	1910 Subpart E	Exit Routes, Emergency Action Plans, and Fire Prevention Plans
O-AR.25	1910 Subpart E App	Exit Routes, Emergency Action Plans, and Fire Prevention Plans
O-AR.26	1910.33	Table of Contents
O-AR.27	1910.34	Coverage and Definitions
O-AR.28	1910.35	Compliance with *NFPA 101®: Life Safety Code®–2000 edition*
O-AR.29	1910.36	Design and Construction Requirements for Exit Routes
O-AR.30	1910.37	Maintenance, Safeguards, and Operational Features for Exit Routes

(Continued on next page)

Table A-2. *(Continued)*

CD File Number	Source Publication No.	Document Title
O-AR.31	1910.38	Emergency Action Plans
O-AR.32	1910.39	Fire Prevention Plans
O-AR.33	1910 Subpart F	Powered Platforms, Manlifts, and Vehicle-Mounted Work Platforms
O-AR.34	1910.66	Powered Platforms for Building Maintenance
O-AR.35	1910.66 App A	Guidelines (Advisory)
O-AR.36	1910.66 App B	Exhibits (Advisory)
O-AR.37	1910.66 App C	Personal Fall Arrest System (Section I – Mandatory; Sections II and III – Non-Mandatory
O-AR.38	1910.66 App D	Existing Installations (Mandatory)
O-AR.39	1910.67	Vehicle-Mounted Elevating and Rotating Work Platforms
O-AR.40	1910.68	Manlifts
O-AR.41	1910 Subpart G	Occupational Health and Environment Control
O-AR.42	1910.94	Ventilation
O-AR.43	1910.95	Occupational Noise Exposure
O-AR.44	1910.95 App A	Noise Exposure Computation
O-AR.45	1910.95 App B	Methods for Estimating the Adequacy of Hearing Protector Attenuation
O-AR.46	1910.95 App C	Audiometric Measuring Instruments
O-AR.47	1910.95 App D	Audiometric Test Rooms
O-AR.48	1910.95 App E	Acoustic Calibration of Audiometers
O-AR.49	1910.95 App F	Calculations and Application of Age Corrections to Audiograms
O-AR.50	1910.95 App G	Monitoring Noise Levels Non-mandatory Informational Appendix
O-AR.51	1910.95 App H	Availability of Referenced Documents
O-AR.52	1910.95 App I	Definitions
O-AR.53	1910.97	Nonionizing Radiation
O-AR.54	1910.98	Effective Dates
O-AR.55	1910 Subpart H	Hazardous Materials
O-AR.56	1910.101	Compressed Gases (General Requirements)

(Continued on next page)

Table A-2. *(Continued)*

CD File Number	Source Publication No.	Document Title
O-AR.57	1910.102	Acetylene
O-AR.58	1910.104	Oxygen
O-AR.59	1910.105	Nitrous Oxide
O-AR.60	1910.106	Flammable and Combustible Liquids
O-AR.61	1910.120	Hazardous Waste Operations and Emergency Response
O-AR.62	1910.120 App A	Personal Protective Equipment Test Methods
O-AR.63	1910.120 App B	General Description and Discussion of the Levels of Protection and Protective Gear
O-AR.64	1910.120 App C	Compliance Guidelines
O-AR.65	1910.120 App D	References
O-AR.66	1910.120 App E	Training and Curriculum Guidelines (Non-mandatory)
O-AR.67	1910. Subpart I	Personal Protective Equipment
O-AR.68	1910.132	General Requirements
O-AR.69	1910.133	Eye and Face Protection
O-AR.70	1910.134	Respiratory Protection
O-AR.71	1910.134 App A	Fit Testing Procedures (Mandatory)
O-AR.72	1910.134 App B-1	User Seal Check Procedures (Mandatory)
O-AR.73	1910.134 App B-2	Respirator Cleaning Procedures (Mandatory)
O-AR.74	1910.134 App C	OSHA Respirator Medical Evaluation Questionnaire (Mandatory)
O-AR.75	1910.134 App D	(Mandatory) Information for Employees Using Respirators When Not Required under Standard
O-AR.76	1910.135	Head Protection
O-AR.77	1910.136	Occupational Foot Protection
O-AR.78	1910.137	Electrical Protective Devices
O-AR.79	1910.138	Hand Protection
O-AR.80	1910 Subpart I App A	References for Further Information (Non-mandatory)
O-AR.81	1910 Subpart I App B	Non-mandatory Compliance Guidelines for Hazard Assessment and Personal Protective Equipment Selection
O-AR.82	1910 Subpart J	General Environmental Controls

(Continued on next page)

Table A-2. *(Continued)*

CD File Number	Source Publication No.	Document Title
O-AR.83	1910.141	Sanitation
O-AR.84	1910.144	Safety Color Code for Marking Physical Hazards
O-AR.85	1910.145	Specifications for Accident Prevention Signs and Tags
O-AR.86	1910145(f) App A	Recommended Color Coding
O-AR.87	1910.145(f) App B	References for Further Information
O-AR.88	1910.146	Permit-required Confined Spaces
O-AR.89	1910.146 App A	Permit-required Confined Space Decision Flow Chart
O-AR.90	1910.146 App B	Procedures for Atmospheric Testing
O-AR.91	1910.146 App C	Examples of Permit-required Confined Space Programs
O-AR.92	1910.146 App D	Confined Space Pre-entry Check List
O-AR.93	1910.146 App E	Sewer System Entry
O-AR.94	1910.146 App F	Non-mandatory Appendix F—Rescue Team or Rescue Service Evaluation Criteria
O-AR.95	1910.147	The Control of Hazardous Energy (Lockout/Tagout)
O-AR.96	1910.147 App A	Typical Minimal Lockout Procedures
O-AR.97	1910 Subpart K	Medical and First Aid
O-AR.98	1910.151	Medical Services and First Aid
O-AR.99	1910.151 App A	Appendix A to 1910.151—First Aid kits (Non-mandatory)
O-AR.100	1910 Subpart L	Fire Protection
O-AR.101	1910.155	Scope, Application and Definitions Applicable to This Subpart
O-AR.102	1910.156	Fire Brigades
O-AR.103	1910.157	Portable Fire Extinguishers
O-AR.104	1910.158	Standpipe and Hose Systems
O-AR.105	1910.159	Automatic Sprinkler Systems
O-AR.106	1910.160	Fixed Extinguishing Systems, General
O-AR.107	1910.161	Fixed Extinguishing Systems, Dry Chemical
O-AR.108	1910.162	Fixed Extinguishing Systems, Gaseous Agent
O-AR.109	1910.163	Fixed Extinguishing Systems, Water Spray and Foam
O-AR.110	1910.164	Fire Detection Systems

(Continued on next page)

Table A-2. *(Continued)*

CD File Number	Source Publication No.	Document Title
O-AR.111	1910.165	Employee Alarm Systems
O-AR.112	1910 Subpart L App A	Fire Protection
O-AR.113	1910 Subpart L App B	National Consensus Standards
O-AR.114	1910 Subpart L App C	Fire Protection References for Further Information
O-AR.115	1910 Subpart L App D	Availability of Publications Incorporated by Reference in Section 1910.156 Fire Brigades
O-AR.116	1910 Subpart L App E	Test Methods for Protective Clothing
O-AR.117	1910 Subpart M	Compressed Gas and Compressed Air Equipment
O-AR.118	1910 Subpart N	Materials Handling and Storage
O-AR.119	1910.176	Handling Materials—General
O-AR.120	1910.178	Powered Industrial Trucks
O-AR.121	1910.178 App A	Powered Industrial Trucks
O-AR.122	1910.183	Helicopters
O-AR.123	1910 Subpart O	Machinery and Machine Guarding
O-AR.124	1910.211	Definitions
O-AR.125	1910.212	General Requirements for All Machines
O-AR.126	1910.213	Woodworking Machinery Requirements
O-AR.127	1910.215	Abrasive Wheel Machinery
O-AR.128	1910.217	Mechanical Power Presses
O-AR.129	1910.217 App A	Mandatory Requirements for Certification/Validation of Safety Systems for Presence Sensing Device Initiation of Mechanical Power Presses
O-AR.130	1910.217 App B	Non-mandatory Guidelines for Certification/Validation of Safety Systems for Presence Sensing Device Initiation of Mechanical Power Presses
O-AR.131	1910.217 App C	Mandatory Requirements for OSHA Recognition of Third-party Validation Organizations for the PSDI Standard

(Continued on next page)

Table A-2. *(Continued)*

CD File Number	Source Publication No.	Document Title
O-AR.132	1910.217 App D	Non-mandatory Supplementary Information
O-AR.133	1910 Subpart P	Hand and Portable Powered Tools and Other Hand-Held Equipment
O-AR.134	1910.241	Definitions
O-AR.135	1910.242	Hand and Portable Powered Tools and Equipment, General
O-AR.136	1910.243	Guarding of Portable Powered Tools
O-AR.137	1910.244	Other Portable Tools and Equipment
O-AR.138	1910 Subpart Q	Welding, Cutting, and Brazing
O-AR.139	1910.251	Definitions
O-AR.140	1910.252	General Requirements
O-AR.141	1910.253	Oxygen-fuel Gas Welding and Cutting
O-AR.142	1910.254	Arc Welding and Cutting
O-AR.143	1910.255	Resistance Welding
O-AR.144	1910.264	Laundry Machinery and Operations
O-AR.145	1910 Subpart S	Electrical
O-AR.146	1910.301	Introduction
O-AR.147	1910.302	Electric Utilization Systems
O-AR.148	1910.303	General Requirements
O-AR.149	1910.304	Wiring Design and Protection
O-AR.150	1910.305	Wiring Methods, Components, and Equipment for General Use
O-AR.151	1910.306	Specific Purpose Equipment and Installations
O-AR.152	1910.332	Training
O-AR.153	1910.333	Selection and Use of Work Practices
O-AR.154	1910.334	Use of Equipment
O-AR.155	1910.335	Safeguards for Personal Protection
O-AR.156	1910.399	Definitions Applicable to This Subpart
O-AR.157	1910 Subpart S App A	Reference Documents
O-AR.158	1910 Subpart A App B	Explanatory Data
O-AR.159	1910 Subpart S App C	Tables, Notes, and Charts

(Continued on next page)

Table A-2. *(Continued)*

CD File Number	Source Publication No.	Document Title
O-AR.160	1910 Subpart Z	Toxic and Hazardous Substances
O-AR.161	1910.1000	Air Contaminants
O-AR.162	1910.1000 TABLE Z-1	Table Z-1 Limits for Air Contaminants
O-AR.163	1910.1000 TABLE Z-2	Table Z-2
O-AR.164	1910.1000 TABLE Z-3	Table Z-3 Mineral Dusts
O-AR.165	1910.1001	Asbestos
O-AR.166	1910.1001 App A	OSHA Reference Method—Mandatory
O-AR.167	1910.1001 App C	Qualitative and Quantitative Fit Testing Procedures—Mandatory
O-AR.168	1910.1001 App D	Medical Questionnaires; Mandatory
O-AR.169	1910.1001 App H	Medical Surveillance Guidelines for Asbestos—Non-mandatory
O-AR.170	1910.1020	Access to Employee Exposure and Medical Records
O-AR.171	1910.1020 App A	Sample Authorization Letter for the Release of Employee Medical Record Information to a Designated Representative (Non-mandatory)
O-AR.172	1910.1020 App B	Availability of NIOSH Registry of Toxic Effects of Chemical Substances (RTECS) (Non-mandatory)
O-AR.173	1910.1025	Lead
O-AR.174	1910.1025 App A	Substance Data Sheet for Occupational Exposure to Lead
O-AR.175	1910.1025 App B	Employee Standard Summary
O-AR.176	1910.1025 App C	Medical Surveillance Guidelines
O-AR.177	1910.1025 App D	Qualitative Fit Test Protocols
O-AR.178	1910.1028	Benzene
O-AR.179	1910.1028 App A	Substance Safety Data Sheet, Benzene
O-AR.180	1910.1028 App B	Substance Technical Guidelines, Benzene
O-AR.181	1910.1028 App C	Medical Surveillance Guidelines for Benzene
O-AR.182	1910.1028 App D	Sampling and Analytical Methods for Benzene Monitoring and Measurement Procedures

(Continued on next page)

Table A-2. *(Continued)*

CD File Number	Source Publication No.	Document Title
O-AR.183	1910.1028 App E	Qualitative and Quantitative Fit Testing Procedures
O-AR.184	1910.1030	Bloodborne Pathogens
O-AR.185	1910.1030 App A	Hepatitis B Vaccine Declination (Mandatory)
O-AR.186	1910.1047	Ethylene Oxide
O-AR.187	1910.1047 App A	Substance Safety Data Sheet for Ethylene Oxide (Non-mandatory)
O-AR.188	1910.1047 App B	Substance Technical Guidelines for Ethylene Oxide (Non-mandatory)
O-AR.189	1910.1047 App C	Medical Surveillance Guidelines for Ethylene Oxide (Non-mandatory)
O-AR.190	1910.1047 App D	Sampling and Analytical Methods for Ethylene Oxide (Non-mandatory)
O-AR.191	1910.1048	Formaldehyde
O-AR.192	1910.1048 App A	Substance Technical Guidelines for Formalin
O-AR.193	1910.1048 App B	Sampling Strategy and Analytical Methods for Formaldehyde
O-AR.194	1910.1048 App C	Medical Surveillance—Formaldehyde
O-AR.195	1910.1048 App D	Non-mandatory Medical Disease Questionnaire
O-AR.196	1910.1048 App E	Qualitative and Quantitative Fit Testing Procedures
O-AR.197	1910.1052	Methylene Chloride
O-AR.198	1910.1052 App A	Substance Safety Data Sheet and Technical Guidelines for Methylene Chloride
O-AR.199	1910.1052 App B	Medical Surveillance for Methylene Chloride
O-AR.200	1910.1052 App C	Questions and Answers—Methylene Chloride Control in Furniture Stripping
O-AR.201	1910.1096	Ionizing Radiation
O-AR.202	1910.1200	Hazard Communication
O-AR.203	1910.1200 App A	Health Hazard Definitions (Mandatory)
O-AR.204	1910.1200 App B	Hazard Determination (Mandatory)
O-AR.205	1910.1200 App C	Information Sources (Advisory)
O-AR.206	1910.1200 App D	Definition of "Trade Secret" (Mandatory)

(Continued on next page)

Table A-2. *(Continued)*

CD File Number	Source Publication No.	Document Title
O-AR.207	1910.1200 App E	Guidelines for Employer Compliance (Advisory)
O-AR.208	1910.1450	Occupational Exposure to Hazardous Chemicals in Laboratories
O-AR.209	1910.1450 App A	National Research Council Recommendations Concerning Hygiene in Laboratories (Non-Mandatory)
O-AR.210	1910.1450 App B	References (Non-Mandatory)

Part 1960: Basic Program Elements for Federal Employees OSHA

O-AR.211	1960 Subpart I	Basic Program Elements for Federal Employee Occupational Safety and Health Programs and Related Matters; Subpart I for Recordkeeping and Reporting Requirements—69: 68793–68805

Part 1904: Recording and Reporting Occupational Injuries and Illnesses

O-AR.212	1904; 1952	Occupational Injury and Illness Recording and Reporting Requirements—66: 5916–6135
O-AR.213	1904 Subpart B App A	Partially Exempt Industries
O-AR.214	1904	Table of Contents/Authority for 1904
O-AR.215	1904.0	Purpose
O-AR.216	1904.2	Partial Exemption for Establishments in Certain Industries
O-AR.217	1904.3	Keeping Records for More than One Agency
O-AR.218	1904.4	Recording Criteria
O-AR.219	1904.5	Determination of Work-Relatedness
O-AR.220	1904.6	Determination of New Cases
O-AR.221	1904.7	General Recording Criteria
O-AR.222	1904.8	Recording Criteria for Needlestick and Sharps Injuries
O-AR.223	1904.10	Recording Criteria for Cases Involving Occupational Hearing Loss
O-AR.224	1904.11	Recording Criteria for Work-Related Tuberculosis Cases
O-AR.225	1904.29	Forms
O-AR.226	1904.30	Multiple Business Establishments
O-AR.227	1904.31	Covered Employees
O-AR.228	1904.32	Annual Summary
O-AR.229	1904.33	Retention and Updating
O-AR.230	1904.34	Change in Business Ownership
O-AR.231	1904.35	Employee Involvement
O-AR.232	1904.36	Prohibition against Discrimination

(Continued on next page)

Table A-2. *(Continued)*

CD File Number	Source Publication No.	Document Title
O-AR.233	1904.37	State Recordkeeping Regulations
O-AR.234	1904.38	Variances from the Recordkeeping Rule
O-AR.235	1904.39	Reporting Fatalities and Multiple Hospitalization Incidents to OSHA
O-AR.236	1904.40	Providing Records to Government Representatives
O-AR.237	1904.41	Annual OSHA Injury and Illness Survey of Ten or More Employers
O-AR.238	1904.42	Requests from the Bureau of Labor Statistics for Data
O-AR.239	1904.43	Summary and Posting of 2001 Data
O-AR.240	1904.44	Retention and Updating of Old Forms
O-AR.241	1904.45	OMB Control Numbers under the Paperwork Reduction Act
O-AR.242	1904.46	Definitions
O-AR.243	1904	Entry FAQ—Injury and Illness—Recordkeeping

Part 1926: Safety and Health Regulations for Construction

CD File Number	Source Publication No.	Document Title
O-AR.244	1926	Table of Contents
O-AR.245	1926.101	Hearing Protection
O-AR.246	1926.300	General Requirements
O-AR.247	1926.431	Maintenance of Equipment
O-AR.248	1926.432	Environmental Deterioration of Equipment
O-AR.249	1926.441	Batteries and Battery Charging
O-AR.250	1926.449	Definitions Applicable to This Subpart
O-AR.251	1926 Subpart D	Authority for 1926 Subpart D—1926 Subpart D
O-AR.252	1926.52	Occupational Noise Exposure
O-AR.253	1926.65	Hazardous Waste Operations and Emergency Response
O-AR.254	1926 Subpart J	Authority for 1926 Subpart J—1926 Subpart J
O-AR.255	1926.350	Gas Welding and Cutting
O-AR.256	1926 Subpart K	Authority for 1926 Subpart K—1926 Subpart K
O-AR.257	1926.400	Introduction
O-AR.258	1926.402	Applicability
O-AR.259	1926.403	General Requirements
O-AR.260	1926.404	Wiring Design and Protection
O-AR.261	1926.405	Wiring Methods, Components, and Equipment for General Use
O-AR.262	1926.406	Specific Purpose Equipment and Installations
O-AR.263	1926.407	Hazardous (Classified) Locations
O-AR.264	1926.408	Special Systems

(Continued on next page)

Table A-2. *(Continued)*

CD File Number	Source Publication No.	Document Title
O-AR.265	1926.416	General Requirements
O-AR.266	1926.417	Lockout and Tagging of Circuits
Part 1913: Rules Concerning OSHA Access to Employee Medical Records		
O-AR.267	1913.10	Rules of Agency Practice and Procedure Concerning OSHA Access to Employee Medical Records

Table A-3. Select NIOSH, Federal OSHA, and State OSHA Documents in Spanish

CD File Number	Source Publication No.	Spanish Document Title	English Title or Translation
NIOSH			
N-SR.1	2004-165 (Sp2005)	Prevención de la exposición ocupacional a los antineoplásticos y otras medicinas peligrosas en centros de atención médica	Preventing Occupational Exposure to Antineoplastic and Other Hazardous Drugs in Health Care Settings
N-SR.2	2004-137Sp	Accidentes viales relacionados con el trabajo: ¿Quién corre peligro?	Work-Related Roadway Crashes: Who's at Risk?
N-SR.3	2003-144	Hoja informativa sobre respiradores	Respirator Fact Sheet
N-SR.4	2003-128	Alerta de NIOSH: Prevención de muertes, lesiones y enfermedades de trabajadores adolescentes	NIOSH Alert: Preventing Deaths, Injuries, and Illnesses of Young Workers
N-SR.5	2002-101 (Sp2006)	Violencia: Peligros ocupacionales en los hospitales	Violence: Occupational Hazards in Hospitals
N-SR.6	2001-115	El glutaraldehído: Los peligros ocupacionales en los hospitales	Glutaraldehyde: Occupational Hazards in Hospitals
N-SR.7	2001-103	La pérdida del oído relacionada con el trabajo	Work-Related Hearing Loss
N-SR.8	2000-135	Lo que todo trabajador debe saber sobre cómo protegerse de los pinchazos (piquetes de aguja)	What Every Worker Should Know: How to Protect Yourself from Needlestick Injuries
N-SR.9	2000-108	Alerta de NIOSH: Prevención de lesiones por pinchazos (piquetes de aguja) en entornos clínicos	NIOSH Alert: Preventing Needlestick Injuries in Health Care Settings
N-SR.10	99-110	Alerta de NIOSH: Prevención de muertes de trabajadores por descargas no controladas de energía eléctrica, mecánica y otros tipos de energía peligrosa	NIOSH Alert: Preventing Worker Deaths from Uncontrolled Release of Electrical, Mechanical, and Other Types of Hazardous Energies
N-SR.11	1999-104	Efectos de los riesgos ocupacionales en la salud reproductiva de la mujer	The Effects of Workplace Hazards on Female Reproductive Health
N-SR.12	99-101	El estrés en el trabajo	Stress at Work

(Continued on next page)

Table A-3. *(Continued)*

CD File Number	Source Publication No.	Spanish Document Title	English Title or Translation
OSHA—Federal			
O-1F-SR.1	3167	Usted tiene el derecho a un lugar de trabajo seguro y saludable. ¡Lo establece la ley!	You Have a Right to a Safe and Healthful Workplace. It's the Law!
O-1F-SR.2		Responsabilidades del empleado	Responsibilities of the Employee
O-1F-SR.3	3173-05R	Todo sobre OSHA: Administración de Seguridad y Salud Ocupacional	All About OSHA: Occupational Safety and Health Administration
O-1F-SR.4	3155	Protéjase del estrés por calor	Heat Stress Card
O-1F-SR.5	3158	La ecuación del frío	Cold Stress Card
OSHA—California			
O-CA-SR.1		Levantando con mayor seguridad	Lifting Safer
O-CA-SR.2		Protección de seguridad y salud en el trabajo	Safety and Health Protection on the Job
O-CA-SR.3	2004-164	Ergonomía fácil: Una guía para la selección de herramientas de mano no-energizadas	Easy Ergonomics: A Guide to Selecting Non-Powered Hand Tools
O-CA-SR.4		Trabajando en forma segura y facil: Para limpiadores, bedeles y amas de llaves	Working Safer and Easier: For Janitors, Custodians, and Housekeepers
O-CA-SR.5		¡No ponga en peligro su salud!	Don't Risk Your Health!
O-CA-SR.6		Use su fuerza con inteligencia	Use Your Strength Intelligently (poster)
O-CA-SR.7		Programa modelo para la prevencion de lesiones y enfermedades en el trabajo para los empleadores con trabajadores temporales	Model Program for the Prevention of Injuries and Illnesses on the Job for Employers with Seasonal Workers
O-CA-SR.8		Compensación del trabajador de California	Workers' Compensation in California
O-CA-SR.9	S-515	Cierre con candado y etiqueta/bloqueo	Lockout/Tagout

(Continued on next page)

Table A-3. *(Continued)*

CD File Number	Source Publication No.	Spanish Document Title	English Title or Translation
O-CA-SR.10	S-1001-91S	Seguridad en el trabajo: Lo que usted debe saber	Job Safety: What You Should Know
O-CA-SR.11	3204	Acceso a los archivos medicos y registros de la exposición a sustancias tóxicas	Access to the Medical Archives and Records of Exposure to Toxic Substances (poster)
O-CA-SR.12	S-503-01/03	Reglamentos para la operación de vehículos industriales	Rules for Operating Industrial Trucks (poster)
O-CA-SR.13		¿Eres un trabajador joven? Protege tu salud, conoce tus derechos	Are You a Working Teen? Protect Your Health, Know Your Rights
O-CA-SR.14		Proyecto de Cal/OSHA para Inspecciones de Seguridad y Salud en Construcción	Cal/OSHA Construction Safety and Health Inspection Project
O-CA-SR.15		Programa modelo para la prevención de lesiones y enfermedades en el trabajo para los patrones con trabajadores temporales en la agricultura	Model Program for the Prevention of Injuries and Illnesses on the Job for Employers with Seasonal Workers in Agriculture
O-CA-SR.16	S-507-S	Como Levantar	How to Lift

OSHA—Michigan

CD File Number	Source Publication No.	Spanish Document Title	English Title or Translation
O-MI-SR.1	CET 0101-S	Sus derechos y responsibilidades de acuerdo a MI OSHA	Your Rights and Responsibilities According to MI OSHA
O-MI-SR.2	CET 0116bs	Exámen de un camión montacarga industrial	Powered Industrial Truck Operator's Test
O-MI-SR.3	CET 0301s	Olvidese de ponerse su casco y usted no podría vivir para contarlo	Forget to Wear Your Hard Hat and You May Never Live to Tell About It
O-MI-SR.4	CET 0304s	Cómo la mayoría de los extinguidores de fuego trabajan	How Most Fire Extinguishers Work
O-MI-SR.5	CET 0305s	¡Ciérrelo fuera! Salve Una vida	Lock It Out! Save a Life!
O-MI-SR.6	CET 0306s	La seguridad primero. ¡Siempre!	Safety First. Always!

(Continued on next page)

Table A-3. *(Continued)*

CD File Number	Source Publication No.	Spanish Document Title	English Title or Translation
O-MI-SR.7	CET 0312s	¡Esté preparado! Segundos pueden salvar vidas	Be Prepared! Seconds Can Save Lives
O-MI-SR.8	CET 2010-S	Protección de seguridad y salud en el trabajo del estado de Michigan	Michigan Safety and Health Protection on the Job (poster)

OSHA—Minnesota

CD File Number	Source Publication No.	Spanish Document Title	English Title or Translation
O-MN-SR.1		Conozca sus derechos	Know Your Rights
O-MN-SR.2		Usted tiene el derecho a un lugar de trabajo seguro y saludable	You Have the Right to a Safe and Healthful Workplace
O-MN-SR.3		Seguridad y protección de la salud en el trabajo	Safety and Health Protection on the Job
O-MN-SR.4		Información sobre el Sistema de Compensación a trabajadores por accidentes en Minnesota	Information about the Workers' Compensation System for Accidents in Minnesota
O-MN-SR.5		Seguro de compensación a trabajadores por accidentes en el trabajo de Minnesota. Derechos y responsabilidades de los empleados	Workers' Compensation Insurance for Accidents in Minnesota: Employees' Rights and Responsibilities

OSHA—North Carolina

CD File Number	Source Publication No.	Spanish Document Title	English Title or Translation
O-NC-SR.1	1400	Leyes ocupacionales de Carolina del Norte: Información a los empleados	North Carolina Workplace Laws: Information for Employees (poster)

OSHA—Oregon

CD File Number	Source Publication No.	Spanish Document Title	English Title or Translation
O-OR-SR.1		Programa en español de seguridad e higiene en el trabajo de OR-OSHA	OR-OSHA Occupational Safety and Health Program in Spanish
O-OR-SR.2		Culturas, idiomas y la seguridad	Cultures, Languages, and Safety
O-OR-SR.3	3124	Comités de seguridad: Una guía para lugares de trabajo con 10 empleados o menos	Safety Committees: A Guide for Workplaces with 10 or Fewer Employees

(Continued on next page)

Table A-3. *(Continued)*

CD File Number	Source Publication No.	Spanish Document Title	English Title or Translation
O-OR-SR.4	1910.134	Cuestionario de evaluación médico por la OSHA: Mandatorio para Proteccion del Sistema Respiratorio	OSHA Medical Evaluation Questionnaire: Respiratory Protection
O-OR-SR.5	3906	Una guía del trabajador para OR-OSHA	A Worker's Guide to OR-OSHA
O-OR-SR.6	440-1507	Usted tiene el derecho a un lugar de trabajo seguro e higiénico. ¡Es la ley!	You Have the Right to a Safe and Healthy Workplace. It's the Law!

OSHA—Puerto Rico

CD File Number	Source Publication No.	Spanish Document Title	English Title or Translation
O-PR-SR.1	56.235	Exposición ocupacional a patogenos hematotransmitidos; norma	Occupational Exposure to Bloodborne Pathogens: Standard
O-PR-SR.2	66.12	Exposición ocupacional a patógenos hematotransmitidos; pinchazos de aguja y otras lesiones con objetos afilados; regla final	Occupational Exposure to Bloodborne Pathogens, Needlesticks, and Other Sharps Injuries: Final Rule
O-PR-SR.3	63.5	Protección respiratoria; norma	Respiratory Protection: Standard
O-PR-SR.4	55.21	Exposición ocupacional químicos peligrosos en laboratorios; norma	Occupational Exposure to Hazardous Chemicals in Laboratories: Standard
O-PR-SR.5	54.169	Control de energía peligrosa (cierre/rotulación); norma	Control of Hazardous Energy (Lockout/Tagout): Standard
O-PR-SR.6	53.66	Exposición ocupacional a óxido de etileno; norma	Occupational Exposure to Ethylene Oxide: Standard
O-PR-SR.7	53.143	Exposición ocupacional a óxido de etileno	Occupational Exposure to Ethylene Oxide
O-PR-SR.8	59.27	Comunicación de riesgos (norma)	Hazard Communication (Standard)
O-PR-SR.9	3186-06N 2003	Planes y programa modelo para las normas de patógenos hematotransmitidos y comunicación de riesgos de OSHA	Plans and Model Program for OSHA Bloodborne Pathogens and Risk Communication Standards

OSHA—Washington

CD File Number	Source Publication No.	Spanish Document Title	English Title or Translation
O-WA-SR.1		Actos inseguros	Unsafe Behavior
O-WA-SR.2		Análisis de tareas	Task Analysis

(Continued on next page)

Table A-3. *(Continued)*

CD File Number	Source Publication No.	Spanish Document Title	English Title or Translation
O-WA-SR.3		Comunicaciones personales	Personal Communications
O-WA-SR.4		Presuntos riesgos de salud y seguridad	Alleged Safety and Health Hazards
O-WA-SR.5		Lista de comprobación de la zona de precaución	Caution Zone Checklist
O-WA-SR.6		Lista de comprobación para el uso seguro de la escalera	Ladder Safety Checklist

Select Bibliography

Listed here are the primary writings that have been used in the making of this book. This bibliography is by no means a complete record of all the works and sources consulted. It indicates the substance and range of reading upon which I have formed my ideas. It is intended to serve as a convenience for those who wish to pursue the study of how employee health and safety, the environment employees work in, patient care, the well-being of health care workers' families, and the corporate bottom line are all connected.

A

Agency for Toxic Substances and Disease Registry (ATSDR). *Mercury.* U.S. Department of Health and Human Services, Public Health Service, Atlanta, GA, 1995. Available at www.atsdrl.atsdr.cdc.gov.

———. *National Alert: A Warning about Continuing Patterns of Metallic Mercury Exposure.* July 11, 1997.

American Hospital Association (AHA). *12 Steps to Sharps Safety.* Available at www.healthsafetyinfo.com

American Institute of Architects. *The Guidelines for Design and Construction of Hospital and Health Care Facilities,* 2001. AIA Bookstore, 1735 New York Avenue, NW, Washington DC 20006.

American Medical Association (AMA). *Alternative Medicine.* Report 12 of the Council on Scientific Affairs (A-97) (last updated September 16, 2005). Available at www.ama-assn.org.

American National Standards Institute (ANSI). *American National Standard for Personal Protection—Protective Footwear.* Z41.1-1991. Available at www.ansi.org.

———. *Emergency Eye Wash and Shower Equipment.* Z358.1.

———. *Hazardous Industrial Chemicals—Precautionary Labeling.* Z129.1-1988.

———. *Personnel Protection—Protective Headwear for Industrial Workers—Requirements.* Z89.1-1986.

———. *Practice for Occupational and Educational Eye and Face Protection.* Z87.1-1989.

———. *Safeguarding: Are ANSI Standards Really Voluntary?*

American Nurses Association (ANA). *Health & Safety Survey.* September 2001. Available at www.NursingWorld.org.

American Osteopathic Association. *Healthcare Facilities Accreditation Requirements for Healthcare Facilities.* February 2005. Chicago.

American Society of Health-System Pharmacists. *ASHP Technical Assistance Bulletin on Handling Cytotoxic and Hazardous Drugs.* Available at www.ashp.org.

American Society of Heating, Refrigerating and Air-Conditioning Engineers (ASHRAE). *The HVAC Design Manual for Hospitals and Clinics.* ASHRAE Bookstore, 1791 Tullie Circle, N.E., Atlanta, GA 30329. Available at www.ashrae.org.

American Society of Safety Engineers. *White Paper Addressing the Return on Investment for Safety, Health, and Environmental (SH&E) Management Programs.* 2002. Available at www.asse.org.

Americans with Disabilities Act (ADA). *ADA Regulations and Technical Assistance Materials.* Available at www.usdoj.gov.

Arson Prevention Advice. Available at www.afs-firewise.co.uk.

B

Bachman, Ronet. *Violence and Theft in the Workplace.* U.S. Department of Justice, Washington, DC, July 1994.

Beebe, Chad E. *Am I Ready for My CMS Survey?* Available at www.wsshe.org.

Best Practices, LLC. *Benchmarks for Establishing and Measuring Successful Health & Safety Functions.* August 31, 2004. Available at www.3.best-in-class.com.

Bongers, Hank. "Critical Incidents Are Incidents That Overwhelm Normal Coping Mechanisms." *SafetyFocus Newsletter*, January/February 2000. National Safety Council, Itasca, IL.

Booth, Bonnie. "IOM Report Spurs Momentum for Patient Safety Movement." *American Medical News.* January 24, 2000. Available at www.ama-assn.org.

Bowman, Dave. *Workplace Violence—A Real Killer.* Lincolnshire International. Available at www.thejobgame.com.

Broan, Elissa, Beatrice A. Yorker, and Catherine F. Kane. *Testimony Presented to: Joint Commission on the Accreditation of Healthcare Organizations Behavioral Healthcare Restraint Task Force.* Executive summary (1999). Available at www.nursingworld.org.

Bureau of Labor Statistics (BLS). *Accidents Involving Head Injuries.* Report 605. U.S. Government Printing Office, Washington, DC, July 1980. Available at bls.gov.

———. *Incidence Rates of Nonfatal Occupational Illness, by Industry and Category of Illness, 2003.* Table SNR08.

———. *Number of Nonfatal Occupational Injuries and Illnesses Involving Days Away from Work by Industry and Selected Events or Exposures Leading to Injury or Illness, 2003.* Table R4.

———. *Percent of Nonfatal Workplace Injuries and Illnesses by Industry, 2003.*

C

Cable, Josh. "The Multicultural Work Force: The Melting Pot Heats Up," *Occupational Hazards* (March 13, 2006). Available at www.occupationalhazards.com.

Canadian Centre for Occupational Health and Safety (CCOHS). *Prevention of Slips, Trips and Falls.* Available at ccohs.ca.

Canadian Initiative on Workplace Violence. *Profit Through Prevention.* Available at www.workplaceviolence.ca.

Carroll, Lewis. *Alice's Adventures in Wonderland.* A facsimile edition of the First Edition. New York, 1941.

Centers for Disease Control and Prevention (CDC). "About the Fourth Decennial International Conference on Nosocomial and Healthcare-Associated Infections." *Emerging Infectious Diseases* Vol. 7, No. 2, March–April 2001.

———. *Biosafety in Microbiological and Biomedical Laboratories,* 4th ed. Atlanta, GA. Available at www.cdc.gov.

————. *Core Curriculum on Tuberculosis: What the Clinician Should Know,* 4th ed. 2000, pp. 225–230.

————. *The Costs of Fall Injuries Among Older Adults.*

————. "Guideline for Hand Hygiene in Health-Care Settings." *MMWR* 51 (RR16), October 25, 2002, pp. 1–44.

————. *Guideline for Infection Control in Health Care Personnel, 1998.*

————. "Guidelines for Environmental Infection Control in Health-Care Facilities." *MMWR* 52 (RR10), June 6, 2003, pp. 1–42.

————. "Guidelines for Preventing Health-Care–Associated Pneumonia." *MMWR* 53 (RR03), March 26, 2004, pp. 1–36.

————. "Guidelines for Preventing the Transmission of *Mycobacterium tuberculosis* in Health-Care Settings, 2005." *MMWR* 54 (RR17), December 30, 2005, pp. 1–141.

————. *Key Facts About Pandemic Influenza.*

————. *An Ounce of Prevention: Keeps the Germs Away.*

————. *A Public Health Action Plan to Combat Antimicrobial Resistance.* Interagency Task Force. Available at www.cdc.gov/drugresistance.

————. *Workbook for Designing, Implementing, and Evaluating a Sharps Injury Prevention Program.*

Chaff, Linda. *Health & Safety Management for Medical Practices.* American Medical Association, Chicago, IL, 2002. Available at www.amapress.org.

————. *Managing Healthcare Hazards: Environmental Strategies.* Labelmaster, Chicago, IL.

————. "The Role of the Hospital Security Department in Safety and Health in the New Millennium." *Journal of Healthcare Protection Management* Vol. 21, No. 2. Publication of the International Association for Healthcare Security and Safety.

————. *Safety Guide for Health Care Institutions,* 5th ed. American Hospital Association, Chicago, IL.

Chaff, Linda, and Meserve, Evelyn. *Health and Safety Training Manual and Study Guide for Healthcare Security Officers.* International Association for Healthcare Security and Safety, Lombard, IL, 2002. Available at www.iahss.org.

Chemical Reactivity Worksheet. Office of Response and Restoration, National Ocean Service, National Oceanic and Atmospheric Administration. Available at www.response.restoration. noaa.gov.

Compressed Gas Association (CGA). *Characteristics and Safe Handling of Medical Gases.* CGA-P-2, 1996. Available at cganet.com.

————. *Handbook of Compressed Gases.* CGA HB, 1999.

————. *Pressure Relief Device Standards, Part 1: Cylinders for Compressed Gases,* 12th ed. CGA S-1.1, 2005.

————. *Safe Handling of Compressed Gas in Containers,* 9th ed. CGA P-1, 2000.

Conner, Marcia L. *Learning: The Critical Technology (an Industry White Paper).* Wave Technologies International, St. Louis, February 1995. Available at marciaconner.com.

D

Donne, John. *The Complete Poetry and Selected Prose of John Donne* (Modern Library Series). Random House, New York, 1994.

E

Ennis, Steve. *Emergency Management Program.* SME Consulting, Fredericksburg, VA, 2003.

————. *Emergency Operations Plan.* 2003.

F

Federal Emergency Management Agency (FEMA). *Emergency Response to Terrorism Job Aid—Edition 2.0*. Joint Publication of the Department of Homeland Security, Federal Emergency Management Agency, United States Fire Administration, the Department of Homeland Security Office for Domestic Preparedness (ODP), and United States Department of Justice Office of Justice Programs, February 2003. Available at www.usfa.fema.gov.

Fire Net International. *Arson Alert! 24 Ways to Stop Your Building Becoming an Arson Statistic.* Available at www.fire.org.uk.

G

Getting in the Door: Language Barriers to Health Services at New York City's Hospitals. City of New York, Office of the Comptroller. Office of Policy Management, January 2005.

H

Haley R.W., D.H. Culver, J. White, W.M. Morgan, T.G. Amber, V.P. Mann, et al. "The Efficacy of Infection Surveillance and Control Programs in Preventing Nosocomial Infections in US Hospitals." *American Journal of Epidemiology* 121, 1985, pp. 182–205.

Hayes, Casey. "Emergency Response for the Multicultural Work Force," *Occupational Hazards* (March 20, 2006). Available at www.occupationalhazards.com.

"Heal Thyself: Once Seen as Risky, One Group of Doctors Changes Its Ways." *Wall Street Journal.* June 21, 2005.

Health Care Without Harm. www.noharm.org.

Healthcare Environmental Resource Center. www.hercenter.org.

Heinlein, Robert A. *Stranger in a Strange Land.* First published in 1961; latest ed. 1995. Ace Books.

Hoel, Helge, Kate Sparks, and Cary L. Cooper. *The Cost of Violence/Stress at Work and the Benefits of a Violence/Stress-Free Working Environment.* Report Commissioned by the International Labour Organization (ILO), Geneva. University of Manchester Institute of Science and Technology.

Hospitals for a Healthy Environment (H2E). www.h2e.org.

I

"Industry Profile: Healthcare Hazards of the Healthcare Profession." *Occupational Health & Safety,* February 1993 (adapted).

International Union of Pure and Applied Chemistry (IUPAC). IUPAC Secretariat, P.O. Box 13757, Research Triangle Park, NC 27709-3757, USA.

J

Joint Commission on Accreditation of Healthcare Organizations. "Crosswalks of 2003 Standards to 2004 Standards." *Comprehensive Accreditation Manual for Hospitals: The Official Handbook.* Oakbrook Terrace, IL. Available at www.jcaho.org.

———. *Comprehensive Accreditation Manual for Hospitals: The Official Handbook*, 2004, with appropriate updates.

———. *Environment of Care Essentials*, 6th ed. 2006.

———. *Environment of Care Handbook*. 2005.

———. *Environment of Care News*. Monthly newsletter discussing health and safety issues in the environment of care. Subscribe at www.jcrinc.com.

———. *Facts about Patient Safety*. Available at http://www.jcaho.org/accredited+organizations/patient+safety/facts+about+patient+safety. . . . (accessed 12/9/2005).

———. "Joint Commission Accreditation Process, The."

———. "Leadership (LD)."

———. "Management of Human Resources (HR)."

———. "Management of Information (IM)."

———. "Management of the Environment of Care (EC)."

———. "National Patient Safety Goals (2006)."

———. "Provision of Care, Treatment, and Services (PC)."

———. *Protecting Those Who Serve: Health Care Worker Safety*, 2005.

———. "Revisions to the CAMH Manual Effective July 1, 2006."

———. "Surveillance, Prevention, and Control of Infection."

———. Survey Activity Guides (January 2006).

———. *Three Things You Can Do to Prevent Infection: A Speak Up™ Safety Initiative*.

K

Kentucky Pollution Prevention Center. *Hospital Pollution Prevention. Benefits of Hospital Pollution Prevention*. Available at www.kppc.org.

———. *Pollution Prevention Techniques*.

L

Laramie, Angela, and Letitia Davis. *The Link Between Workplace and Public Health Surveillance: Example of a Web-Based Surveillance System for Sharps Injuries Among Health Care Workers in Massachusetts*. Available at www.cdc.gov/niosh.

Leigh, J.P., et al. *Costs of Occupational Injuries and Illnesses*. University of Michigan Press, Ann Arbor, 2000. Available at pbs.org.

M

Moss, Jacqueline. "Technological System Solutions to Clinical Communication Error." *Journal of Nursing Administration* 35(2), February 2005.

Mulry, Ray. *In the Zone: Making Winning Moments Your Way of Life*. Great Ocean Publishers, Arlington, VA, 1995.

N

National Fire Protection Association (NFPA). *NFPA 30: Flammable and Combustible Liquids*. Quincy, MA.

———. Free online access. www.nfpa.org/freecodes/free_access_document.asp.

————. *NFPA 70*, National Electrical Code.

————. *70E: Standard for Electrical Safety in the Workplace.*

————. *NFPA 99: Health Care Facilities*, 1999 ed.

————. *NFPA 101: Life Safety Code*, 2000 ed.

————. *NFPA 600: Standard on Industrial Fire Brigades*, 2000 ed.

————. *NFPA 1600: Disaster/Emergency Management and Business Continuity Programs.*

National Institutes of Health. *Recommendations for the Safe Handling of Cytotoxic Drugs* (NIH 2002). Available at www.nih.gov.

National Institute of Occupational Safety and Health (NIOSH). *Backbelts: Do They Prevent Injury?* DHHS (NIOSH) Publication No. 94-127. Available at www.cdc.gov/niosh.

————. *Elements of Ergonomics Programs.* DHHS (NIOSH) Publication No. 97-117.

————. *Guide to the Selection and Use of Particulate Respirators.* DHHS (NIOSH) Publication No. 96-101.

————. *Guidelines for Protecting the Safety and Health of Health Care Workers.* DHHS (NIOSH) Publication No. 88-119.

————. *Musculoskeletal Disorders and Workplace Factors* (second printing). DHHS (NIOSH) Publication No. 97-141.

————. *NIOSH Alert: Preventing Occupational Exposures to Antineoplastic and other Hazardous Drugs in Health Care Settings.* DHHS (NIOSH) Publication No. 2004-165.

————. *NIOSH Pocket Guide to Chemical Hazards.* DHHS (NIOSH) Publication No. 1005-149.

————. *Occupational Hazards in Hospitals.* 2000.

————. *Preventing Occupational Exposure to Antineoplastic and other Hazardous Drugs in Health Care Settings.* DHHS (NIOSH) Publication No. 2005-111.

————. *Respiratory Protective Devices: Final Rules and Notice.* 42 CFR Part 84.

————. *Stress at Work.* DHHS (NIOSH) Publication No. 99-101.

————. *Understanding Respiratory Protection Against SARS.*

————. *Worker Health Chartbook, 2004.* DHHS (NIOSH) Publication No. 2004-146.

————. *Work-Related Roadway Crashes: Prevention Strategies for Employers.* DHHS (NIOSH) Publication No. 2004-136.

National Safety Council (NSC). *Injury Facts*, 2004 ed. Itasca, IL.

New Jersey Association of Non-Profit Homes for the Aging (NJANPHA). "CMS Issues Final Rule on Fire Safety Requirements." *NJANPHA News*, Issue 2, 2003. Available at www.njanpha.org.

New Jersey Department of Health & Senior Services. Office of Minority and Multicultural Health. *Cultural Competency Information and Resources.* Available at www.nj.gov.

Newman, Mary A., and John B. Kachuba. *An Asbestos Abatement Program for Healthcare Institutions.* Healthcare Environments, Inc., Cincinnati, 1990.

Next-Generation Environment, Health and Safety Goals. Baxter Worldwide. Available at www.quickfind.baxter.com.

O

Occupational Safety and Health Administration (OSHA). *Access to Employee Exposure and Medical Records.* Standard 29 CFR 1910.1020. Available at www.osha.gov.

————. *Access to Medical and Exposure Records.* U.S. Department of Labor. OSHA 3110, 2001 (revised).

————. *All About OSHA.* OSHA 2056-07R, 2003.

————. *Appropriateness of Computer-Based Interactive Training Programs to Satisfy Requires OSHA Training: Standard Interpretations.* June 11, 1997.

————. *Bloodborne Pathogens.* Standard 29 CFR 1910.1030.

————. *Compressed Gases (General Requirements).* 1910.101.

————. *The Control of Hazardous Energy (Lockout/Tagout).* 1910.147.

————. "Controlling Occupational Exposure to Hazardous Drugs." *OSHA Technical Manual*, Section VI, Chapter 2.

————. *Electrical.* 1910 Subpart S.

————. *Ergonomics.* 1999.

————. *Ethylene Oxide.* Standard 29 CFR 1910.1047.

————. *Exit Routes, Emergency Action Plans, and Fire Prevention Plans.* 1910 Subpart E.

————. *Eye and Face Protection.* 1910.133.

————. *Fire Protection.* 1910 Subpart L.

————. *Fire Protection.* 1910 Subpart L Appendix A.

————. *Fire Protection: National Consensus Standards.* 1910 Subpart L Appendix B.

————. *Flammable and Combustible Liquids.* 1910.106.

————. *Guidelines for Nursing Homes: Ergonomics for the Prevention of Musculoskeletal Disorders.* OSHA 3182, 2003.

————. *Guidelines for Preventing Workplace Violence for Health Care and Social Service Workers.* OSHA 3148-01R, 2004.

————. *Hand and Portable Powered Tools and Other Hand-Held Equipment.* 1910 Subpart P.

————. *Hand Protection.* 1910.138.

————. *Handling Materials—General.* 1910.176.

————. *Hazard Comunication.* Standard 29 CFR 1910.1200.

————. *Hazard Communication: Hazard Determination (Mandatory).* Standard 29 CFR 1910.1200 Appendix B.

————. *Hazard Communication: Health Hazard Definitions (Mandatory).* Standard 29 CFR 1910.1200 Appendix A, August 14, 1987.

————. *Hazardous Materials.* 1910 Subpart H.

————. *Hazardous Waste Operations and Emergency Response (HAZWOPER).* 1910.120.

————. *Head Protection.* 1910.135.

————. *Helicopters.* 1910.183.

————. "Hospital Investigations: Health Hazards." *OSHA Technical Manual*, Section VI, Chapter 1.

————. *Hospitals, Healthcare-Wide Hazards, Ergonomics.* OSHA eTool.

————. *Incorporation by Reference.* Standard 29 CFR 1910.6.

————. *Industrial Hygiene.* OSHA 3143.

————. *Job Hazard Analysis.* OSHA 3071, 2002 (revised).

————. *Laundry Machinery and Operations.* 1910.264.

————. *Machinery and Machine Guarding.* 1910 Subpart O.

————. *Medical and First Aid.* 1910 Subpart K.

————. *Medical Services and First Aid.* 1910.151.

————. *Nitrous Oxide.* 1910.105.

————. *Non-mandatory Compliance Guidelines for Hazard Assessment and Personal Protective Equipment Selection.* 1910 Subpart I Appendix B.

————. *Occupational Foot Protection.* 1910.136.

————. *Occupational Noise Exposure.* 1910.95.

————. *OSHA Hazard Awareness Advisor*. Version 1.0, September 1999.

————. *OSHA Standards for General Industry*. 29 CFR Part 1910.

————. *Personal Protective Equipment*. 1910 Subpart I.

————. *Powered Industrial Trucks*. 1910.178.

————. *Powered Platforms, Manlifts, and Vehicle-Mounted Work Platforms*. 1910 Subpart F.

————. *Protocol for Developing Industry-Specific and Task Specific Ergonomics Guidelines*. Revised December 16, 2002.

————. *Recording and Reporting Occupational Injuries and Illnesses*. 29 CFR 1904.

————. *Recordkeeping Policies and Procedures Manual*. 29 CFR 1904, 1913.10. OSHA Instruction. Directive Number CPL 02-00-135. December 30, 2004.

————. *Respiratory Protection*. 1910.134.

————. "Respiratory Protection." *OSHA Technical Manual*, Section VIII, Chapter 2.

————. *Safety and Health Achievement Recognition Program (SHARP)*.

————. *Safety and Health Program Management Guidelines: Issuance of Voluntary Guidelines* (54 FR 3904-3916).

————. *Safety and Health Regulations for Construction*. Standard 29 CFR 1926.32.

————. *Safety Color Code for Marking Physical Hazards*. 1910.144.

————. *Sanitation*. 1910.141.

————. *Screening and Surveillance: A Guide to OSHA Standards*. OSHA 3162, 2000 (reprinted).

————. *Specifications for Accident Prevention Signs and Tags*. 1910.145.

————. *Tools for a Safety and Health Program Assessment*. Office of Training and Education.

————. *Toxic and Hazardous Substances*. 1910 Subpart Z.

————. *Training Requirements in OSHA Standards and Training Guidelines*. OSHA 2254, 1998 (revised).

————. *Ventilation*. 1910.94

————. "Voluntary Protection Programs (VPP)."

————. *Walking-Working Surfaces*. 1910 Subpart D.

————. *Welding, Cutting, and Brazing*. 1910 Subpart Q.

————. *Working Safely with Video Display Terminals*. OSHA 3092 1997 (Revised).

Old, Leo. "Is Your Fire Brigade Up to Snuff?" *Hospital Engineering Trends*, August 2005. Smith Seckman Reid, Inc., Nashville, TN.

Oregon Occupational Safety and Health Administration (OR-OSHA). *Developing Your Safety and Health Program: Suggestions for Business Owners and Managers*. Available at www.osha.gov.

Osgood, William R. *Where Is my Business Headed and Why?* Available at www.buzgate.org.

P

Paracelsus. *Selected Writings* (J. Jacobi, ed.; N. Guterman, trans.). Pantheon, New York, 1951.

R

Ramazzini, Bernardino. *Diseases of Workers*. Translated from the Latin text *De Morbis Artificum Diatriba* (1713) by Wilmer Cave Wright. OH&S Press, 1993.

RCRA Orientation Manual. EPA 530-R-02-016. January 2003.

S

"Safety Is the Flavor Every Day at Edy's." *Compliance Magazine*, July 2004. Richmond, VA.

Sagan, Carl. *Cosmos*. Novel and film series.

Silverstein, Shel. *Where the Sidewalk Ends: The Poems and Drawings of Shel Silverstein*. HarperCollins Children's Books, New York, 2004.

South Carolina Department of Labor. *Best Practices in Workplace Security*. Homeland Security guide developed by the South Carolina Department of Labor, Licensing and Regulation (which operates an OSHA-approved state plan).

Standard Industrial Classification Manual, 1972. Executive Office of the President of the United States, Office of Management and Budget. U.S. Government Printing Office, Washington, DC.

Sugrue, Brenda, and Ray J. Rivera. *2005 State of the Industry: ASTD's Annual Review of Trends in Workplace Learning and Performance*. American Society for Training and Development, Alexandria, VA.

Sustainable Hospitals. www.sustainablehospitals.org.

T

Tackling Arson: Evaluated Options. Available at www.crimereduction.gov.uk.

Terkel, Studs. *Working*. New Press, New York, 1974.

U

U-M Health System Implements Straight Talk at Hurley Medical Center in National Crusade to Prevent Burn Injuries: Fire Safety Program Extinguishes the Desire for Kids to Set Fires. Available at www.med.umich.edu.

USASBCCOM. *Guidelines for Mass Casualty Decontamination During a Terrorist Chemical Agent Incident*. January 2000; Revision 1, August 2003.

U.S. Congress (91st) *The Occupational Health and Safety Act of 1970*. Public Law 91-596, specifically: *Duties*, Sections 5(a)(1) and 5(a)(2). Washington, DC, December 29, 1970.

U.S. Department of Agriculture, Animal and Plant Health Inspection Service. *Agricultural Bioterrorism Protection Act of 2002; Possession, Use, and Transfer of Biological Agents and Toxins*. Interim final rule (9 CFR Part 121). *Federal Register* 667 (2240), December 13, 2002, pp. 76907–76938.

U.S. Department of Health and Human Services (HHS). *Healthy People 2010*. Managed by the Office of Disease Prevention and Health Promotion. Available at www.healthypeople.gov.

———. Office of Inspector General. *Possession, Use, and Transfer of Select Agents and Toxins*. Interim final rule (42 CFR Part 73). *Federal Register* 67 (240), December 13, 2002, pp. 76885–76905.

U.S. Department of Justice. *Stalking in America: Findings from the National Violence Against Women Survey*. National Institutes of Justice. Available at www.ojp.usdoj.gov.

———. *Terrorism 1980–2001*. Available at www.fbi.gov.

U.S. Environmental Protection Agency. *Resource Conservation and Recovery Act of 1976* (40 CFR Parts 260–290).

———. *Tools for Schools: IAQ Coordinator's Guide*. Publication Number EPA 402-K-95-001.

U.S. Fire Administration. *Topical Fire Research Series*. Volume 2, Issue 8, October 2001 (rev. March 2002). Available at www.usfa.fema.gov.

U.S. Nuclear Regulatory Commission. *Radioactive Waste: Production, Storage, Disposal*. Available at www.nrc.gov.

U.S. Small Business Administration. *Common Sense Strategic Analysis*. Strategic Management Learning System (SMLS). Available at www.bdki.com.

V

Veit, Lori. "A Closer Look at Waste Management." *Housekeeping Solutions*, March 2004. Cleanlink. Available at www.cleanlink.com.

W

Weinstein, Robert A. "Nosocomial Infection Update." *Emerging Infectious Diseases*, special issue. CDC, Atlanta, GA. Available at www.cdc.gov.

———. "SHEA Consensus Panel Report: A Smooth Takeoff." *Infection Control and Hospital Epidemiology* 19:91–93, 1998.

Wenzel, R.P., and M.B. Edmond. "The Impact of Hospital-Acquired Bloodstream Infections." *Emerging Infectious Diseases* Vol. 7, No. 2, March–April 2001. CDC, Atlanta, GA.

Workers' Comp Insider. *Keeping the Multicultural Workforce Safe*. (March 14, 2006) Available at www.workerscompinsider.com.

Worksafe Australia. *Benchmarking Occupational Health and Safety: Team Leader's Manual*. Commonwealth of Australia, 1996. Available at www.worksafe.gov.au.

———. *Beyond Lost Time Injuries: Positive Performance Indicators for OHS Summary Paper*. National Occupational Health & Safety Commission (Australia).

———. *Caring for People in the Workplace*.

———. *Coping with Violence Against Human Service Workers*.

World Health Organization. *Safe Management of Wastes from Healthcare Activities*. WHO International, Geneva, 1999. Available at www.who.int.org.

———. *WHO Global Influenza Preparedness Plan: The Role of WHO and Recommendations for National Measures Before and During Pandemics*.

Index